Optical Coherence Tomography in Glaucoma

Ahmet Akman • Atilla Bayer
Kouros Nouri-Mahdavi

Editors

Optical Coherence Tomography in Glaucoma

A Practical Guide

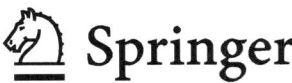 Springer

Editors
Ahmet Akman
Department of Ophthalmology
School of Medicine
Başkent University
Ankara
Turkey

Atilla Bayer
Department of Glaucoma
Dünyagöz Eye Hospital
Ankara
Turkey

Kouros Nouri-Mahdavi
Stein Eye Institute
University of California Los Angeles
Los Angeles, CA
USA

ISBN 978-3-030-06935-3   ISBN 978-3-319-94905-5   (eBook)
https://doi.org/10.1007/978-3-319-94905-5

This Springer imprint is published by Springer Nature, under the registered company Springer International Publishing AG
The registered company address is: Gewerbestrasse 11, 6330 Cham, Switzerland

To my amazing parents, Bilge and Ethem, it's impossible to thank you adequately for everything you've done for us; I am so lucky to be your son, To my brother, Arda, thanks for all those childhood memories we shared together, To my wonderful wife, Beril, and my terrific children, Defne and Sarp, you are real wonders of my life, and thanks for your support, encouragement, and love.

Ahmet Akman

To the memory of my father, and to my mother, for supporting and encouraging me to believe in myself, To my dear wife, Ülkü, for her endless help, patience, and motivation, And to my son, Emir, for the many borrowed hours. With love.

Atilla Bayer

In memory of my grandfather, Ataollah Daneshvar, MD, to whom I owe where I am today! To my parents, who led me to be who I am and taught me to seek excellence in whatever I do! To Maryam, Ava, and Tina, the 3 most precious people in my life, who have given and continue to give meaning to my life! Thank you for being so kind, generous, and understanding!

Kouros Nouri-Mahdavi

Foreword

Optical coherence tomography (OCT) is changing the way clinicians diagnose and monitor glaucoma. In fact, it is fair to say that the impact of OCT on clinical practice rivals the impact that MRI and CAT have had on medical specialties, such as neurology and neurosurgery. Further, the OCT scans have far better resolutions, by a factor of 100 or so, than an MRI has, providing the clinician with a wealth of information. Thus, it is not surprising that most glaucoma specialists now consider OCT to be the main structural tool for detecting and monitoring glaucoma in patients with suspected or established disease. However, this wonderful technology also creates a problem for the glaucoma clinician.

Unlike neurologists and neurosurgeons, who have radiologists to interpret their MRI scans, ophthalmologists must learn to interpret OCT scans themselves. In an attempt to help solve this problem, OCT manufacturers offer a plethora of reports, each with a variety of plots and summary statistics. However, now the clinician is faced with the problem of which report to use, and which aspect of a report to focus on. This has led many clinicians to depend heavily upon pie charts and summary statistics; the "red means bad and green means good" approach. While this is an easy method to use and teach, it leads to too many mistakes, both false positives and false negatives. And, equally important, it does not come close to making optimal use of this wonderful technology. Thus, it is essential for anyone diagnosing and treating glaucoma to learn to make better use of OCT.

To date, there is no book that provides the clinician with a comprehensive review of how to use OCT in everyday management of glaucoma. This book *Optical Coherence Tomography in Glaucoma: A Practical Guide* meets this critical need.

This book first covers the basics of OCT technology in understandable language and then addresses the specific features of the most commonly used commercial OCT devices today. The next few chapters address the utility of OCT in diagnosing glaucoma. While it is important to know what to look for in OCT reports, it is also essential to know what to ignore. Or in other words, to understand artifacts seen on OCT images. This subject is thoroughly addressed so that even veteran OCT users will benefit from this chapter. Once diagnosed, the clinician faces the challenge of monitoring the progression of the glaucomatous damage. Progression is discussed in a number of chapters. The authors also discuss masqueraders of glaucoma and end with a chapter that provides an introduction to the current state of OCT angiography.

There are three features that make this book particularly valuable. First, throughout the book, the importance of using OCT information from different layers (e.g., retinal nerve fiber and ganglion cell layers) and different regions (e.g., optic disc and macular regions) of the eye is emphasized as well as the complementary nature of this information. The authors emphasize the importance of reviewing OCT printout in their entirety instead of just concentrating on summary statistics (e.g., pie charts and global thickness measures) provided by the device. Second, the importance of comparing structural and functional damage is emphasized. Third, and most important pedagogically, throughout the book there are numerous clinical case presentations with a large number of figures to illustrate important concepts.

Finally, all this is made possible because the authors are experienced glaucoma specialists with years of experience in using OCT for daily management of glaucoma patients. I am confident that this book will serve ophthalmologists at various stages of their careers, from residents and fellows to general ophthalmologists and glaucoma specialists. We should commend the authors for undertaking this important task. This book is a wonderful addition to the current literature on OCT and I look forward to future editions.

Donald C. Hood
Columbia University
New York, NY, USA

Preface

The development and widespread acceptance of optical coherence tomography (OCT) in ophthalmology has significantly changed the paradigm in glaucoma diagnosis and monitoring during the last two decades. OCT has not only enabled clinicians to diagnose glaucoma in the very early stages, but given its high resolution and reproducibility, it has also facilitated objective detection of early structural progression. As such, OCT has replaced previous imaging systems used for the diagnosis and monitoring of glaucoma. It is now the most important diagnostic tool for the detection and monitoring of early glaucoma. Worsening of pre-perimetric glaucoma can now be identified with OCT and it can also be used as an adjunct to visual field analysis in moderate and advanced stages of the disease.

While there have been many books published on the theoretical and practical aspects of perimetry, there are few published resources dedicated only to the use of OCT in glaucoma. Most books published on the role of OCT in ophthalmology are mainly focused on retinal disorders and usually only a chapter or two summarize the use of OCT in glaucoma. The scattered resources for clinicians using OCT for managing glaucoma in their daily practice have been a major obstacle to the widespread adoption of OCT imaging. We believe that the lack of a comprehensive book on the utility of OCT in glaucoma is one of the reasons that has restricted its full potential among both general and glaucoma specialists.

The goal of *Optical Coherence Tomography in Glaucoma: A Practical Guide* is to provide a comprehensive yet practical text to the interested readers on various applications of OCT for the diagnosis and monitoring of glaucoma. The text is divided into five parts. Part I includes the history, basics, and role of OCT in glaucoma management. Part II concentrates on the interpretation of OCT in glaucoma diagnosis with sample case presentations. A special emphasis is given to artifacts, anatomical variations, and glaucoma masqueraders that can confound the diagnosis of glaucoma. We also discuss the role of OCT in myopic eyes and its utility in imaging the anterior segment in this part. Part III focuses on the role of OCT for the detection of structural progression in glaucoma. Part IV consists of a chapter on the structure and function relationships in glaucoma. Finally, the last part (Part V) provides a review of current knowledge on OCT angiography, which is a recent addition to our diagnostic armamentarium.

Since all the authors are familiar with either the Cirrus HD-OCT, Spectralis OCT, or both, all the material presented uses images from these two devices. However, all OCT machines utilize similar principles and approaches to glaucoma diagnosis and monitoring, and therefore we believe that users of other OCT devices will also find this book beneficial.

This book incorporates the work and ideas of many people, to whom we are extremely thankful. In particular, we would like to thank the imaging technicians at the Department of Ophthalmology, School of Medicine, Başkent University, Suat Çıtak, Hakan Noyan, Metin Zengin, and Emrah Kasıkçı and those at Dünyagöz Ankara Hospital Imaging Department, Kemal Ataseven, Erkan Kıymaz, and Nabi Yavaş, who have carried out many of the OCTs, visual field tests, and fundus photographs presented in this book. We are also grateful to the research coordinator, Sharon Henry, and ophthalmic imaging/perimetry technicians, Michon Rozier, Marlene Traynor, Kathy Johns, and Wendy Torres, for their assistance and diligence in performing OCT imaging and visual field exams at Stein Eye Institute's Glaucoma Division.

We certainly hope this text will help glaucoma specialists, comprehensive ophthalmologists, and ophthalmology residents and glaucoma fellows better understand and use OCT imaging in their practice and, therefore, improve patient care for glaucoma patients around the world.

Ankara, Turkey   Ahmet Akman
Ankara, Turkey   Atilla Bayer
Los Angeles, CA, USA   Kouros Nouri-Mahdavi

Contents

Abbreviations

AOD	Angle opening distance
APS	Automatic positioning system
ARA	Angle recess area
AS-OCT	Anterior segment optical coherence tomography
BM	Bruch's membrane
BMO	Bruch's membrane opening
C/D	Cup to disc ratio
DOB	Date of birth
FoBMO	Fovea to center of bruch's membrane opening
FoDi	Fovea to disc
GCC	Ganglion cell complex
GCIPL	Ganglion cell layer + inner plexiform layer
GCL	Ganglion cell layer
GMPE	Glaucoma module premium edition
GPA	Guided progression analysis
ILM	Internal limiting membrane
IOP	Intraocular pressure
IPL	Inner plexiform layer
IR	Infrared reflectance
IT	Iris thickness
MRW	Minimum rim width
OCT	Optical coherence tomography
OCTA	Optical coherence tomography angiography
ONH	Optic nerve head
RGC	Retinal ganglion cell
RNFL	Retinal nerve fiber layer
RPE	Retinal pigment epithelium
SD	Spectral domain
SS	Swept source

TD	Time domain
TIA	Trabecular-iris angle
TISA	Trabecular-iris space area
TSNIT	Temporal-superior-nasal-inferior-temporal
VF	Visual field
VFI	Visual field index

Part I
Optical Coherence Tomography in Glaucoma, Basics

Chapter 1
Optical Coherence Tomography: Introduction, History and Current Status

Ahmet Akman

1.1 Introduction

Optical coherence tomography (OCT) is one of the most significant advances in the field of ophthalmology in the last two decades. OCT has become an essential tool for retina specialists in the diagnosis and follow-up of macular diseases. Modern anti-VEGF treatments might not have become so successful and widespread without the use of OCT imaging. Glaucoma is the second specialty in ophthalmology the practice of which OCT revolutionized. Currently, it is the main test used for early diagnosis and monitoring of glaucoma. As OCT provides various parameters and biomarkers with regard to the optic nerve head (ONH), retinal nerve fiber layer (RNFL) and inner macular health with high reproducibility, it has replaced previous technologies such as confocal scanning laser ophthalmoscopy and scanning laser polarimetry. With the use of OCT, it has become possible to diagnose glaucoma at a very early stage, even years before the visual field defects emerge. OCT is widely used by ophthalmologists worldwide in daily practice, but interpretation of OCT results in glaucoma requires familiarity with how the device works and interprets images. A wide range of artifacts and inter-individual variations can lead to diagnostic errors, if the reader is not well-acquainted with the technology.

While several books and chapters are available on visual field testing, most books on OCT are focused on its utility in retinal disorders and only a limited amount of space is dedicated to the role of OCT in glaucoma. As a result, current ophthalmic literature lacks a detailed book on the use of OCT in glaucoma. The goal of this book is to provide the reader with an overview of the role of OCT in glaucoma management and demonstrate how best to interpret OCT images for diagnosis and monitoring of glaucoma in everyday practice.

A. Akman
Department of Ophthalmology, School of Medicine, Başkent University,
Ankara, Turkey

© Springer International Publishing AG, part of Springer Nature 2018
A. Akman et al. (eds.), *Optical Coherence Tomography in Glaucoma*,
https://doi.org/10.1007/978-3-319-94905-5_1

1.2   History

Early studies regarding application of light interferometry for imaging ocular tissues date back to the late 1980s. Fercher and Roth published some of the earliest articles on the use of laser interferometry for imaging retinal tissues and measuring the eye length [1–3]. Other researchers studied similar techniques during late 1980's with additional papers about light interferometry being published soon after [4, 5].

In 1990, two independent groups, Naohiro Tanno et al. from Yamagata University in Japan and James G. Fujimoto and collaborators from the Massachusetts Institute of Technology in the United States developed the first OCT systems, and patent applications were submitted at about the same time in Japan and the United States during 1991 [6–8]. David Huang et al. from James G. Fujimoto's laboratory published their landmark article on OCT in the journal *Science* in 1991 [8]. Fercher and colleagues published the first in vivo retinal OCT images in 1993 [9]. Subsequently, many publications related to OCT imaging of the posterior and anterior segments of the eye were published [10–13]. The original paper on imaging of the macula with Fourier domain OCT was published by Fercher and colleagues in 1995. First papers on clinical OCT imaging of the ONH and RNFL were published in 1995 and 1996 [14–16].

The first commercial OCT company, Advanced Ophthalmic Devices (AOD), was founded in 1992 by James G. Fujimoto, Carmen Puliafito, and Eric Swanson, who started the OCT research at the Massachusetts Institute of Technology, Massachusetts Eye and Ear Infirmary, and Tufts University New England Eye Center. Humphrey Instruments, which is now owned by Carl Zeiss Meditec (Dublin, CA), acquired AOD in 1993. Swanson in a 2009 article stated that "Zeiss, through a combination of market foresight, good engineering, marketing, distribution, and a strong patent position got a head start and enjoyed a virtual monopoly on the market for a decade" [17]. In 1997, Zeiss introduced the first commercial time domain optical coherence tomography (TD-OCT) platform, OCT-1, for clinical use in ophthalmology, which was followed by OCT-2. With the introduction of Zeiss Stratus TD-OCT, OCT became a crucial device in both retina and glaucoma clinics. A few years later, spectral domain OCT (SD-OCT) systems became available with higher resolution, faster image acquisition capabilities, and advanced segmentation software. Cirrus HD-OCT by Zeiss, Spectralis OCT by Heidelberg Engineering (Heidelberg Engineering, Heidelberg, Germany), RTvue OCT by Optovue (Optovue Inc., Fremont, CA) and 3D-OCT 2000 by Topcon (Topcon Medical Systems, Oakland, NJ) were the first SD-OCT systems introduced to clinical practice. Many hardware and software upgrades including, better segmentation algorithms and enhanced depth imaging (EDI) protocols subsequently increased the performance of these systems.

Swept Source OCT (SS-OCT) and Adaptive Optics OCT (AD-OCT) systems followed SD-OCT based platforms. Apart from retinal imaging, SS-OCT based systems became commercially available for biometric measurements such as in Zeiss' IOLMaster 700 [18]. Retinal angiography is another field into which OCT has branched in recent years. OCT angiography is a non-invasive imaging technique, which does not require injection of a dye, and is capable of generating fundus angiography images in a very short time. Apart from retinal vascular diseases, it has the potential to become a useful tool for investigating ONH circulation in glaucoma.

References

1. Fercher AF, Roth E. Ophthalmic laser interferometry. Proc. SPIE. 1986;658:48–1.
2. Fercher AF, Mengedoht K, Werner W. Eye-length measurement by interferometry with partially coherent light. Opt Lett. 1988;13:186–8.
3. Fercher AF. Ophthalmic interferometry. In: von Bally G, Khanna S, editors. Proceedings of the international conference on optics in life sciences. Germany: Garmisch-Partenkirchen; 1990. p. 221–8.
4. Fujimoto JG, De Silvestri S, Ippen EP, Puliafito CA, Margolis R, Oseroff A. Femtosecond optical ranging in biological systems. Opt Lett. 1986;11:150–2.
5. Youngquist RC, Carr S, Davies DE. Optical coherence-domain reflectometry: a new optical evaluation technique. Opt Lett. 1987;12:158–60.
6. Naohiro T, Tsutomu I, Akio S. Lightwave reflection measurement, Japanese Patent # 2010042 (1990) (in Japanese).
7. Chiba S, Tanno N. Backscattering optical heterodyne tomography. In: 14th laser sensing symposium; 1991. (in Japanese).
8. Huang D, Swanson EA, Lin CP, Schuman JS, Stinson WG, Chang W, Hee MR, Flotte T, Gregory K, Puliafito CA, Fujimoto JG. Optical coherence tomography. Science. 1991;254(5035):1178–81.
9. Fercher AF, Hitzenberger CK, Drexler W, Kamp G, Sattmann H. In vivo optical coherence tomography. Am J Ophthalmol. 1993;116:113–4.
10. Swanson EA, Izatt JA, Hee MR, Huang D, Lin CP, Schuman JS, Puliafito CA, Fujimoto JG. In vivo retinal imaging by optical coherence tomography. Opt Lett. 1993;18:1864–6.
11. Puliafito CA, Hee MR, Lin CP, Reichel E, Schuman JS, Duker JS, Izatt JA, Swanson EA, Fujimoto JG. Imaging of macular diseases with optical coherence tomography. Ophthalmology. 1995;102:217–29.
12. Hee MR, Izatt JA, Swanson EA, Huang D, Schuman JS, Lin CP, Puliafito CA, Fujimoto JG. Optical coherence tomography of the human retina. Arch Ophthalmol. 1995;113:325–32.
13. Izatt JA, Hee MR, Swanson EA, Lin CP, Huang D, Schuman JS, Puliafito CA, Fujimoto JG. Micrometer-scale resolution imaging of the anterior eye in vivo with optical coherence tomography. Arch Ophthalmol. 1994;112:1584–9.
14. Schuman JS, Hee MR, Arya AV, Pedut- Kloizman T, Puliafito CA, Fujimoto JG, Swanson EA. Optical coherence tomography: a new tool for glaucoma diagnosis. Curr Opin Ophthalmol. 1995;6:89–95.
15. Schuman JS, Hee MR, Puliafito CA, Wong C, Pedut-Kloizman T, Lin CP, Hertzmark E, Izatt JA, Swanson EA, Fujimoto JG. Quantification of nerve fiber layer thickness in normal and glaucomatous eyes using optical coherence tomography. Arch Ophthalmol. 1995;113:586–96.
16. Schuman JS, Pedut-Kloizman T, Hertzmark E, Hee MR, Wilkins JR, Coker JG, Puliafito CA, Fujimoto JG, Swanson EA. Reproducibility of nerve fiber layer thickness measurements using optical coherence tomography. Ophthalmology. 1996;103:1889–98.
17. Swanson E. Ophthalmic optical coherence tomography market: past, present, & future. OCTnews. http://www.octnews.org/articles/1027616/ ophthalmic-optical-coherence-tomography-market-pas/.
18. Akman A, Asena L, Güngör SG. Evaluation and comparison of the new swept source. OCT-based IOLMaster 700 with the IOLMaster 500. Br J Ophthalmol. 2016 Sep;100(9):1201–5.

Chapter 2
Optical Coherence Tomography: Basics and Technical Aspects

Ahmet Akman

2.1 What Is Optical Coherence Tomography?

Optical Coherence Tomography (OCT) is a diagnostic imaging technique based on optical reflectometry, which acquires high resolution, in vivo images from transparent or semi-transparent tissues, with a resolution in the order of a low power microscope with a penetration depth of 2–4 mm [1, 2]. It is analogous to ultrasound imaging, the only difference being that laser light is used. Use of light instead of ultrasound improves the image resolution considerably although tissue penetration is limited only to a few millimeters. OCT measures the intensity and echo delay time of the back scattered light from transparent or semi-transparent biological tissues and provides in vivo, non-invasive, cross sectional imaging. As the echo delay time from different tissues cannot be quantified directly due to technical reasons, interferometry is used to overcome this problem [2, 3].

OCT is used intensively in the field of ophthalmology as many commercial OCT systems are available for diagnostic purposes. With modern OCT systems, high-resolution 3D images of target tissues can be acquired within few seconds. These properties have made OCT an indispensable tool for the diagnosis and monitoring of retinal diseases and glaucoma.

2.2 How Does OCT Work?

In a biological imaging system, tissue properties must be detected in order to specify the type of tissue and the relative position of tissues of interest so as to construct the final image [2, 3]. Different biological tissues have different light reflecting

A. Akman
Department of Ophthalmology, School of Medicine, Başkent University,
Ankara, Turkey

© Springer International Publishing AG, part of Springer Nature 2018
A. Akman et al. (eds.), *Optical Coherence Tomography in Glaucoma*,
https://doi.org/10.1007/978-3-319-94905-5_2

(back reflectance) properties resulting in different echo magnitudes. These relative differences enable OCT to differentiate layers of the target tissue. In order to replicate the tissue architecture, the system must determine the relative positions of different layers to each other. This depends on the echo delay time. Hence, the longer the distance traveled, the longer the time delay for the light to return to the detector. Because of the speed of the light, the measurement of distances with a 10 µm resolution in retina requires an echo delay time of 30 femtoseconds (30 × 10^{-15} or 1/1,000,000,000,000,000 of a second) which is very difficult to measure with the current detectors [3]. In order to detect such small delays in a reflected signal, interferometry techniques are required. These techniques started with Time Domain-OCT and evolved over time to the Fourier Domain-OCTs.

2.3   OCT System Designs

The two main techniques for detecting and comparing the back scattered light from target tissues consist of time domain and Fourier domain analysis. Fourier domain analysis can be of two subtypes known as spectral domain and swept source.

2.3.1   Time Domain OCT

Time domain-OCT (TD-OCT) was the first technique used in the early years of OCT research and OCT 1 by Carl Zeiss Meditec was the first commercial TD-OCT device available for ophthalmological use in 1997 [4–6]. Technically, in order to measure the light intensity and echo delay time, the light from the broadband source is split with a beam splitter into two different paths. The first beam is projected into the eye (the sample arm), and the other part of the light beam is conveyed to a movable reference mirror (the reference arm). The light beam reflected back from the sample tissue, and the one form the reference mirror are compared using a low coherence interferometry system which requires the mechanical movement of the reference mirror closer to and farther from the beam splitter in time, in order to estimate the depth or axial distance within the tissue (Fig. 2.1). Multiple axial scans (A-scans) are combined to construct individual B-scans. Computer systems in the OCT devices then construct the final 2D or 3D images either in gray scale or false color using proprietary algorithms.

Due to the need for continuing movements of the reference mirror, time domain systems can acquire a maximum of 400 A-scans per second, which limits the axial resolution of TD-OCT systems to around 10–15 µm.

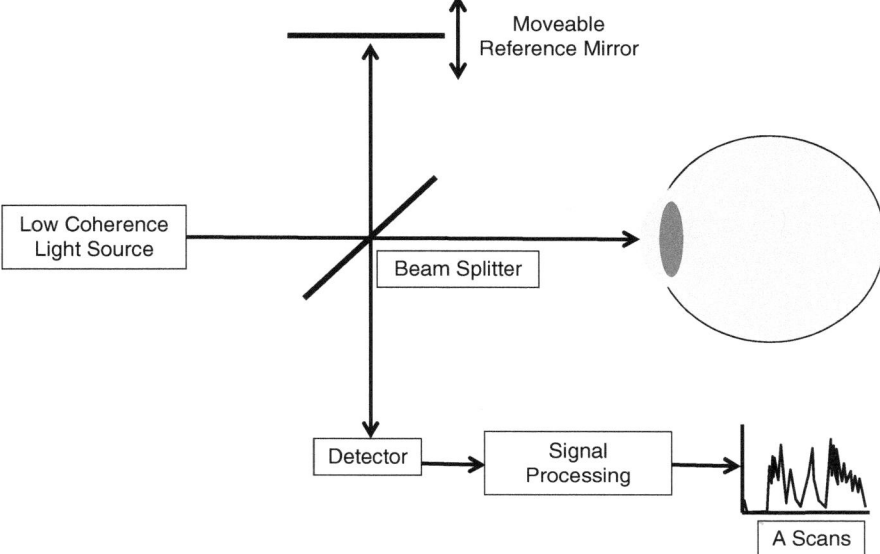

Fig. 2.1   Basic principle of Time Domain OCT

2.3.2   *Spectral Domain OCT*

Spectral Domain OCT (SD-OCT) is one of the OCT techniques that use Fourier domain transformation. This method is also called spatially encoded frequency domain OCT. Leitgeb et al. described the adaptation of Fourier domain-OCT spectroscopic measurements to OCT in 2000 [7]. SD-OCTs do not require a moving reference mirror like TD-OCTs. This increases the scanning speed exponentially [8]. Commercially available SD-OCT systems have scanning speeds of 18,000–70,000 A scans/second making them 200–400 times faster than TD-OCT systems.

In spectral domain technique, the light source is a broad-bandwidth light source. In addition, unlike to the TD-OCT which utilizes an interferometer with a scanning reference arm using mechanically moving reference mirror for detecting echo delay times, SD-OCT uses a fixed mirror and a spectrometer and linear CCD for analyzing interferences between sample beam and reference beam using Fourier transformation. Absence of mechanically movable mirror speeds up the image acquisition up to 200–400 times. The spectral interference patterns between the reference and the sample beams are dispersed by a spectrometer and collected simultaneously with an array detector in SD-OCT systems (Fig. 2.2). This method, essentially measures all echoes of the light simultaneously, thus the acquired

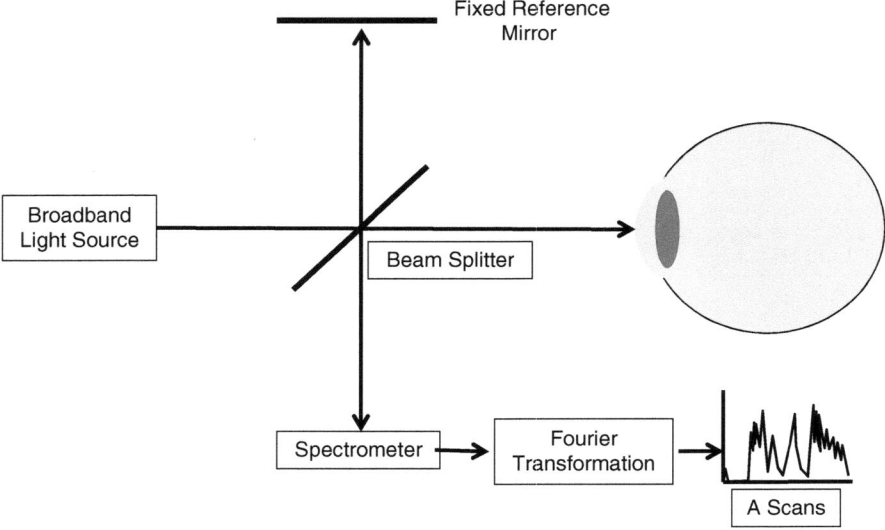

Fig. 2.2 Basic principle of Spectral Domain OCT

spectra can be immediately converted to depth data (A-scans) [3]. Increasing scanning speed reduces artifacts caused by eye movements and results in higher resolution [8]. The axial resolution of current SD-OCT systems is around 5 μm. After the development of SD-OCT systems, they quickly became the standard for leading OCT manufacturers. Zeiss Cirrus HD-OCT (Carl Zeiss Meditec, Dublin, CA), Heidelberg Engineering Spectralis OCT (Heidelberg Engineering, Heidelberg, Germany) Optovue RT-Vue (Optovue Inc., Fremont, CA) and Topcon 3D OCT 2000 (Topcon Medical Systems, Oakland, NJ) are the most commonly used SD-OCT platforms worldwide.

2.3.3 Swept-Source OCT

Swept-Source OCT (SS-OCT) is another type of OCT that uses the Fourier domain principles. It is also called time encoded frequency domain OCT, and it combines the advantages of standard TD-OCT and SD-OCT. SS-OCT does not need a moving mirror like TD-OCT and does not require a spectrometer like SD-OCT.

SS-OCT uses a narrow bandwidth light source, which changes the wavelength and sweeps across a narrow band of wavelengths in time. The variation in frequency with time, encodes different echo delay times in the light beam. Hence, SS-OCT labels spectral components in time instead of spatial separation [9]. In SS-OCT, as the light source is already divided into a spectrum through the swept source laser, a spectroscope is unnecessary and instead, a high-speed detector detects the interference signal as a function of time and a Fourier transformation is used for measuring

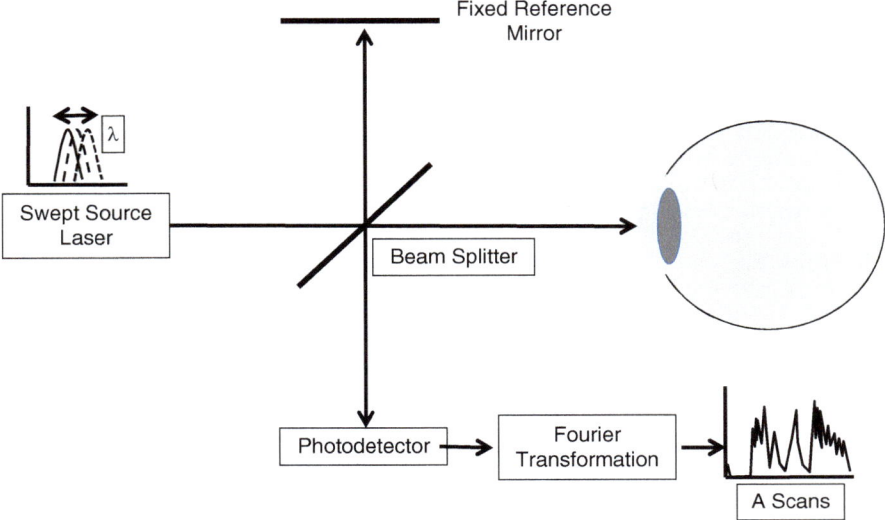

Fig. 2.3 Basic Principle of Swept Source OCT

the echo delay times and echo magnitudes [10–12] (Fig. 2.3). Like SD-OCT, SS-OCT measures all the light echoes at the same time, which dramatically improves the detection sensitivity [3].

In addition to being less technically complex, SS-OCTs can reach scan speeds up to 100,000 A-scans/second. Improved signal to noise ratio (SNR), deeper tissue penetration and wider imaging field are other advantages of SS-OCT although the axial resolution of current SS-OCT systems is lower than SD-OCTs [13].

In summary, TD-OCT, the first commercial OCT system, revolutionized the field of ophthalmology. Fourier domain-OCT subsequently improved the speed and imaging quality of OCT systems, and made the OCT an indispensable tool for the management of retinal disease and glaucoma. SS-OCT platforms and OCT Angiography are newer technologies and will likely become more widely available in near future.

References

1. Huang D, Swanson EA, Lin CP, Schuman JS, Stinson WG, Chang W, Hee MR, Flotte T, Gregory K, Puliafito CA, Fujimoto JG. Optical coherence tomography. Science. 1991;254(5035):1178–81.
2. Fercher AF, Drexler W, Hitzenberger CK, Lasser T. Optical coherence tomography-principles and applications. Rep Prog Phys. 2003;66(2):239.
3. Drexler W, Fujimoto JG. Introduction to optical coherence tomography. In: Drexler W, Fujimoto JG, editors. Optical coherence tomography: technology and applications: Springer; 2008. p. 1–40.

4. Schuman JS, Hee MR, Arya AV, Pedut- Kloizman T, Puliafito CA, Fujimoto JG, Swanson EA. Optical coherence tomography: a new tool for glaucoma diagnosis. Curr Opin Ophthalmol. 1995;6:89–95.
5. Fercher AF, Hitzenberger CK, Drexler W, Kamp G, Sattmann H. In vivo optical coherence tomography. Am J Ophthalmol. 1993;116:113–4.
6. Swanson EA, Izatt JA, Hee MR, Huang D, Lin CP, Schuman JS, Puliafito CA Fujimoto JG. In vivo retinal imaging by optical coherence tomography. Opt Lett. 1993;18:1864–6.
7. Leitgeb R, Wojtkowski M, Kowalczyk A, Hitzenberger CK, Sticker M, Fercher AF. Spectral measurement of absorption by spectroscopic frequency-domain optical coherence tomography. Opt Lett. 2000;25:820–2.
8. de Boer JF, Cense B, Park BH, Pierce MC, Tearney GJ, Bouma BE. Improved signal-to-noise ratio in spectral-domain compared with time-domain optical coherence tomography. Opt Lett. 2003;28:2067–9.
9. Choma MA, Hsu K, Izatt JA. Swept source optical coherence tomography using an all-fiber 1300-nm ring laser source. J Biomed Opt. 2005;10:44009.
10. Choma M, Sarunic M, Yang C, Izatt J. Sensitivity advantage of swept source and Fourier domain optical coherence tomography. Opt Express. 2003;11:2183–9.
11. Yun SH, Tearney G, de Boer J, Bouma B. Pulsed-source and swept-source spectral-domain optical coherence tomography with reduced motion artifacts. Opt Express. 2004;12:5614–24.
12. Zhang J, Rao B, Chen Z. Swept source based fourier domain functional optical coherence tomography. Conf Proc IEEE Eng Med Biol Soc. 2005;7:7230–3.
13. Munk MR, Giannakaki-Zimmermann H, Berger L, Huf W, Ebneter A, Wolf S, Zinkernagel MS. OCT-angiography: a qualitative and quantitative comparison of 4 OCT-A devices. PLoS One. 2017;12(5):e0177059.

Chapter 3
Role of Optical Coherence Tomography in Glaucoma

Ahmet Akman

3.1 Introduction

Retinal ganglion cells (RGC) are large, complex neurons, which are the main cells affected in glaucoma. Dendrites of the RGCs make synapses with bipolar and amacrine cells in the inner plexiform layer (IPL) of the retina. Cell bodies of the RGCs make up the ganglion cell layer (GCL) and their axons form the retinal nerve fiber layer (RNFL). All the axons in the RNFL converge at the optic nerve head (ONH) to form the neuro-retinal rim. The RGC axons synapse in the lateral geniculate body with the third neuron of the visual pathway.

Optical Coherence Tomography (OCT) has revolutionized the diagnosis and monitoring of glaucoma as it can detect RGC damage objectively and quantitatively [1]. As structural damage frequently precedes functional damage, methods that are able to identify structural damage are of utmost importance for early diagnosis of glaucoma [2–4]. For decades, the only tool available for diagnosing glaucoma with structural means was clinical observation of the changes on ONH photographs. With the advent of digital imaging methods such as scanning laser polarimetry and confocal scanning laser systems, objective and quantitative evaluation of the ONH and RNFL became possible [5–7]. OCT has replaced these systems over the last decade and has become the gold standard for detecting early structural glaucomatous damage, as it can evaluate RNFL, macular ganglion cell and ONH changes at the same time with high reproducibility and reliability [7–11]. Kuang et al. demonstrated that OCT could detect glaucomatous damage 5 years prior to appearance of the first visual field (VF) defects in one third of patients based on average RNFL thickness measurements [12].

The 10th World Glaucoma Association Consensus publication, published in 2016, stated that, detecting progressive glaucomatous RNFL thinning and neuroretinal

A. Akman
Department of Ophthalmology, School of Medicine, Başkent University, Ankara, Turkey

© Springer International Publishing AG, part of Springer Nature 2018
A. Akman et al. (eds.), *Optical Coherence Tomography in Glaucoma*,
https://doi.org/10.1007/978-3-319-94905-5_3

13

rim narrowing are the best available gold standards for glaucoma diagnosis. Detection of VF defects is not imperative for the diagnosis of glaucoma and OCT is the best currently available digital imaging technology for detecting structural damage in glaucoma [13].

Figure 3.1 summarizes the timeline of changes in glaucomatous eyes demonstrating disease progression. In the preperimetric stages of the disease, RNFL loss is the first sign of structural damage followed by or accompanied by ONH changes. Animal data have shown that neuroretinal changes may precede RNFL loss although clinical evidence is still lacking [14]. As the disease progresses to the perimetric stage, VF changes start to emerge. The relationship of these structural and functional tests in glaucoma will be discussed in detail in Chap. 16.

Among the three parameters that can be evaluated with OCT, RNFL thickness measurements are the most widely studied. RNFL thickness parameters were the main outcome to be measured in the TD-OCT era. With the higher resolution and denser sampling capabilities of SD-OCT, reliable Ganglion Cell Analysis became a possibility. Finally, SD-OCT allowed imaging of the ONH anatomic features with great precision and led to development of newer outcome measures such as the Bruch's membrane opening (BMO) based minimum rim width (MRW). The aim of this chapter is to summarize the role of these three approaches in clinical practice for the diagnosis of glaucoma.

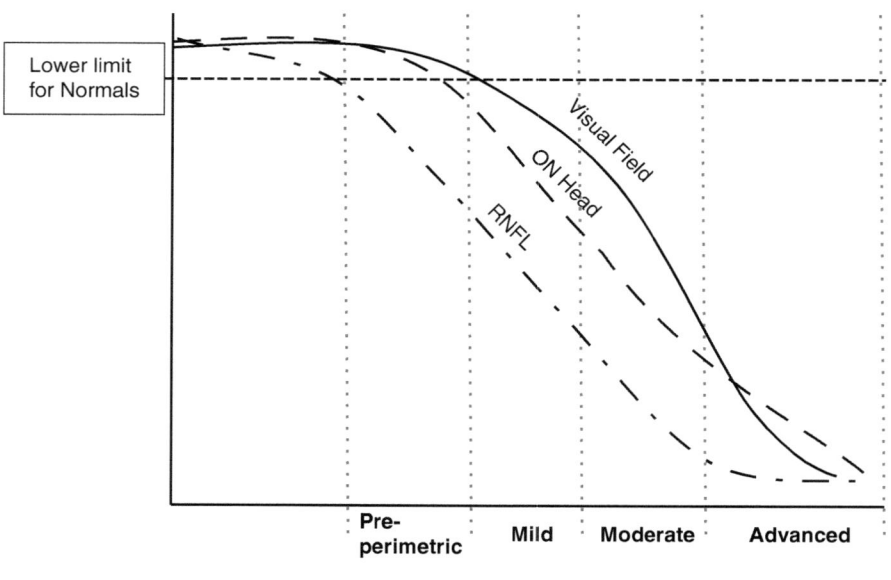

Fig. 3.1 Timeline of structural and functional changes in glaucoma. (Modified form original slide by Weinreb RN, Robert N. Shaffer Lecture at the 105th Annual Meeting of the American Academy of Ophthalmology, New Orleans, 2001, with permission from Robert N. Weinreb)

3.2 RNFL Analysis

Quigley and associates showed that RNFL changes frequently preceded ONH changes [10]. However, RNFL thinning is difficult to identify on routine fundus examination. To overcome this obstacle, various imaging modalities have been used in the past to detect peripapillary RNFL loss, including red free photography, scanning laser polarimetry and confocal scanning laser ophthalmoscopy. Since the availability of OCT, it has become the preferred technique for RNFL analysis in eyes with suspected or established glaucoma [15].

There are two basic strategies for peripapillary RNFL analysis with OCT. The first one is to scan and construct a three-dimensional map of the RNFL around the ONH. Current Carl Zeiss Meditec (Dublin, CA), Topcon Medical Systems (Oakland, NJ) and Optovue Inc. (Fremont, CA) SD-OCT systems construct these maps, which provide a detailed analysis of RNFL changes included in the cube. The second and most studied strategy is to measure the peripapillary RNFL thickness on a 3.46 mm scan circle centered on the ONH or BMO. This circle is called the calculation circle in Zeiss Cirrus HD-OCT as it is calculated from the 6 × 6mm Optic Disc Cube. On the other hand, Heidelberg Spectralis OCT (Heidelberg Engineering, Heidelberg, Germany) does not use a scan cube for RNFL measurements. It uses data from a single 3.46 mm circular scan around the ONH and names this circle the scan circle. The newer software on the Heidelberg Spectralis OCT (Glaucoma Module Premium Edition, GMPE) now measures the RNFL on 3 concentric circles centered on the BMO at 3.46, 4.1, and 4.7 mm diameters. Also, other instruments and some other authors use the term 'measurement circle' for this. As the calculation circle, measurement circle and scan circle are terms that define the same 3.46 mm circle, they are used interchangeably depending on the OCT device throughout this book.

3.2.1 RNFL Thickness Map

SD-OCT devices can scan the ONH area in a few seconds and construct three-dimensional maps of the RNFL around the ONH with high precision. Figure 3.2 shows RNFL thickness map scans from different OCT devices. Different OCT devices use different scan cube sizes; Cirrus HD-OCT scans a 6 × 6 mm area comprised of 200 horizontal scans each consisting of 200 A-scans resulting in a three-dimensional RNFL thickness map with a resolution of 200 × 200 A-scans. Each A-scan corresponds to a 30-micron square of the retina in an emmetropic eye. RNFL changes across the 6 × 6 mm (200 × 200 pixel) area around the ONH may detect RNFL loss better compared to a single 3.46 mm circumpapillary RNFL scan [16–18].

Leung et al. compared the RNFL thickness map with the circumpapillary RNFL calculation circle data and concluded that the former significantly improved diagnostic sensitivity by providing additional spatial and morphologic information

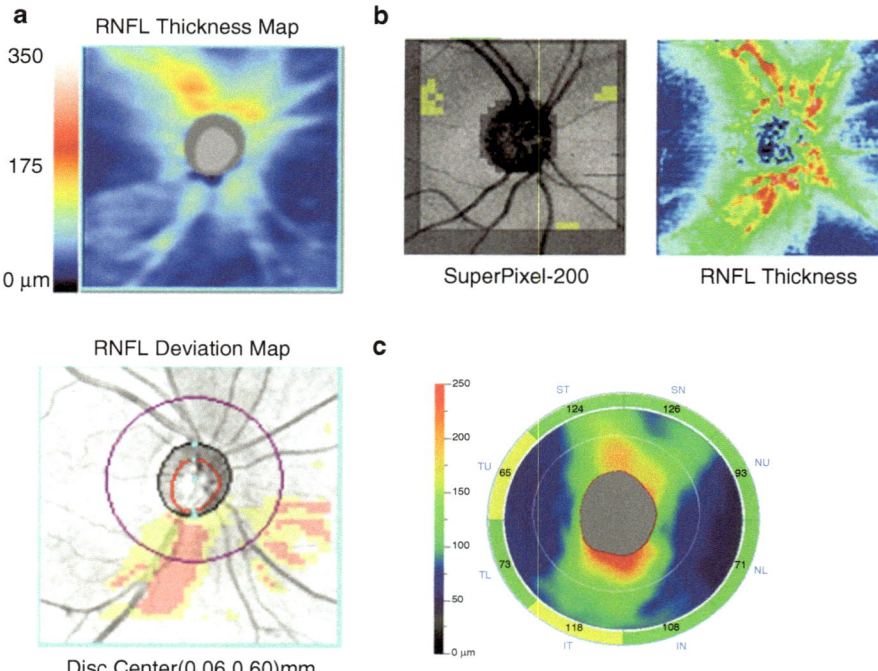

Fig. 3.2 RNFL thickness maps from three SD-OCT devices. (**a**). Zeiss Cirrus HD-OCT (pseudo-color RNFL thickness map, RNFL deviation map), (**b**) Topcon 3D OCT 2000 (RNFL deviation map, pseudo-color thickness map), and (**c**) Optovue (pseudo-color thickness map)

about RNFL damage [18]. In another study, the same group showed that the most common location for RNFL thinning was at the infero-temporal meridians approximately 2 mm from the disc center. As the radius of the 3.46 mm calculation circle is 1.73 mm, RNFL thickness map scan is required to show changes in this region, which is outside the confines of the 3.46 mm calculation circle [17].

3.2.2 The RNFL Calculation Circle

Peripapillary RNFL measurement based on the calculation circle is the most frequently used method for evaluating RNFL loss. In the early days of OCT, TD-OCT systems did not have enough resolution and scan speed to construct RNFL thickness maps; hence, only a single circumpapillary RNFL scan centered on the ONH was utilized. The scan circle was set to an arbitrary 3.4 mm diameter based on an earlier study by Schuman et al. [19]. Subsequently, all OCT manufacturers adopted the 3.46 mm scan circle and it became the standard for glaucoma diagnostic studies in the literature. Apart from this 3.46 mm scan circle, which is available in all current

OCT devices, the GMPE software of Spectralis OCT has 4.1 and 4.7 mm scan circle options although their clinical significance is yet to be determined. Current SD-OCT devices center the 3.46 mm scan circle on the ONH Bruch's membrane opening (BMO) centroid automatically. The role of BMO in glaucoma diagnostics will be discussed in detail under ONH analysis in Sect. 3.4.

3.2.2.1   The RNFL Calculation Circle and TSNIT Plots

Circumpapillary RNFL calculation or circular scan data can be presented in many different formats. Each manufacturer has their own preferred format for this purpose. Most OCT devices provide average, hemifield, quadrant and clock hour sector thickness measurements. In addition, the numeric data are often presented on false color (pseudo-color) maps or with pie graphs.

One common plot used by all OCT platforms is the TSNIT plot for reporting the RNFL thickness values along the calculation or scan circle. TSNIT maps were originally used to display RNFL thickness measurements on GDx device (Laser Diagnostic Technologies, San Diego, CA), which measures RNFL thicknesses based on scanning laser polarimetry. With the evolution of OCT, scanning laser polarimetry lost its popularity but many of the presentation concepts for RNFL measurements and analysis were adopted for OCT reports.

The segmentation algorithm of the OCT software identifies the RNFL and measures the RNFL thickness on the circular peripapillary scan. The RNFL measurements along the calculation or scan circle are then plotted starting from temporal quadrant (9 o'clock in the right eye, 3 o'clock in the left eye) in a clockwise fashion for the right eye and counterclockwise fashion for the left eye as TSNIT plot. TSNIT stands for **T**emporal **S**uperior **N**asal **I**nferior **T**emporal locations (Fig. 3.3). The RNFL thickness values are displayed along the calculation circle starting temporally, moving superiorly, nasally, inferiorly and ending temporally. The direction is clockwise for the right eye and counterclockwise for the left eye. Normally, a double hump pattern is visible on the TSNIT plot with the peak RNFL areas located in the superior and inferior quadrants. Comparisons to the normative database of any given OCT device is performed and the probability values for abnormality along the RNFL thickness measurements are presented on the TSNIT plots. The probability levels for the RNFL thickness on the TSNIT plot are displayed on a four-color scale with white, green, yellow and red colors displaying progressively thinner RNFL. RNFL measurements at or below the thinnest 1%ile of the measurements from the normative database fall into the red area and are considered to be outside normal limits. RNFL measurements within the thinnest 1–5%ile of the normative database are considered borderline abnormal and are flagged as yellow. Eyes with RNFL measurements within the middle 90%ile of the normative database measurements are considered within normal limits and marked in green. RNFL thickness measurements beyond the 95%ile of the normative database measurements are considered higher than normal and are flagged as white [20].

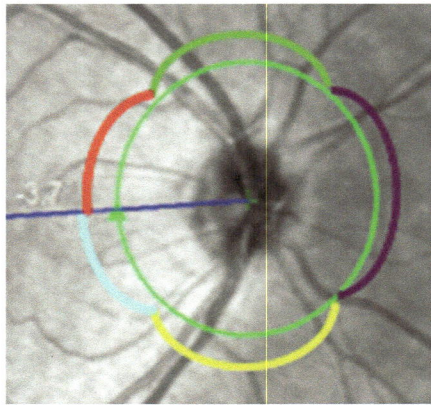

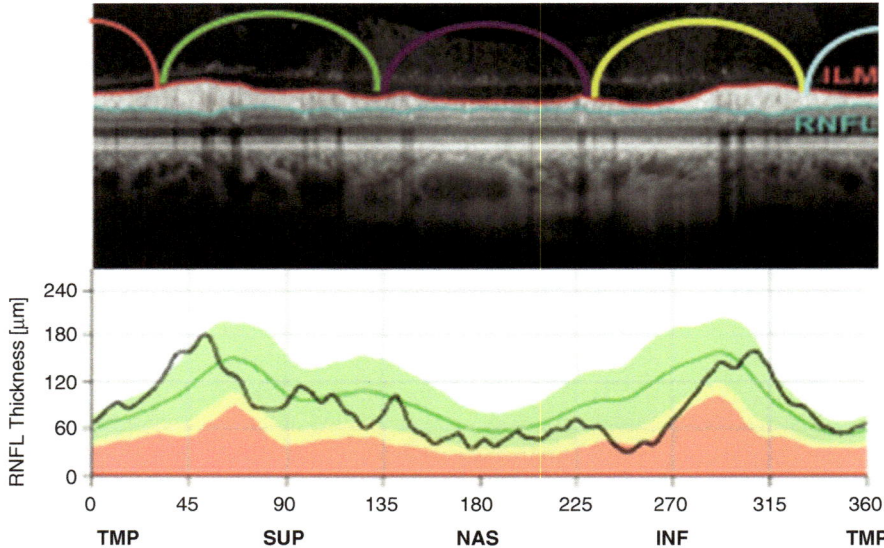

Fig. 3.3 Schematic representation for calculation of a TSNIT map for an RNFL scan from Spectralis OCT

Each manufacturer uses its own normative database values for defining the green, yellow and red areas on the TSNIT maps. Although the layout looks similar, the results cannot be used interchangeably among different devices.

Most of the published papers about the diagnostic capability of OCT in glaucoma use the average and sectorial RNFL thickness data from the calculation circle. In general, the average and inferior quadrant peripapillary RNFL thickness values are the OCT parameters with the best diagnostic accuracy, followed by the superior quadrant RNFL thickness [1, 17, 21, 22]. The test-retest variability of the current SD-OCT systems for the average RNFL thickness is under 5 μm making the average RNFL thickness parameter the most reproducible OCT parameter [23–27]. Using the quadrant and sector RNFL thickness data for glaucoma diagnosis may increase the sensitivity but decreases the specificity. Average RNFL thickness abnormalities can detect glaucoma with 95% specificity in up to 35% of glaucoma suspect eyes 4 years prior to detectable VF loss and in up to 19% of the eyes, 8 years prior to detectable VF loss [12].

RNFL thickness slowly decreases with age. Normative databases of the commercial OCT systems include RNFL thickness data from different age groups and the RNFL thickness results of each patient is compared with age-matched normative values. In addition to age, axial length and race can influence the distribution of normal RNFL thickness measurements. To overcome this problem, some of the OCT devices include normative data from individuals from different races and varying levels of myopia.

3.3   Macular Ganglion Cell Analysis

More than 50% of the eye's RGCs are located at the macula [28]. The GCL, which is composed of 6 to 8 layers of RGCs constitutes up to 30% to 35% of the total retinal thickness in the macula [27]. RGC loss can be detected in the macula at early stages of glaucoma [28–30]. Importance of the macular region in glaucoma is underestimated as the most frequently used VF testing algorithms such as 30–2 or 24–2 may miss evidence of early glaucomatous damage in the macula and the 10–2 strategy is not commonly used in early disease [31–33]. The reason for the underestimation of early macular damage in glaucoma before SD-OCT became available was the lack of clinical examination methods or imaging techniques that could detect macular damage in glaucoma. TD-OCT's focus was on RNFL thickness measurements, as segmentation of the inner retinal layers was not reliable with the relatively low resolution and the poor sampling density of TD-OCT devices [34]. SD-OCTs overcame the technical difficulties in segmenting macular layers, and macular imaging protocols became an essential part of the diagnostic tools for glaucoma detection. Macular imaging has significant advantages over peripapillary RNFL and ONH parameters in diagnosing glaucoma as it has very low variability and is less prone to artifacts and anatomical variations.

Low reflectivity of the ganglion cell layer is the main challenge for the SD-OCT segmentation algorithms. Since it is difficult to differentiate the GCL and inner plexiform layer (IPL) boundary, and the GCL from RNFL internally, various manufacturers have used different inner retinal layer combinations for diagnosis of glaucoma. Optovue's RT-Vue OCT introduced Ganglion Cell Complex (GCC) thickness measurements. The GCC includes the three innermost layers of the retina; the RNFL, ganglion cell layer and IPL, hence, the GCC contains the axons, cell bodies and dendrites of the ganglion cells that are preferentially affected by glaucoma. Therefore, measuring GCC thickness would be expected to be more sensitive and specific to the disease [35]. Zeiss' Cirrus HD-OCT provides the ganglion cell and inner plexiform layers (GCL + IPL) in its Ganglion Cell Analysis (GCA) software.

This is based on the premise that excluding RNFL from the inner retinal thickness measurements could decrease variability [36].

Heidelberg Engineering Spectralis OCT Posterior Pole Asymmetry analysis was originally able to measure only the total retinal thickness in the macula instead of segmenting different layers of the macula. An intra-eye asymmetry analysis compares the inferior and superior half of the macula [37]. In addition, an inter-eye asymmetry comparison presents one-to-one between-eye differences in superpixel thickness. This method also has a high sensitivity and specificity [38]. The current version of the Spectralis OCT (GMPE) is able to segment individual macular layers separately, but no statistical analysis is provided in the current software.

Topcon Medical Systems manufactures both SD and SS-OCT systems. The SS-OCT system of Topcon, called the DRI-OCT Triton, can scan the peripapillary area and macula in a single 9 × 12mm scan and can measure both GCC and GCL + IPL thickness concurrently.

Introduction of these different segmentation algorithms enhanced the utility and importance of macular OCT imaging. Multiple studies have shown that GCC and GCL + IPL thickness measurements are able to differentiate glaucomatous eyes from normal control eyes with high accuracy [39–42]. Yang et al. showed that both SS-OCT and SD-OCT devices could detect glaucoma with comparable accuracy when compared to peripapillary RNFL measurements [43].

The inferior temporal sector is the most common region displaying GCL + IPL thinning in the macula, which is consistent with the peripapillary area demonstrating RNFL defects most frequently (inferior sectors) [16, 44–46]. As glaucoma deteriorates, arcuate defects and more diffuse damage can be observed in the macula [29, 47].

Although macular ganglion cell OCT compares well to peripapillary RNFL thickness measurements for detection of glaucoma, macular diseases are common in the elderly and disorders such as senile macular degeneration, diabetic maculopathy, and epiretinal membranes may limit the usefulness of macular OCT in glaucoma diagnosis and monitoring. In addition, as the macula contains only 50% of the eye's RGCs, the health of the remaining 50% of RGCs can only be gauges with peripapillary RNFL measurements.

3.4 Optic Nerve Head Analysis

All OCT devices scan the ONH area and provide some information about the ONH health. The scan area and scan properties vary among different OCT devices. Depending on the software algorithm and technical capabilities of the device, different ONH parameters including the cup-to-disc ratio, neuroretinal rim area, and neuroretinal rim volume are provided.

For the ONH analysis, the OCT machine needs to first identify the ONH border. Most current OCT devices consider the BMO as a proxy for the ONH boundary. One reason is the relative ease of identifying the Bruch's membrane on OCT scans.

The segmentation algorithm can fairly easily find the BMO for all available B scans. Identification of the BMO enables the software to determine the centroid of the ONH, which is subsequently used for proper centration of the calculation ring used for RNFL analysis. This method is used by all manufacturers and has a very high repeatability and reproducibility [48, 49]. In addition, identification of the BMO allows the devices to define the optic disc border. After placement of the optic disc border ring, the cup boundary was determined by internal limiting membrane (ILM) termination in some of the earlier OCT devices.

A new definition of the neuroretinal rim area measures the minimum distance from the BMO to ILM and the resulting parameter is called the BMO-MRW (Fig. 3.4) [50, 51].

Zeiss' Cirrus HD-OCT extracts the ONH data from the 200 × 200 Optic Disc Cube scan and has used a concept similar to BMO-MRW since Cirrus HD-OCT optic nerve software was released in 2010. Although this method is widely named as MRW measurement, Cirrus' software minimizes areas instead of distance to determine the neuro-retinal rim border. Cirrus' ONH normative significance limits are corrected for optic disc size and disc tilt. The results are reported in TSNIT type graphs and a summary table for key parameters. On the other hand, Spectralis' original report did not present any information about ONH parameters. ONH analysis became available with the introduction of the GMPE software, which uses the BMO-MRW concept for determining the neuroretinal rim boundaries (Fig. 3.4). The GMPE software can provide geometrically accurate measurements based on 24 radial measurements centered on the BMO centroid (48 data points); this is in contrast to older systems such scanning laser ophthalmoscopy that measured the neuroretinal rim area along or parallel to the fixed plane of the clinical disc margin. The BMO-MRW based approach has a higher diagnostic accuracy for glaucoma and demonstrates a stronger structure-function relationship [51, 52].

The superiority of ONH parameters to RNFL outcomes for diagnosis of early glaucoma is still controversial. While some studies showed ONH parameters to per-

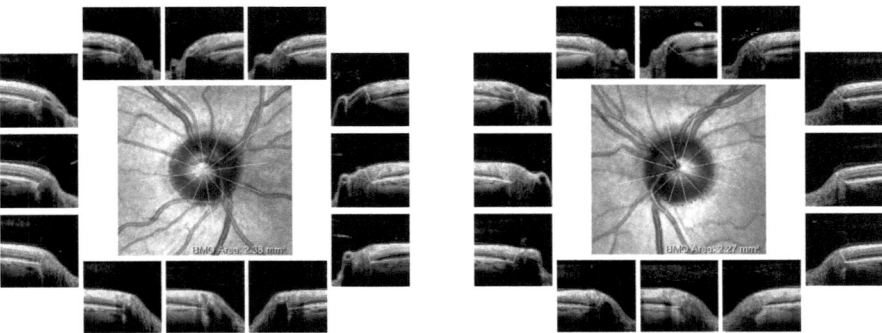

Fig. 3.4 Identification of Bruch's Membrane Opening (BMO) and the BMO-Minimum Rim Width (BMO-MRW) by the GMPE module of Spectralis OCT. The green arrows represent the minimum distance between the termination of the Bruch's membrane and ILM

form better for diagnosing early glaucoma, others found RNFL and macular parameters to perform better [53–55]. ONH parameters are very useful for differential diagnosis of non-glaucomatous optic neuropathies. If an OCT print-out shows RNFL and GCC or GCL + IPL damage while the ONH parameters such as cup-to-disc ratio are within normal limits, non-glaucomatous optic neuropathies must be considered in the differential diagnosis. Chap. 9 will discuss the OCT findings in these glaucoma masqueraders in detail.

Apart from diagnosing glaucoma, SD-OCT technology has greatly improved our understanding of the ONH anatomy. Chauhan and Burgoyne proposed that SD-OCT data represented a paradigm shift for clinical assessment of the ONH [56]. The authors emphasized that a SD-OCT based approach to neuroretinal rim evaluation utilizing the BMO-MRW concept and taking into account the fovea-to-BMO axis angle is anatomically and geometrically more accurate and may enhance glaucoma detection.

Using a combination of RNFL, ONH and macular measurement modalities together can increase the chances of identifying glaucomatous damage early during the disease process. Any one of these parameters can be affected earlier than the others and therefore, taking into account the findings from the RNFL, ONH and macula can enhance early diagnosis of glaucoma [1].

References

1. Dong ZM, Wollstein G, Schuman JS. Clinical utility of optical coherence tomography in Glaucoma. Invest Ophthalmol Vis Sci. 2016:57–67.
2. Quigley HA, Addicks EM, Green WR. Optic nerve damage in human glaucoma III. Quantitative correlation of nerve fiber loss and visual field defect in glaucoma, ischemic neuropathy, papilledema, and toxic neuropathy. Arch Ophthalmol. 1982;100:135–46.
3. Hood DC, Kardon RH. A framework for comparing structural and functional measures of glaucomatous damage. Prog Retina Eye Res. 2007;26:688–710.
4. Sommer A, Katz J, Quigley HA, Miller NR, Robin AL, Richter RC, Witt KA. Clinically detectable nerve fiber atrophy precedes the onset of glaucomatous field loss. Arch Ophthalmol. 1991;109:77–83.
5. Kamal DS, Viswanathan AC, Garway-Heath DF, Hitchings RA, Poinoosawmy D, Bunce C. Detection of optic disc change with the Heidelberg retina tomograph before confirmed visual field change in ocular hypertensives converting to early glaucoma. Br J Ophthalmol. 1999;83:290–4.
6. Philippin H, Unsoeld A, Maier P, Walter S, Bach M, Funk J. Ten-year results: detection of long-term progressive optic disc changes with confocal laser tomography. Graefes Arch Clin Exp Ophthalmol. 2006;244:460–4.
7. Sehi M, Greenfield DS. Assessment of retinal nerve fiber layer using optical coherence tomography and scanning laser polarimetry in progressive glaucomatous optic neuropathy. Am J Ophthalmol. 2006;142:1056–9.
8. Wollstein G, Schuman JS, Price LL, Aydin A, Stark PC, Hertzmark E, Lai E, Ishikawa H, Mattox C, Fujimoto JG, Paunescu LA. Optical coherence tomography longitudinal evaluation of retinal nerve fiber layer thickness in glaucoma. Arch Ophthalmol. 2005;23:464–70.

9. Strouthidis NG, Scott A, Peter NM, Garway-Heath DF. Optic disc and visual field progression in ocular hypertensive subjects: detection rates, specificity, and agreement. Invest Ophthalmol Vis Sci. 2006;47:2904–10.
10. Quigley HA, Katz J, Derick RJ, Gilbert D, Sommer A. An evaluation of optic disc and nerve fiber layer examinations in monitoring progression of early glaucoma damage. Ophthalmology. 1992;99:19–28.
11. Medeiros FA, Alencar LM, Zangwill LM, Bowd C, Sample PA, Weinreb RN. Prediction of functional loss in glaucoma from progressive optic disc damage. Arch Ophthalmol. 2009;127:1250–6.
12. Kuang TM, Zhang C, Zangwill LM, Weinreb RN, Medeiros FA. Estimating lead ime gained by optical coherence tomography in detecting Glaucoma before development of visual field defects. Ophthalmology. 2015;122:2002–9.
13. Weinreb RN, Garway-Heath DF, Leung C, Mederios FA, Liebmann J. Diagnosis of primary open angle glaucoma, World Glaucoma association Consesus Series, vol. 10. Amsterdam, The Netherlands: Kugler Publications; 2016.
14. Fortune B, Burgoyne CF, Cull GA, Reynaud J, Wang L. Structural and functional abnormalities of retinal ganglion cells measured in vivo at the onset of optic nerve head surface change in experimental glaucoma. Invest Ophthalmol Vis Sci. 2012;53:3939–50.
15. Huang D, Swanson EA, Lin CP, Schuman JS, Stinson WG, Chang W, Hee MR, Flotte T, Gregory K, Puliafito CA, Fujimoto JG. Optical coherence tomography. Science. 1991;254(5035):1178–81.
16. Leung CK. Diagnosing glaucoma progression with optical coherence tomography. Curr Opin Ophthalmol. 2014;25:104–11.
17. Leung CK, Yu M, Weinreb RN, Lai G, Xu G, Lam DS. Retinal nerve fiber layer imaging with spectral-domain optical coherence tomography: patterns of retinal nerve fiber layer progression. Ophthalmology. 2012;119:1858–66.
18. Leung CK, Lam S, Weinreb RN, Liu S, Ye C, Liu L, He J, Lai GW, Li T, Lam DS. Retinal nerve fiber layer imaging with spectral-domain optical coherence tomography: analysis of the retinal nerve fiber layer map for glaucoma detection. Ophthalmology. 2010;117:1684–91.
19. Schuman JS, Pedut-Kloizman T, Hertzmark E, Hee MR, Wilkins JR, Coker JG, Puliafito CA, Fujimoto JG, Swanson EA. Reproducibility of nerve fiber layer thickness measurements using optical coherence tomography. Ophthalmology. 1996;103:1889–98.
20. Zeiss Cirrus HD-OCT User Manual – Models 500, 5000 Instrument and Review Software 8.1, 2015, p. 179.
21. Wang X, Li S, Fu J, Wu G, Mu D, Li S, Wang J, Wang N. Comparative study of retinal nerve fiber layer measurement by RTVue OCT and. GDx VCC Br J Ophthalmol. 2011;95:509–5.
22. Rao HL, Zangwill LM, Weinreb RN, Sample PA, Alencar LM, Medeiros FA. Comparison of different spectral domain optical coherence tomography scanning areas for glaucoma diagnosis. Ophthalmology. 2010;117:1692–9.
23. Leung CK, Cheung CY, Weinreb RN, Qiu Q, Liu S, Li H, Xu G, Fan N, Huang L, Pang CP, Lam DS. Retinal nerve fiber layer imaging with spectral-domain optical coherence tomography: a variability and diagnostic performance study. Ophthalmology. 2009;116:1257–63.
24. Mwanza J, Chang R, Budenz D, et al. Reproducibility of peripapillary retinal nerve fiber layer thickness and optic nerve head parameters measured with Cirrus HD-OCT in glaucomatous eyes. Invest Ophthalmol Vis Sci. 2010;51:5724–30.
25. Horne MR, Callan T, Durbin M, Abunto T. Inter-visit and Inter-instrument variability for CIRRUS HD-OCT Peripapillary retinal nerve Fiber layer thickness measurements. ARVO 2008 Abstracts, Invest Ophthalmol Vis Sci. 2008;49:4624.
26. Tan BB, Natividad M, Chua KC, Yip LW. Comparison of retinal nerve fiber layer measurement between 2 spectral domain OCT instruments. J Glaucoma. 2012;21:266–73.
27. Wu H, de Boer JF, Chen TC. Reproducibility of retinal nerve Fiber layer thickness measurements using spectral domain optical coherence tomography. J Glaucoma. 2011;20:470–6.

28. Curcio CA, Allen KA. Topography of ganglion cells in human retina. J Comp Neurol. 1990;300:5–25.
29. Hood DC, Slobodnick A, Raza AS, de Moraes CG, Teng CC, Ritch R. Early glaucoma involves both deep local, and shallow widespread, retinal nerve fiber damage of the macular region. Invest Ophthalmol Vis Sci. 2014;55:632–6.
30. Hood DC, Raza AS, de Moraes CG, Liebmann JM, Ritch R. Glaucomatous damage of the macula. Prog Retin Eye Res. 2013;32:1–21.
31. Traynis I, De Moraes CG, Raza AS, Liebmann JM, Ritch R, Hood DC. Prevalence and nature of early glaucomatous defects in the central 10 degrees of the visual field. JAMA Ophthalmol. 2014;132:291–29.
32. Grillo LM, Wang DL, Ramachandran R, Ehrlich AC, De Moraes CG, Ritch R, Hood DC. The 24-2 visual field test misses central macular damage confirmed by the 10-2 visual field test and optical coherence tomography. Translational Vision Science & Technology. 2016;5:15.
33. De Moraes CG, Hood DC, Thenappan A, Girkin CA, Medeiros FA, Weinreb RN, Zangwill LM, Liebmann JM. 24-2 visual fields miss central defects shown on 10-2 tests in glaucoma suspects, ocular hypertensives, and early glaucoma. Ophthalmology. 2017;124:1449–56.
34. Medeiros FA, Zangwill LM, Bowd C, Vessani RM, Susanna R Jr, Weinreb RN. Evaluation of retinal nerve fiber layer optic nerve head, and macular thickness measurements for glaucoma detection using optical coherence tomography. Am J Ophthalmol. 2005;139:44–55.
35. Tan O, Chopra V, Lu AT, Schuman JS, Ishikawa H, Wollstein G, Varma R, Huang D. Detection of macular ganglion cell loss in glaucoma by Fourier-domain optical coherence tomography. Ophthalmology. 2009;116:2305–14.
36. Mwanza JC, Oakley JD, Budenz DL, Chang RT, Knight OJ, Feuer WJ. Macular ganglion cell–inner plexiform layer: automated detection and thickness reproducibility with spectral domain–optical coherence tomography in Glaucoma. Invest Ophthalmol Vis Sci. 2011;52:8323–9.
37. Asrani S, Rosdahl JA, Allingham RR. Novel software strategy for glaucoma diagnosis: asymmetry analysis of retinal thickness. Arch Ophthalmol. 2011;129:1205–11.
38. Seo JH, Kim TW, Weinreb RN, Park KH, Kim SH, Kim DM. Detection of localized retinal nerve fiber layer defects with posterior pole asymmetry analysis of spectral domain optical coherence tomography. Invest Ophthalmol Vis Sci. 2012;53:4347–53.
39. Mwanza JC, Durbin MK, Budenz DL, Sayyad FE, Chang RT, Neelakantan A, Godfrey DG, Carter R, Crandall AS. Glaucoma diagnostic accuracy of ganglion cell-inner plexiform layer thickness: comparison with nerve fiber layer and optic nerve head. Ophthalmology. 2012;119:1151–8.
40. Schulze A, Lamparter J, Pfeiffer N, Berisha F, Schmidtmann I, Hoffmann EM. Diagnostic ability of retinal ganglion cell complex, retinal nerve fiber layer, and optic nerve head measurements by Fourier-domain optical coherence tomography. Graefes Arch Clin Exp Ophthalmol. 2011;249:1039–10.
41. Sung KR, Wollstein G, Kim NR, Na JH, Nevins JE, Kim CY, Schuman JS. Macular assessment using optical coherence tomography for glaucoma diagnosis. Br J Ophthalmol. 2012;96:1452–5.
42. Garas A, Vargha P, Hollo G. Diagnostic accuracy of nerve fiber layer macular thickness and optic disc measurements made with the RTVue-100 optical coherence tomograph to detect glaucoma. Eye (Lond). 2011;25:57–65.
43. Yang Z, Tatham AJ, Weinreb RN, Medeiros FA, Liu T, Zangwill LM. Diagnostic ability of macular ganglion cell inner plexiform layer measurements in glaucoma using swept source and spectral domain optical coherence tomography. PLoS One. 2015;10:e0125957.
44. Tan O, Li G, Lu AT, Varma R, Huang D. Advanced imaging for Glaucoma study group. Mapping of macular substructures with optical coherence tomography for glaucoma diagnosis. Ophthalmology. 2008;115:949–56.
45. Hood DC, Raza AS, de Moraes CG, Johnson CA, Liebmann JM, Ritch R. The nature of macular damage in glaucoma as revealed by averaging optical coherence tomography data. Translational Vision Science & Technology. 2012;1:3.

46. Kotera Y, Hangai M, Hirose F, Mori S, Yoshimura N. Three-dimensional imaging of macular inner structures in glaucoma by using spectral-domain optical coherence tomography. Invest Ophthalmol Vis Sci. 2011;52:1412–4.
47. Wang DL, Raza AS, de Moraes CG, Chen M, Alhadeff P, Jarukatsetphorn R, Ritch R, Hood DC. Central glaucomatous damage of the macula can be overlooked by conventional OCT retinal nerve fiber layer thickness analyses. Translational Vision Science & Technology. 2015;4:4.
48. Reis AS, Sharpe GP, Yang H, Nicolela MT, Burgoyne CF, Chauhan BC. Optic disc margin anatomy in patients with glaucoma and normal controls with spectral domain optical coherence tomography. Ophthalmology. 2012;119:738–47.
49. Almobarak FA, O'Leary N, Reis AS, Sharpe GP, Hutchison DM, Nicolela MT, Chauhan BC. Automated segmentation of optic nerve head structures with optical coherence tomography. Invest Ophthalmol Vis Sci. 2014;55:1161–8.
50. Chauhan BC, Danthurebandara VM, Sharpe GP, Demirel S, Girkin CA, Mardin CY, Scheuerle AF, Burgoyne CF. Bruch's's membrane opening-minimum rim width and retinal nerve fibre layer thickness in a normal white population. A multi-Centre study. Ophthalmology. 2015;122:1786–94.
51. Chauhan BC, O'Leary N, Almobarak FA, Reis AS, Yang H, Sharpe GP, Hutchison DM, Nicolela MT, Burgoyne CF. Enhanced detection of open-angle glaucoma with an anatomically accurate optical coherence tomography-derived neuroretinal rim parameter. Ophthalmology. 2013;120:535–43.
52. Pollet-Villard F, Chiquet C, Romanet JP, Noel C, Aptel F. Structure-function relationships with spectral-domain optical coherence tomography retinal nerve fiber layer and optic nerve head measurements. Invest Ophthalmol Vis Sci. 2014;55:2953–62.
53. Kasumovic SS, Pavljasevic S, Cabric E, Mavija M, Dacic-Lepara S, Jankov M. Correlation between retinal nerve fiber layer and disc parameters in glaucoma suspected eyes. Med Arch. 2014;68:113–1.
54. Sung KR, Na JH, Lee Y. Glaucoma diagnostic capabilities of optic nerve head parameters as determined by Cirrus HD optical coherence tomography. J Glaucoma. 2012;21:498–504.
55. Lisboa R, Paranhos A Jr, Weinreb RN, Zangwill LM, Leite MT, Medeiros FA. Comparison of different spectral domain OCT scanning protocols for diagnosing preperimetric glaucoma. Invest Ophthalmol Vis Sci. 2013;54:3417–34.
56. Chauhan BC, Burgoyne CF. From clinical examination of the optic disc to clinical assessment of the optic nerve head: a paradigm change. Am J Ophthalmol. 2013;156:218–27.

Chapter 4
Optical Coherence Tomography: Manufacturers and Current Systems

Ahmet Akman

4.1 Carl Zeiss Meditec

As the manufacturer of the first commercial optical coherence tomography (OCT) systems, Carl Zeiss Meditec (Dublin, CA) is the manufacturer of a diagnostic OCT device called Cirrus HD-OCT, which is an SD-OCT system, marketed by Carl Zeiss Meditec since 2007. During this period, Cirrus HD-OCT undergone numerous upgrades. The OCT angiography (OCTA) module of the Cirrus HD-OCT is called the Angioplex Metrix. Another addition to Zeiss' OCT line is a Swept Source OCT (SS-OCT) system called Plex Elite 9000 SS-OCT, which will be available in the near future. In addition to diagnostic OCT systems, Carl Zeiss Meditec also manufactures IOLMaster 700, a Swept Source OCT-based biometry system for intraocular lens power calculations and Rescan 700 intraoperative OCT imaging system incorporated with Lumera 700 surgical microscope for retinal surgery.

4.1.1 Cirrus HD-OCT 5000 and 500

Cirrus HD-OCT 5000 and 500 devices are both SD-OCT systems, which use 840 nm superluminescent diode laser optical sources. Both devices have scan speeds of 27,000 A-scans/s, and 5 µm axial and 15 µm transverse resolutions. The difference between the 5000 and 500 models is the presence of a line-scanning ophthalmoscope in the 5000 model, which images the fundus during alignment and imaging. The live OCT image is used for alignment in the 500 device. The Angioplex Metrix module for OCTA can be installed on the 5000 model. FastTrac is an eye tracking system available on Cirrus 5000 model,

A. Akman
Department of Ophthalmology, School of Medicine, Başkent University,
Ankara, Turkey

© Springer International Publishing AG, part of Springer Nature 2018
A. Akman et al. (eds.), *Optical Coherence Tomography in Glaucoma*,
https://doi.org/10.1007/978-3-319-94905-5_4

which tracks the patient's eye movements and reduces motion artifacts. Anterior segment modules can be installed on both the 5000 and 500 models. Advanced software for glaucoma diagnostics is one of the most important components of the Cirrus HD-OCT systems.

4.1.2 Primus 200 OCT

Optical coherence tomography is an expensive technology that is mainly afforded by hospitals or large clinics. In recent years, OCT has become an essential instrument for all ophthalmology practices. Hence, OCT manufacturers have started to produce more affordable and practical OCT systems for smaller volume private practices. Primus 200 OCT aims to bring the OCT availability to private practices. It is an SD-OCT based OCT system from Carl Zeiss Meditec, that has a scan speed of 12,000 A-scans/s, and 5 ± 1 μm axial and < 20 μm transverse resolutions. Both macula and glaucoma modules of the Primus system have limited scan patterns compared to Cirrus HD-OCT. Currently, available scan protocols are 5-line raster scan, 1-line HD scan, Macular Cube scan (512 × 32), and optic nerve head (ONH)/ retinal nerve fiber layer (RNFL) cube scan (128 × 128) [1].

4.1.3 Plex Elite 9000 Swept Source OCT

Swept Source OCT is a recent addition to the commercial OCT line. Although the SS-OCT concept was first described in the mid-1990s, these devices have just become commercially available in recent years with developments in tunable laser based swept source light systems. Plex Elite 9000 uses a swept source tunable laser with a wavelength of 1060 nm. The system can reach a speed up to 100,000 A-scans/s. Although the axial resolution of 6.3 μm is lower than the SD-OCT based Cirrus HD-OCTs system, higher scan speeds enabling wider OCT and OCTA scan protocols such as 9 × 9mm and 12 × 12mm cubes are the main advantages [2–4]. A single wide field macular cube scan provides information about fovea and optic disc including ONH topography, RNFL and macular ganglion cell layer. Figures 4.1 and 4.2 show wide field OCT and OCTA scans from this device.

4.2 Heidelberg Engineering Inc.

Heidelberg Engineering (Heidelberg Engineering Inc., Heidelberg, Germany) manufactures Spectralis Modular OCT systems. Spectralis OCT has different modules for various applications. For glaucoma, the basic original module included the

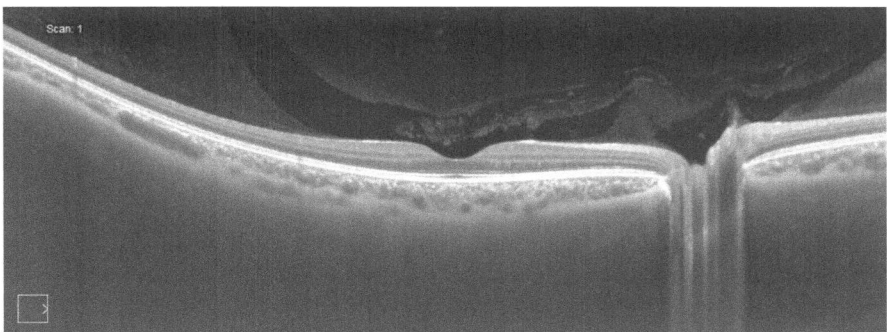

Fig. 4.1 Wide field OCT image of macula and disc in a single scan obtained by Zeiss Elite Plex 9000 SS-OCT system (with permission from Carl Zeiss Meditec)

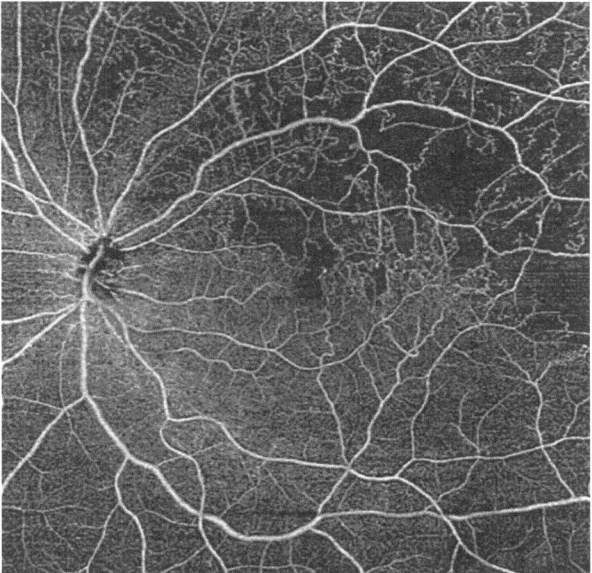

Fig. 4.2 Ultra-Wide 12 × 12mm single shot cubes for flow detection by ZEISS Elite Plex 9000 SS-OCT (with permission from Carl Zeiss Meditec)

RNFL analysis and Posterior Pole Asymmetry analysis software. Glaucoma Module Premium Edition (GMPE) is the newer addition to the Spectralis OCT system, and in addition to some upgrades to the RNFL analysis, detailed ONH analysis is possible with this module. Anterior segment OCT imaging can be performed with the optional anterior segment module. OCTA is one of the recent additions to the Spectralis OCT system but is yet to be available clinically at the time of this writing.

4.2.1 Spectralis OCT

Spectralis OCT includes the retina and glaucoma modules in the standard configuration. The scan rate of Spectralis OCT is 40,000 A-scans/s in the OCT1 device resulting in an axial resolution of 3.9 μm and transverse resolution of 14μm [5]. The OCT 2 module, which is the second generation of the Spectralis OCT increases the scan speed up to 85,000 A-scans/s. Increased scanning speed makes wide field OCT and OCTA possible (Fig. 4.3), hence the OCT 2 module is required for OCTA applications of the Spectralis system (Fig. 4.4). Multimodal imaging, in which fundus photos, fluorescein angiography images and OCT images can be examined in a single output is another feature of the Spectralis system.

IR 30° + OCT 30° (9.8 mm) ART (4) Q: 34 [HS]

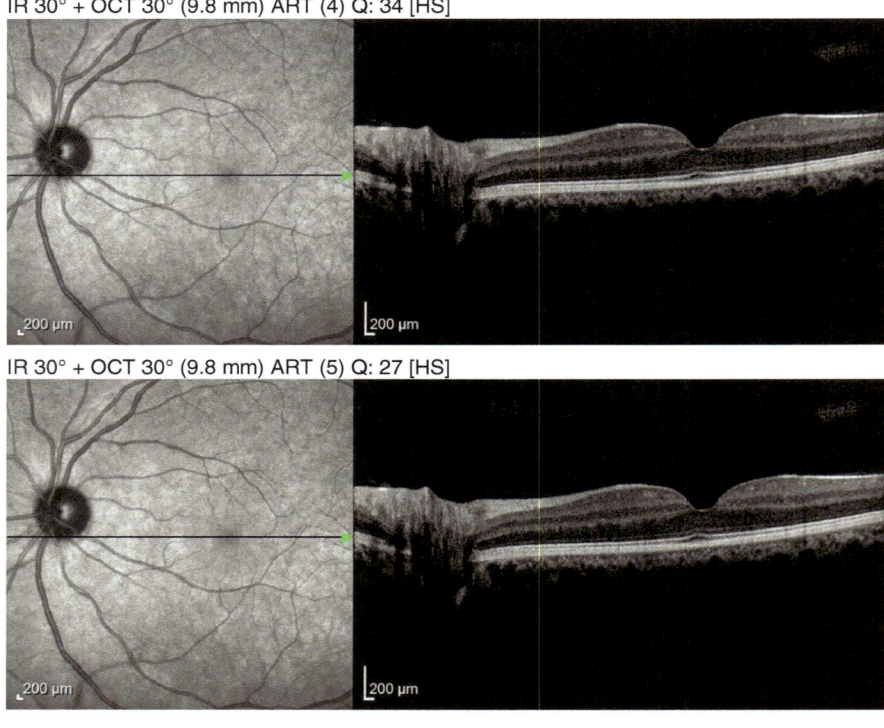

IR 30° + OCT 30° (9.8 mm) ART (5) Q: 27 [HS]

Fig. 4.3 Wide field OCT scans of a healthy eye by the Spectralis OCT with OCT-1 module

4.3   Topcon Medical Systems

Topcon Medical Systems (Oakland, NJ) has been a manufacturer of OCT systems for a long time and is one the companies that first developed commercial SD-OCT systems. Currently, Topcon has two different OCT lines. 3D OCT-1 Maestro is a SD-OCT with fundus camera. DRI OCT Triton is a Swept Source based OCT system capable of performing multimodal imaging and OCTA.

4.3.1   3D OCT-1 Maestro OCT

Maestro is a fully automated SD-OCT based system that can acquire OCT scans by aligning with the pupil automatically. Scan rate is 50,000 A-scans/s with 3 μm axial and 20 μm transverse resolutions. The device simultaneously acquires color fundus photos for multimodal imaging. 12 × 9 mm wide-field OCT imaging is also possible.

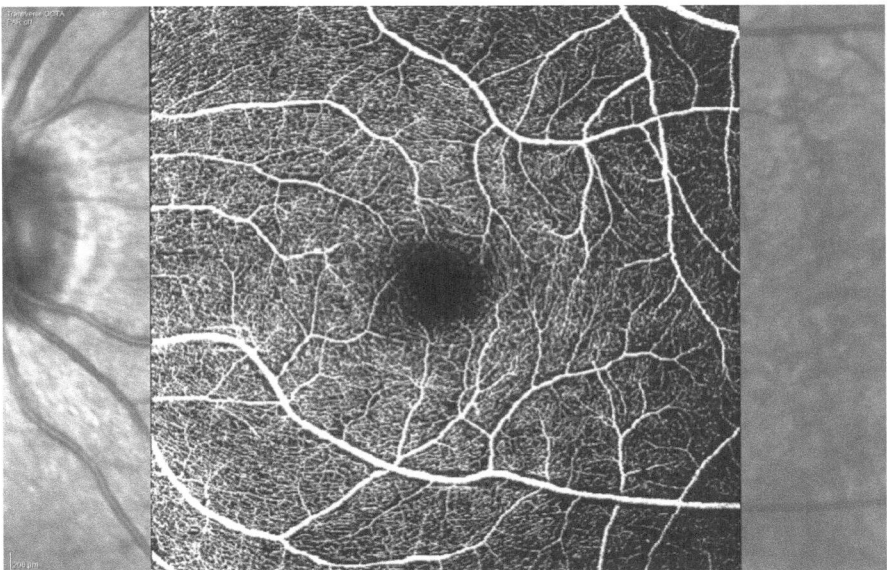

Fig. 4.4 OCTA image from the Spectralis system

4.3.2   DRI OCT Triton Swept Source OCT

DRI OCT Triton SS-OCT is the only commercially available diagnostic SS-OCT system currently in the market. The system uses a 1050 nm scanning light source capable of penetrating deeper layers of the eye. In addition, longer wavelength penetrates better through media opacities like cataract and vitreous hemorrhage. The device has a scan rate of 100,000 A-scans/s with an 8 μm axial and 20 μm transverse resolution [4]. Multimodal imaging is possible as color and red-free fundus photography is a standard option in the Triton system. Anterior segment OCT and OCTA can be added to the Triton system.

The higher scan speed and SMARTtrack eye tracking system enable acquisition of 3D wide-field 12 × 9 mm images, thickness map and B-scans in a very short time. The main advantage of wide field OCT is scanning of a large area of the fundus in a short time concentrating on pathologic regions that can be missed on narrow field scans.

4.4   Optovue

Optovue Inc. (Fremont, CA) was the first company to introduce an FDA-approved SD-OCT system in 2006. The company specializes in manufacturing diagnostic OCT devices and has many different OCT platforms for different patient care settings.

4.4.1   Avanti Wide Field OCT

Avanti Wide field OCT (previously called Avanti RTVue XR) combines the retina, glaucoma and anterior segment OCT capabilities in a single device. The scan rate is 70,000 A-scans/s with a 5 μm axial and 15 μm transverse resolution. The anterior segment module can calculate the total corneal power, which could be used for IOL power calculations specifically in eyes with a history of refractive surgery [6]. The AngioVue OCTA module can be added to the Avanti system.

4.4.2   AngioVue HD

The AngioVue HD is the OCTA system by Optovue, which can produce high density scans on 6 × 6 mm and 3 × 3 cubes [6]. OCTA of the macular (Fig. 4.5) region, peripapillary area (Fig. 4.6) and a combination of the two (Fig. 4.7) is possible with the system.

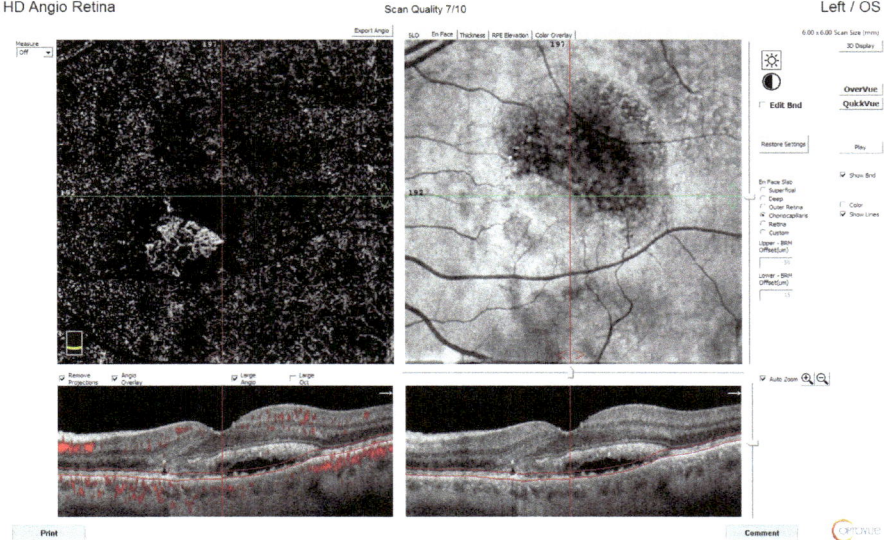

Fig. 4.5 Macular OCTA image of a choroidal neovascular membrane, AngioVue HD OCTA system by Optovue

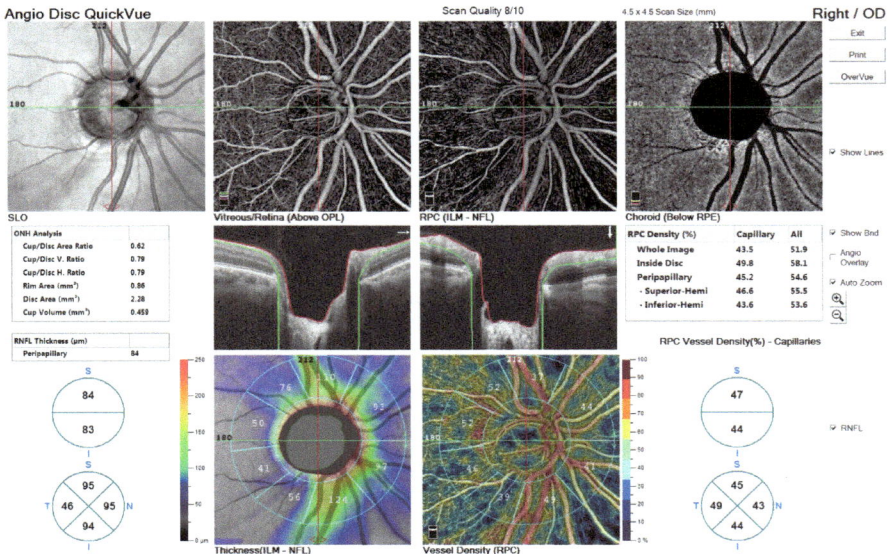

Fig. 4.6 The printout of an optic nerve head and peripapillary optical coherence tomography angiography (OCTA) scan in a glaucoma patient with the AngioVue HD OCTA system by Optovue

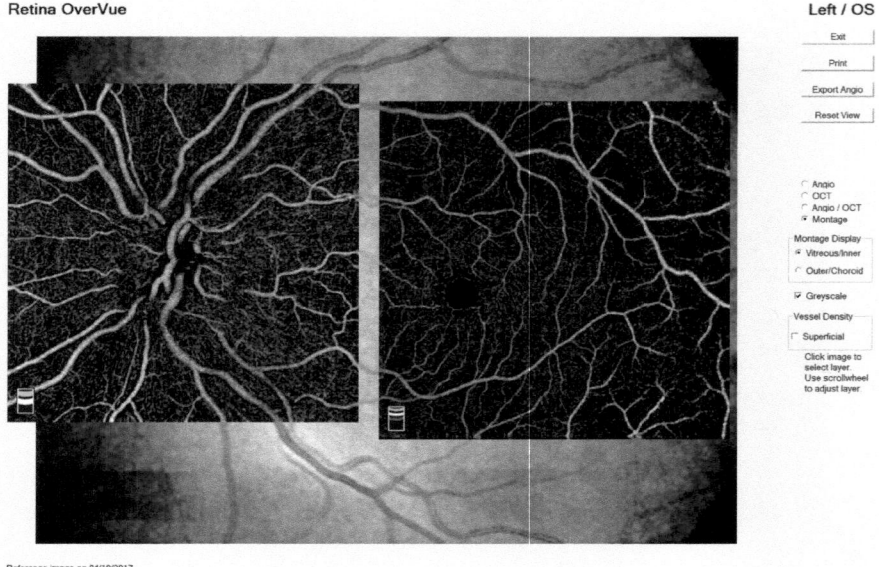

Reference image on 04/19/2017

Fig. 4.7 The combined report of peripapillary and macular optical coherence tomography angiography (OCTA) scans, showing the superficial capillary plexus in a normal eye. The scan was performed with the AngioVue HD OCTA system by Optovue

4.4.3   iVue OCT

iVue is an affordable alternative to Avanti OCT designed for low volume practices. The scan rate is 26000A-scans/s with a 5 μm axial and 15 μm transverse resolution. It can be combined with the iFusion fundus camera system.

4.4.4   iScan OCT

The iScan OCT from Optovue is an automatically aligning OCT device that simplifies image acquisition. The scan rate is 26,000 A-scans/s with a 5 μm axial and 15 μm transverse resolution.

4.5   Other Manufacturers

Many other companies manufacture diagnostic OCT systems for ophthalmic use. In addition to diagnostics, OCT imaging is incorporated into femtosecond laser systems used in cataract and refractive surgery, surgical microscopes for retinal surgery, and biometry devices for IOL power calculations. Table 4.1 provides an overview of the OCT systems available on the market as of this writing.

Table 4.1 Technical specifications of common OCT devices

Manufacturer	Device	Technology	Scan Speed (A-scan/s)	Axial/Transverse Resolution (µm)	Additional Modules	Important points
Zeiss	Cirrus HD-OCT 5000	SD	27,000, 68,000 (only for OCTA)	5/<15	Anterior segment OCTA	Advanced glaucoma statistical software Guided progression analysis Asian eyes database
Zeiss	Cirrus HD-OCT 500	SD	27,000	5/<15	Anterior segment	Advanced glaucoma statistical software Guided progression analysis Asian eyes database
Zeiss	Primus 200	SD	12,000	$5 \pm 1/<20$	Anterior segment	Low cost—Aims private practices Lacks most of the glaucoma scans and analysis of Cirrus
Zeiss	Plex elite 9000	SS	100,000	6.3/<20	Anterior segment OCTA	Wide-field; can scan macula and optic disc on a single scan Deeper tissue penetration
Heidelberg Engineering	Spectralis	SD	40,000 OCT1 80,000 OCT2	3.9–7/14	Anterior segment OCTA	Wide-field scan Higher resolution GMPE module Fastest SD-OCT
Topcon	3D OCT-1 maestro	SD	50,000	2.6–6/20	Fundus camera Anterior segment	Wide-field scan Auto align/capture

(continued)

Table 4.1 (continued)

Manufacturer	Device	Technology	Scan Speed (A-scan/s)	Axial/Transverse Resolution (μm)	Additional Modules	Important points
Topcon	DRI OCT triton	SS	100,000	8/20	Anterior segment OCTA	Wide-field; can scan macula and optic disc on a single scan Deeper tissue penetration Simultaneous fundus photo Multimodal imaging Advanced glaucoma statistics software
Optovue	Avanti	SD	70,000	3–5/15	Anterior segment	Wide-field scan Corneal power calculation for IOL formulas Advanced glaucoma statistics software
Optovue	AngioVue	SD	70,000	3–5/15	Retina Glaucoma	OCTA
Optovue	iVue	SD	26,000	5/15	iCam—Fundus camera	Low cost—Aims private practices Advanced glaucoma statistics software
Optovue	iScan	SD	26,000	5/15	Anterior segment	Low cost—Aims private practices Auto align and scan Advanced glaucoma statistics software

GMPE glaucoma module premium edition, *HD-OCT* high definition optical coherence tomography, *IOL* intraocular lens, *OCT* optical coherence tomography, *OCTA* optical coherence tomography angiography, *SD* spectral domain, *SS* swept source

In addition, OCT is becoming an important tool for other medical specialties such as cardiology, gastroenterology and dermatology. The reader is encouraged to read the original article by James Fujimoto and Eric Swanson titled "The development, commercialization, and impact of optical coherence tomography" to fully understand how OCT technology was developed and what the future of OCT will be [7].

References

1. Carl Zeiss Meditec Primus 200 OCT 501(k) premarket report of FDA. https://www.accessdata. fda.gov/cdrh_docs/pdf16/K163195.pdf. Accessed 11 March 2018.
2. Carl Zeiss Meditec Plex Elite 9000 OCT 501(k) premarket report of FDA. https://www.access-data.fda.gov/cdrh_docs/pdf16/K161194.pdf. Accessed 11 March 2018.
3. Carl Zeiss Meditec Plex Elite 9000 premarket data from Carl Zeiss Meditec website https://www.zeiss.com/content/dam/Meditec/downloads/pdf/ari-network-download/plex-elite-bro-chure_en_31_020_0001v_us_31_020_0001v.pdf. Accessed 11 March 2018.
4. Cole ED, Duker JSOCT. Technology: will we be "swept" away? Rev Ophthalmol. April 2017.; Accessed 11 March 2018
5. Heidelberg Engineering. Spectralis HRA + OCT User manual software version 5.7. 2013.
6. Optovue website data. https://content.optovue.com/hubfs/PDF/300-53141_A_Optovue-Avanti-AngioVue-Brochure_US.pdf. Accessed 11 March 2018.
7. Fujimoto J, Swanson E. The development, commercialization, and impact of optical coherence tomography. Invest Ophthalmol Vis Sci. 2016;57:OCT1–OCT13.

Part II
How to Interpret the Optical Coherence Tomography Results

Chapter 5
Interpretation of Imaging Data from Cirrus HD-OCT

Ahmet Akman

5.1 Introduction

Carl Zeiss Meditec (Dublin, CA) manufactured the first commercial optical coherence tomography (OCT) system as the OCT-1 in 1997, which was followed by OCT-2 in 2000. In 2002, third-generation Time-Domain OCT (TD-OCT), Stratus OCT became available and opened new frontiers in ophthalmic diagnostics. Optic nerve head (ONH) and retinal nerve fiber layer (RNFL) analyses started with Stratus OCT. But the real game-changer for glaucoma diagnosis and follow-up was the introduction of Spectral-Domain OCT (SD-OCT) systems, which showed details of the human eye as never seen before. The current version of the SD-OCT manufactured by Carl Zeiss Meditec is called Cirrus HD-OCT. The glaucoma software of Cirrus HD-OCT has evolved in time with the inclusion of ONH analysis, macular Ganglion Cell Analysis and guided progression analysis (GPA) for both RNFL and macular images. Cirrus HD-OCT has the most advanced progression analysis software among all available OCT systems at this point.

5.2 Scanning Algorithm of Cirrus HD-OCT for the ONH and Peripapillary Area

Cirrus HD-OCT's algorithm for scanning the ONH and peripapillary area is called Optic Disc Cube 200 × 200. It consists of 200 horizontal linear B-scans, each consisting of 200 A-scans, which spans a 6 × 6 mm area in an emmetropic eye (axial length of 24.46 mm). Data extracted from this cube are analyzed and presented as

A. Akman
Department of Ophthalmology, School of Medicine, Başkent University, Ankara, Turkey

© Springer International Publishing AG, part of Springer Nature 2018
A. Akman et al. (eds.), *Optical Coherence Tomography in Glaucoma*,
https://doi.org/10.1007/978-3-319-94905-5_5

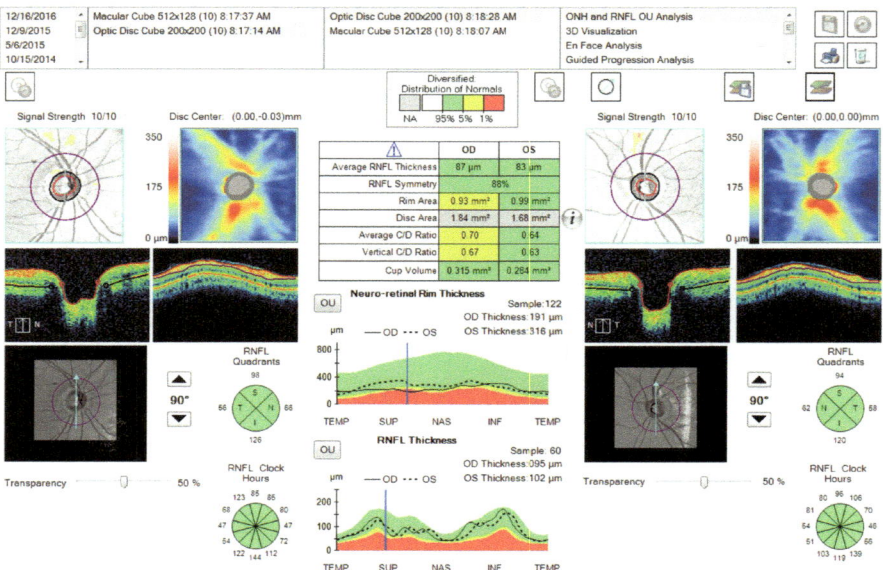

Fig. 5.1 Screenshot of Cirrus' HD-OCT software demonstrates the 200 × 200 ONH and RNFL OU Analysis for a 70-year old male ocular hypertensive patient. The screenshot shows high quality, artifact free scans (signal strength 10/10) and good centration of the scan cubes

200 × 200 ONH and RNFL OU Analysis. Figure 5.1 shows a screenshot of this analysis from the Cirrus' software window and Fig. 5.2 shows the printout page provided to clinicians. This is the most common report used to evaluate the ONH and peripapillary RNFL in patients with suspected or definitive glaucoma. The next section will describe the interpretation of this report.

5.3 How to Read the Cirrus HD-OCT ONH and RNFL Analysis Report?

Cirrus HD-OCT's *ONH and RNFL OU Analysis* is based on the *Optic Disc Cube 200 × 200* report, summarizes the ONH and peripapillary RNFL and compares the patient's results with the normative database of the device. Clinicians who interpret these reports should review them systematically in order not to miss the small details that could be important for the final decision-making and also to identify artifacts or anatomical variations that can lead to misdiagnosis.

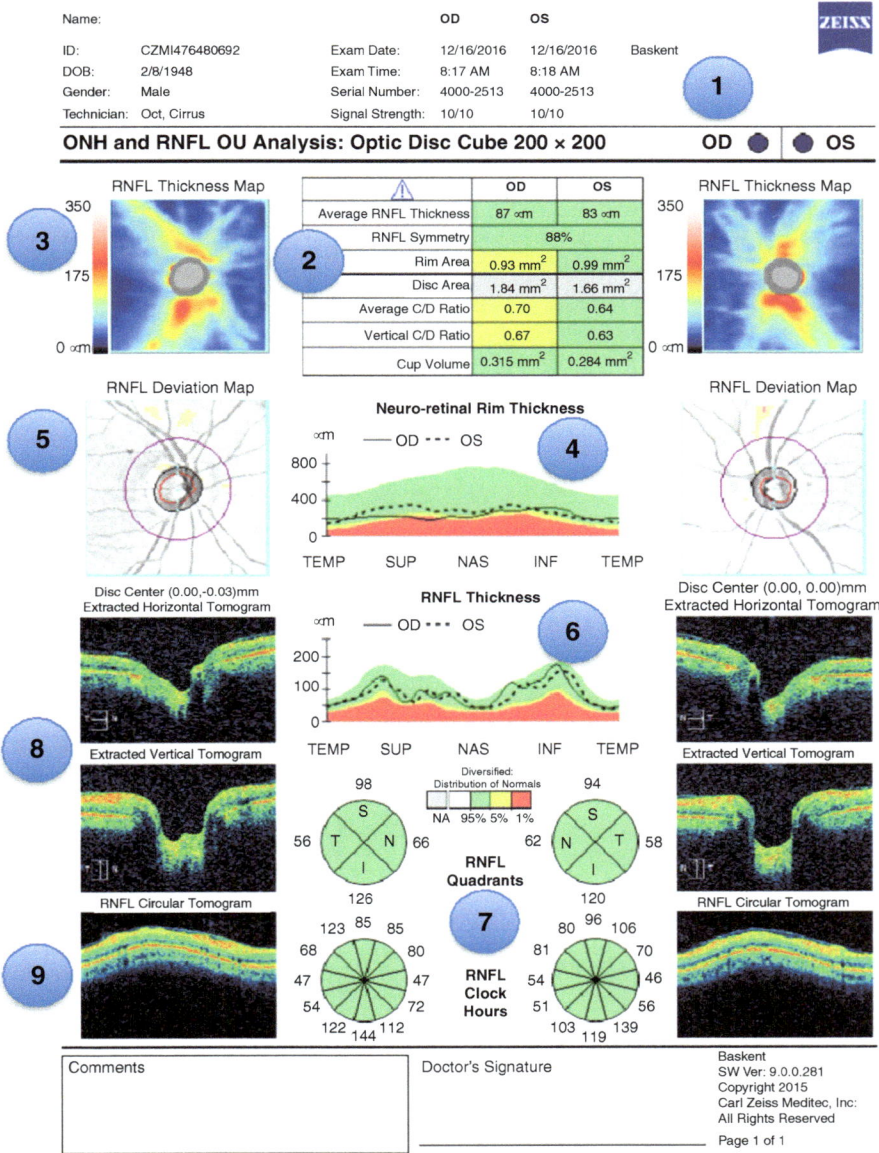

Fig. 5.2 Cirrus HD-OCT's *ONH and RNFL OU Analysis* printout derived from the *Optic Disc Cube 200 × 200* of the same exam in Fig. 5.1. This is the most commonly used report from the Cirrus HD-OCT and summarizes all the important data for ONH and RNFL analysis. Color code schemes used in this printout are described in Sec. 5.3.1. Sections of the printout are explained in the Sec. 5.3.2. The label numbers in blue circles corresponds to the heading numbers used in Sect. 5.3.2

5.3.1   *Color Code Schemes in Cirrus HD-OCT* (Fig. 5.2)

Three different color code schemes are used on Cirrus HD-OCT printouts. The reader needs to thoroughly understand the color code schemes, as same colors have different meanings in different parts of the one-page report. The numbers in parenthesis in the following paragraphs correspond to the label numbers in Fig. 5.2.

Color code A is used in the *RNFL Thickness Map* (3), for representing the RNFL thickness according to the scale on the left side of the map (range: 0-350 µm, color range: blue to white). Cold colors (blue, green) represent thinner RNFL and warm colors (yellow, red) represent regions with thicker RNFL.

Color code B is used in the *Key parameters Table* (2), *Neuro-retinal rim thickness TSNIT plot* (4), *RNFL deviation map* (5), *RNFL thickness TSNIT plot* (6), *RNFL quadrant and clock hour graphs* (7). It is based on the distribution of the same parameters mentioned above in the normative database of Cirrus HD-OCT. The scale range can be seen found above the RNFL quadrants pie graph. Measurements that are beyond the range of the normative database are shaded gray. Measurements that fall within the thickest 5% of normal measurements are displayed as white; those within the 5–95% prediction limits are represented as green (normal); thickness measurements that fall between the 1–5% of the prediction limits of the normative database are considered borderline abnormal and marked in yellow; finally measurements displayed in red are considered outside normal limits and have thickness values below the thinnest 1% of normative database measurements (Fig. 5.3).

Color code C is used in *extracted horizontal and vertical ONH tomograms* (8) and the *circular RNFL tomogram* (9). It is a false color code scheme based on the reflectance of the tissue layers. The hot colors (red, yellow) represent layers with high reflectance and the cold colors (blue-black) represent layers with lower reflectivity. The three different color codes on the printout should be evaluated according to these schemes explained above.

5.3.2   *Sections of the Printout* (Fig. 5.2)

1. **Patient Data and Signal Strength:** Check the name and date of birth (DOB) of the patient, as the results will be compared to the age-matched data from the normative database. Errors in DOB can affect the results significantly. Signal strength is the quality control measure for the scan. Zeiss recommends that scans with signal strength <6 should be repeated. However, in some patients, media

Fig. 5.3 Graph demonstrating the distribution of the color scale of Cirrus HD-OCT used to compare the thickness measurements in individual eyes vs. the normative database of the machine

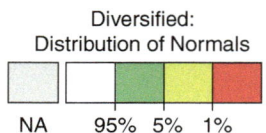

opacities, dry eyes or inability to fixate properly prevents a good quality scan. Poor OCT lens cleaning, older devices, poor centration and inexperienced operator can also result in lower quality scans. If repeated scans still have low signal strength, the results must be evaluated with caution as scans with signal strength <6 could result in thinner RNFL values [1–5]. If it is not possible to obtain a good quality scan, particularly in young patients without cataract or ocular pathology, check the device and contact the manufacturer.

2. **Key Parameters Table:** Summary of the key parameters for both eyes is provided in the Key Parameters Table. The results are compared with the normative database values and color coded according to the distribution of normal scale (color code B) (Fig. 5.3).

3. **RNFL Thickness Map:** This map displays the actual thickness values measured throughout the ONH Cube with the *color code A*. These measurements and the resulting color map are not related in any way to the normative database since they consist of the *raw RNFL thickness data* for the scanned eye. This raw RNFL thickness report is one of the unique features of Cirrus HD-OCT. After verifying the patient data and signal strength, the interpreter should look at the RNFL thickness map for scan quality. Cirrus HD-OCT shows areas that cannot be scanned or where measurements cannot be calculated as black and any black area on RNFL map can significantly affect the results of remaining RNFL analysis data. Besides, other artifacts like eye movements can be observed on this map. A good scan in a healthy eye shows the thick RNFL bundles in the superior and inferior quadrants in yellow, orange and red false color code. This is the only map on the standard printout page without any relation to the normative database.

4. **Neuro-Retinal Rim Thickness Plot:** This plot is in TSNIT configuration (see Chap. 3 for details of TSNIT configuration). The neuro-retinal rim thickness is measured between the Bruch's membrane opening (BMO) that represents the border of the ONH (black circle on RNFL deviation map (5)) and the border of the optic cup (red circle on RNFL deviation map (5)). The thickness values are compared with age- and disc size matched data of the normative database.

5. **RNFL Deviation Map:** The above-mentioned BMO circle (black), cup border (red) and RNFL calculation circle (purple) are superimposed on the OCT's *en face* infrared image. The device measures the RNFL thickness throughout the 200×200 data cube, where each A-scan represents a pixel corresponding to a 30 μm wide square. Sixteen such pixels (4×4 pixels) are combined to create superpixels of 16 A-scans. As a result, each superpixel covers an area of about 120×120 μm. There is a total of 50×50 (2500) superpixels analyzed, except the superpixels at the edge and inside the optic disc. The RNFL thickness at superpixels is compared to the normative database; no overlay color code is used for areas of normal thickness as much of the image would be covered with green superpixels and this would obscure the anatomical detail of the OCT image. Superpixels displaying an RNFL thickness at or below 5%ile are shown in yellow and those thinner than 1%ile cutoff point of the normative database are flagged in red on the en face OCT image. In summary, any region that is not red

or yellow is within or above normal limits (i.e., the RNFL thickness is above the lower 5% of the eyes in the normative database). The borders of the RNFL deviations map may appear as thick green or thin blue lines in Cirrus HD-OCT model 5000 printouts, which incorporates the Fast-Trac retinal tracking system.

6. **RNFL Thickness TSNIT Plot:** This plot is the foundation of RNFL analysis not only in Cirrus HD-OCT but in all OCT systems. Cirrus HD-OCT uses measurements from a 3.46 mm diameter calculation circle centered on the BMO for creating the TSNIT plot. The calculation ring is centered automatically using the BMO centroid identification method that was described in Chap. 3 and used for normative database comparisons. The software extracts 256 data points from the 200 × 200 Disc Cube area for the calculation circle so the TSNIT plots has 256 points on the Y axis. Patient's RNFL thickness measurements are plotted for both eyes on the color-coded background that represents the age-matched normative data. In normal eyes, a typical double hump configuration for the RNFL distribution is observed. Again, the white area represents the thickest 5% of the eyes in the normative database, the green area represents the thickness in the middle 90% of the age-matched normal eyes, yellow area corresponds to borderline values (eyes with thickness measurements falling within the 1–5%ile prediction limits) and red area displays the outside normal range (1% of eyes in the normative database). Some normal variations or artifacts could be classified as abnormal on the TSNIT plot. The interpreter should check the TSNIT plots very carefully to see that if the RNFL thickness measurements are really abnormal or artifacts or anatomical variations are present. The quadrant and clock hour graphs (7) summarize the measurements on the TSNIT plot so they can be easily misleading if an artifact or anatomical variation is affecting the TSNIT plot. Chapter 8 includes sample cases with different kinds of artifacts and anatomical variations.

7. **RNFL Quadrant and RNFL Clock-Hour Thickness Measurements:** These are pie graph summaries of the RNFL Thickness TSNIT plots. The clinician needs to carefully check the RNFL thickness TSNIT plots for artifacts and anatomical variations before reaching conclusions based on these pie graphs. The color code is given according to the distribution of normals scale (*color code B*), which is provided just above the RNFL quadrants graph.

8. **Extracted Vertical and Horizontal Tomograms:** These are the horizontal and vertical B-scans of the optic disc extracted from the 6 × 6 data cube. In these tomograms, the color code C is used for representing tissue reflectance. These tomograms are helpful for verifying the cup configuration and for identifying artifacts related to neuroretinal rim measurements.

9. **RNFL Circular Tomogram:** This is the raw OCT image of the calculation circle from which the segmentation is performed and RNFL thickness values are calculated for the TSNIT plot and pie graphs. The reviewer should check this tomogram for artifacts, segmentation errors and retinal diseases or vitreo-retinal interface problems that can cause a "green disease" misdiagnosis.

5.4   Cirrus HD-OCT's Macula Report

The macular region is scanned and ganglion cell analyses are performed to aid with glaucoma diagnosis and monitoring. This scan generates a 6 × 6 mm macular cube data centered on the fovea. Cirrus HD-OCT has two scan options for the macular cube. The default one is the 512 × 128 grid, which consists of 128 horizontal B-scans each composed of 512 A-scans. A 200 × 200 macular scan algorithm is also available with 200 horizontal B-scans consisting of 200 A-scans each. The 512 × 128 algorithm carries out 65,536 A-scans and has a higher horizontal resolution compared to the 200 × 200 cube scan which consists of 40,000 A-scans with higher resolution in the vertical direction. The 200 × 200 Macular Cube has a shorter acquisition time and can be useful for patients with less than optimal fixation. Figure 5.4 demonstrates a screen shot of the *Ganglion Cell OU Analysis* from the Macular Cube 512 × 128.

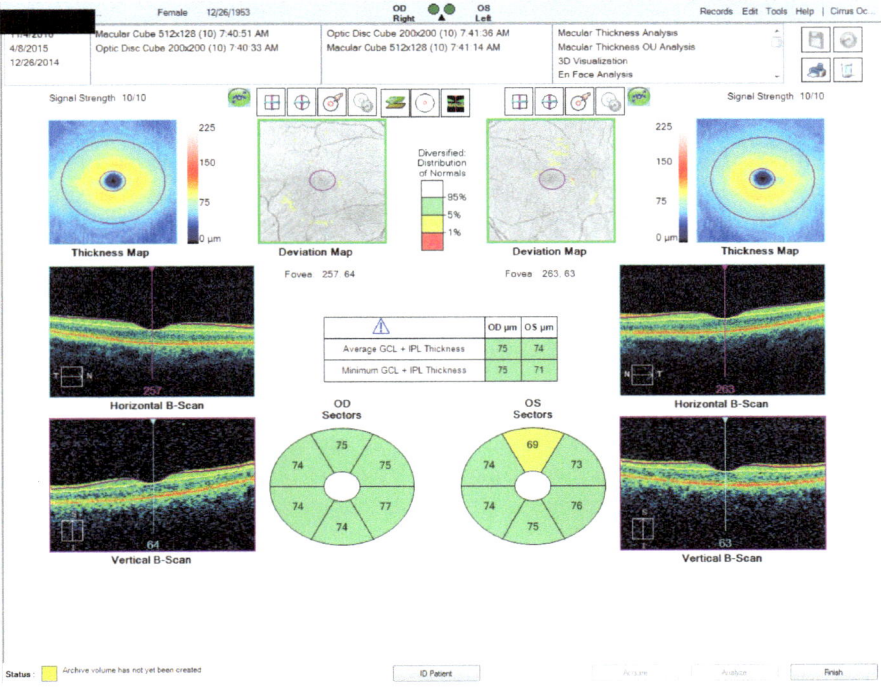

Fig. 5.4   Screenshot of the macular Ganglion Cell OU Analysis: Macular Cube 512 × 128 scan of a 65-year old female ocular hypertensive patient. The screenshot shows high quality, artifact free scans (signal strength 10/10) and good centration of the scan cubes

5.5 How to Read the Cirrus HD-OCT's Ganglion Cell Analysis Report?

Color coding in macular Ganglion Cell Analysis is similar to the ONH and RNFL analysis describes above and follows the same three color code schemes. The details were described in Sect. 5.3.1.

5.5.1 Sections of the Printout (Fig. 5.5)

1. **Patient Data and Signal Strength:** Check the name and DOB of the patient, as the results will be compared to age-matched data from the normative database. Errors in DOB can affect the results significantly similar to the peripapillary RNFL analysis. As described in Sect. 5.3, signal strength is the quality control metric for the scan and the manufacturer recommends that scans with signal strength <6 should be repeated.

2. **Thickness Map:** As Cirrus HD-OCT measures the ganglion cell layer (GCL) and inner plexiform layer (IPL) together, the thickness map shows the GCL+IPL thickness measurements in a 6 × 6 mm cube focusing on an elliptical annulus centered to the fovea. The automatic fovea finder program determines location of the fovea. Interpreter must first check the correct placement of fovea by the automatic finder. The thickness measurements and color codes are not related to the values from the normative database, i.e., these are the *raw GCL+IPL thickness data* for the scanned macula. The color code A is used, but the range of measurements is between 0 and 225 μm instead of 0-350 μm for the ONH and RNFL analysis.

3. **Deviation Map:** This is the GCL+IPL thickness measurements across the 6 × 6 mm cube are compared with the age-matched data from the normative database and overlaid on the *en-face* infrared image of the macula. The approach utilized to calculate the GCL+IPL thickness at superpixels is similar to that used for the RNFL deviation map of the *RNFL and ONH OU analysis* of the Optic Disc Cube. The device measures RNFL thickness throughout the 6 × 6 mm data cube with each A-scan translating into a 30 μm square pixel. Sixteen adjacent pixels are combined to create superpixels of 16 A-scans (4 × 4 pixel squares). As a result, each superpixel covers an area about 120 × 120 μm. These superpixels are compared to the normative database data; no overlay color code is used for areas of normal thickness. Superpixels with GCL+IPL thickness between 1 and 5%ile of the prediction limits for normal subjects are flagged in yellow and superpixels that have a GCL+IPL value thinner than 1%ile cutoff point for the normal subjects are shown in red on the en-face OCT image. In summary, any region that is not red or yellow is within or above normal limits.

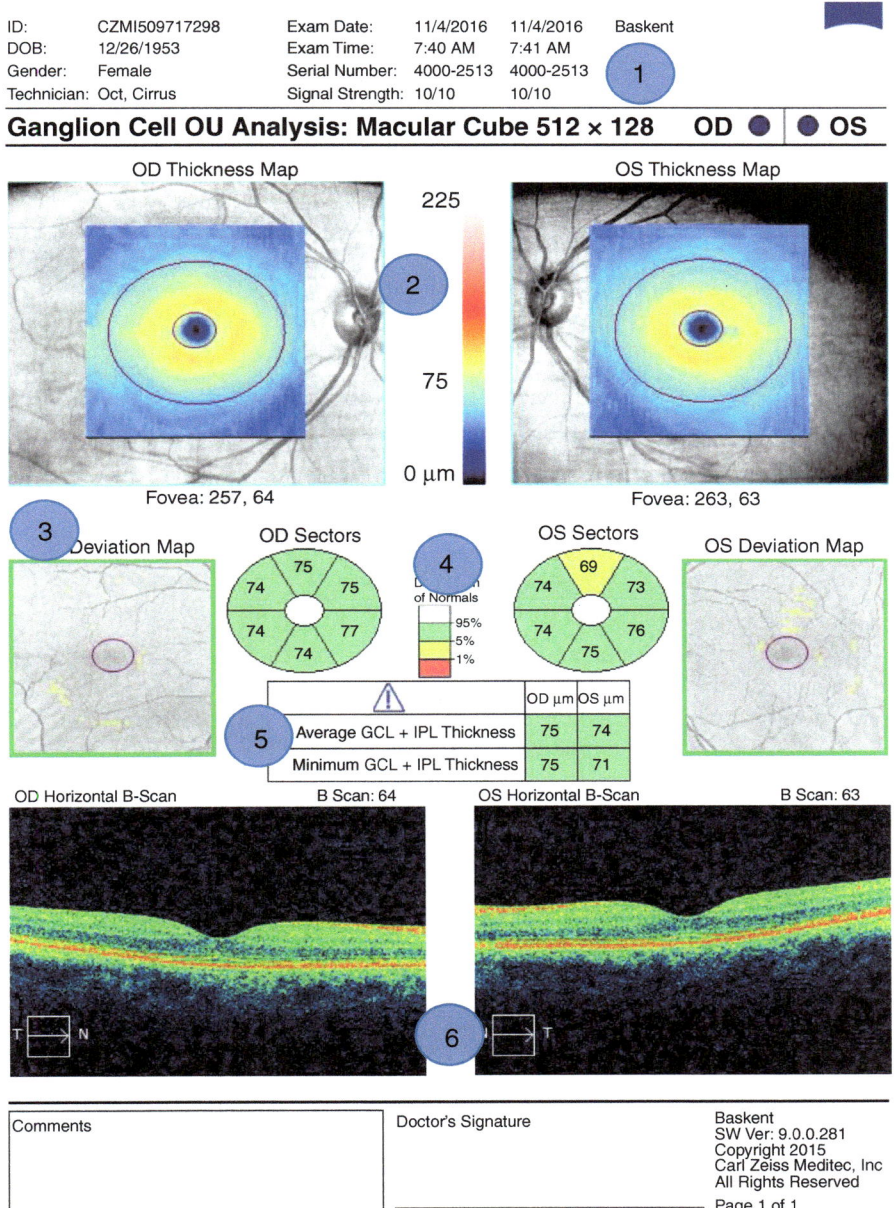

Fig. 5.5 Cirrus HD-OCT's Ganglion Cell OU analysis based on macular cube 512×128 printout of the same exam in Fig. 5.4. Sections of the printout are explained in the Sec. 5.5.1. The label numbers in blue circles corresponds to the heading numbers used in Sect. 5.5.1

4. **The Sector Map:** The oval 4.8 × 4.0 mm region centered on the fovea consists of a central elliptical region 1.2 × 1.0 mm in diameter representing the fovea where the GCL+IPL thickness is minimal and an outer elliptical region where the sectorial measurements are provided. This elliptical annulus is divided into three equally sized pie-shaped sectors in the superior and inferior regions. The color coding is according to color code B described previously.

5. **Thickness Table:** The thickness table shows the average and minimum GCL+IPL thickness measurements in the elliptical annulus again coded according to the color code B.

6. **Horizontal Tomogram of the Macula:** This tomogram (B-scan) serves the following purposes. At first, the interpreter should check if the tomogram passes through the fovea. If that is the case, one can assume that the elliptical annulus is correctly positioned by the automatic fovea finder and the data provided on the aforementioned maps are reliable. Second, macular pathologies that can affect the analysis can be detected on this tomogram. The color code for this tomogram is based on the color code C.

5.6   The PanoMap Analysis

The PanoMap Analysis combines the 512 × 128 Macular Cube or 200 × 200 Macular Cube and the 200 × 200 Optic Disc Cube scans in a single report. Integrating a wide-field view of RNFL and ONH analysis in combination with Ganglion Cell OU analysis and Macular Thickness analysis, gives the interpreter a chance to evaluate the macula, peripapillary area and disc together (Fig. 5.6). The color code and principles of interpretation of the PanoMap report are similar to those for the RNFL/ONH and GCA reports.

5.7   The Normative Databases of Cirrus HD-OCT

All of the OCT systems compare a given patient's data with the normative database of the device. These comparisons are one of the most important factors supporting the clinician in clinical decision-making. Good understanding of the limitations of such comparisons is essential for clinicians.

The normative database of the Cirrus HD-OCT contains the RNFL, GCL+IPL and ONH measurement data of 282 individuals with a refractive error within certain limits and with no known ocular pathologies. The normative database of Cirrus HD-OCT uses age-matched data for RNFL and GCL+IPL comparisons and age and disc size matched data for ONH comparisons for patients aged 18 years or above.

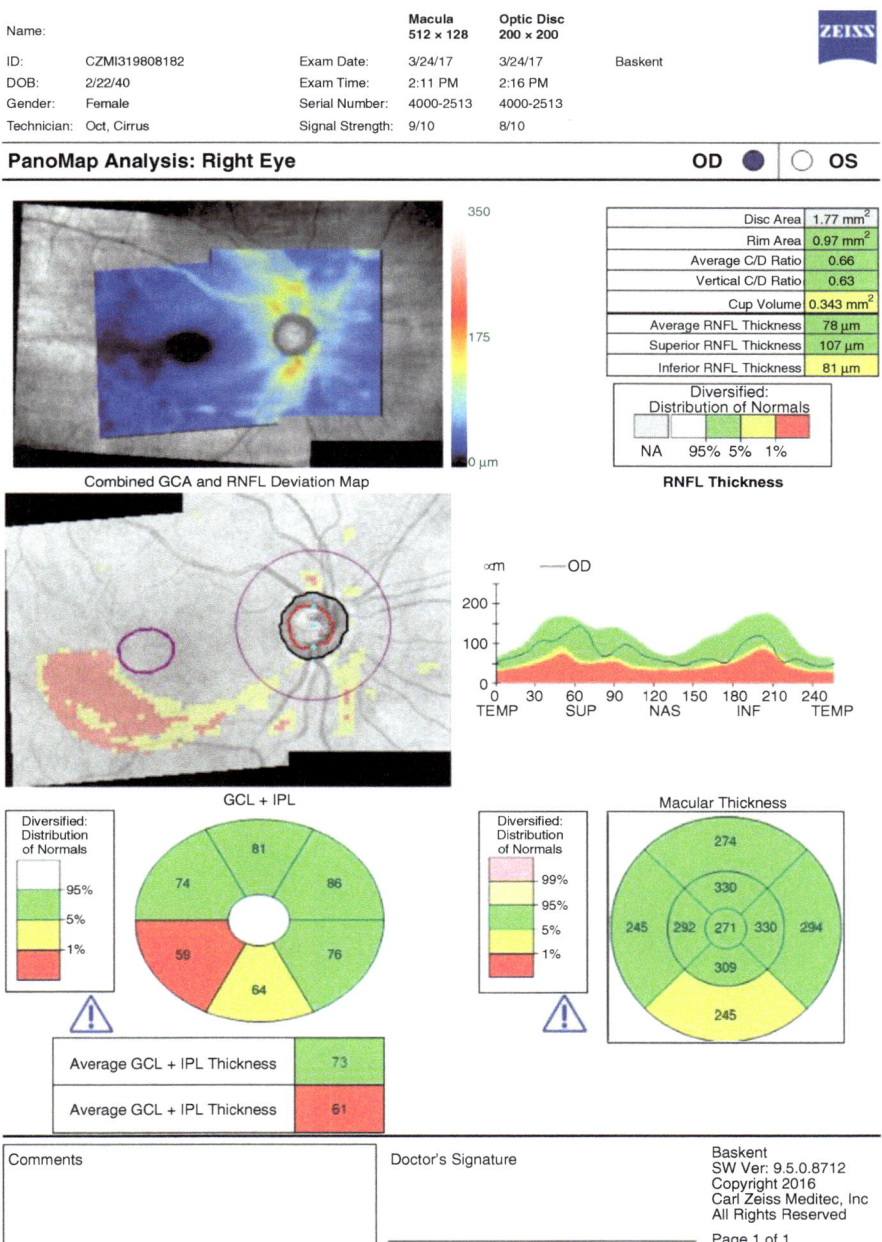

Fig. 5.6 The PanoMap analysis is a combination of 200 × 200 Optic Disc Cube and 512 × 128 Macular Cube scans. In addition, a macular full thickness map is included

Data were not collected from subjects younger than 18 years, so normative database comparisons are not possible for patients younger than 18 years. Measurements from the eyes in the normative database are assumed to have a normal distribution. More information on the normative database of the Cirrus HD-OCT system is available in the user manual for the device.

It is the clinician's responsibility to review results of each patient before interpreting the comparison with the normative data. Normative database comparisons do not provide a definitive diagnosis but demonstrate how this patient's measurements compare to the range of data from age-matched individuals in the normative database. Not every measurement considered to be thinner than normal based on the normative database represents a pathological RNFL or GCL+IPL loss. To emphasize, on the RNFL and macular ganglion cell deviation maps, at each superpixel, 5% of normal eyes will be highlighted in yellow, and 1% of normal eyes will be highlighted as abnormal (red) because of the normal statistical variations. Since each map consists of 2500 superpixels, 125 pixels on average might be expected to be highlighted as yellow or red on each scan [6]. For the RNFL calculation circle based data, such as TSNIT plots, quadrant and clock hour graphs, one eye out of every 20 normal eyes would be expected to demonstrate yellow or red superpixels [6].

In addition to these normal statistical variations, the normative database has its own limitations like limited range of spherical error (-12 to $+6$ Diopters) and axial length (22 to 28 mm). Highly myopic or hyperopic eyes may have different RNFL characteristics and may be flagged more frequently as abnormal when compared to the current normative database. Anatomical variations that are discussed in Chap. 8 can also cause an impression of RNFL loss. An experienced interpreter can easily identify this kind of anatomical variations, and many examples of such variations are presented in Chap. 8.

5.7.1 Cirrus HD-OCT RNFL and ONH Normative Database

Normative database comparisons of RNFL thickness measurements are performed with two different approaches. First, the 200 × 200 cube data, which consists of 2500 super-pixels, are compared with the age matched normative database and results are reported on the RNFL deviation map; second, the thickness data from the RNFL calculation circle are compared to the normative database; such comparisons are used in the remaining analyses including key parameters table, RNFL thickness TSNIT plot, RNFL quadrants and RNFL clock hours graphs.

Normative database comparisons of the ONH parameters are performed for the neuro-retinal rim profile and ONH data, which are presented in the Key Parameters table and the neuro-retinal thickness TSNIT plot.

Table 5.1 Definition of the various color codes for Cirrus HD-OCT RNFL and ONH OU analysis (with permission, Carl Zeiss Meditec, Cirrus HD-OCT User Manual Software 8.1)

Measurement	Matched to Normal Based On	Grey	White	Green	Yellow	Red
RNFL						
Average RNFL Thickness, RNFL Symmetry, RNFL Clock Hours, RNFL Quadrants, RNFL Thickness (graph)	Age	Grey shading does not apply to RNFL measurements	The thickest 5% of measurements fall in the white area (white >95%).	90% of measurements fall in the green area (5% < green ≤ 95%).	The thinnest 5% of measurements fall in the yellow area or below (1% < yellow ≤ 5%, suspect).	The thinnest 1% of measurements. Measurements in red are considered outside normal limits (red ≤ 1%, outside normal limits).
Optic Nerve Head						
Rim Area and Neuroretinal Rim Thickness (graph)	Disc Area and Age	ONH Normative Database is not applicable if: 1) The disc area is larger than 2.5 mm² or smaller than 1.33 mm², or 2) The Vertical C/D Ratio is below 0.25, or 3) The ONH Normative Database license has not been activated.	The largest 5% of measurements fall in the white area (white > 95%).	90% of measurements fall in the green area (5% < green ≤ 95%).	The smallest 5% of measurements fall in the yellow area or below (1% < yellow ≤ 5%, suspect).	The smallest 1% of measurements. Measurements in red are considered outside normal limits (red ≤ 1%, outside normal limits).
Average C/D Ratio, Vertical C/D Ratio, Cup Volume			The smallest 5% of measurements fall in the white area (white > 95%).	90% of measurements fall in the green area (5% < green ≤ 95%).	The largest 5% of measurements fall in the yellow area or below (1% < yellow ≤ 5%, suspect).	The largest 1% of measurements. Measurements in red are considered outside normal limits (red ≤ 1%, outside normal limits).

The RNFL and ONH Normative Database of Cirrus HD-OCT (Table 5.1) uses the white-green-yellow-red color code (Color code B pattern summarized previously in Sect. 5.3.1).

5.7.2 Cirrus HD-OCT Macular GCL+IPL Normative Database

The normative database comparisons for the GCL+IPL thickness measurements are performed with the same two approaches used for the RNFL measurements. First, the 200 × 200 cube area data, consisting of 2500 super-pixels, are compared with the age-matched normative database and reported on the GCL+IPL deviation map; second, the thickness data from the elliptical annulus are used in the remainder of analyses including key parameters table (2) and sector map (4).

5.8   Key Points

- Patient demographic data must be checked in order to prevent clinical errors. Date of birth has to be correct as the normative database comparisons are age dependent.
- Scan quality is very important; poor quality scans results in thinner RNFL and GCL+IPL measurements.
- In a good quality scan, the en face image is artifact free, sharp and clear, the scan is well centered, the illumination needs to be uniform without dark corners and the signal strength should be six or greater.
- Ocular surface problems and dry eyes are one of the most common reasons for poor quality scans, the device should not be placed under air conditioning vents which can accelerate drying of the patient's eyes.
- After confirming the quality of the scans, the physician must rule out the presence of coexisting pathologies, artifacts and anatomical variations that can confound the results and interpretation.
- The physician must determine if the patient's ocular condition merits comparison to a normative database. For Cirrus-HD OCT, the normative database does not include patients younger than 18 years of age and only a few high myopes are included in the normative database.
- It is very important for the clinician to have ready access to the raw acquired images before looking at the interpretation provided in the report.

References

1. Cheung CY, Leung CK, Lin D, Pang CP, Lam DS. Relationship between retinal nerve fiber layer measurement and signal strength in optical coherence tomography. Ophthalmology. 2008;115:1347–51.
2. Vizzeri G, Bowd C, Medeiros FA, Weinreb RN, Zangwill LM. Effect of improper scan alignment on retinal nerve fiber layer thickness measurements using stratus optical coherence tomograph. J Glaucoma. 2008;17:341–9.
3. Wu Z, Vazeen M, Varma R, Chopra V, Walsh AC, LaBree LD, Sadda SR. Factors associated with variability in retinal nerve fiber layer thickness measurements obtained by optical coherence tomography. Ophthalmology. 2007;114:1505–12.
4. Cheung CY, Chen D, Wong TY, Tham YC, Wu R, Zheng Y, Cheng CY, Saw SM, Baskaran M, Leung CK, Aung T. Determinants of quantitative optic nerve measurements using spectral domain optical coherence tomography in a population-based sample of non-glaucomatous subjects. Invest Ophthalmol Vis Sci. 2011;52:9629–35.
5. Wu Z, Huang J, Dustin L, Sadda SR. Signal strength is an important determinant of accuracy of nerve fiber layer thickness measurement by optical coherence tomography. J Glaucoma. 2009;18:213–6.
6. Zeiss Cirrus HD-OCT User Manual–Models 500, 5000 Instrument and Review Software 8.1, 2015, p. 171–6.

Chapter 6
Interpretation of Imaging Data from Spectralis OCT

Atilla Bayer

6.1 Introduction

Advances in spectral-domain optical coherence tomography (SD-OCT) have enabled imaging of the optic nerve head (ONH) anatomic features and more accurate evaluation of the retinal nerve fiber layer (RNFL), and the macular region. Structures such as the lamina cribrosa anterior surface topography [1, 2], termination of Bruch's membrane–retinal pigment epithelium complex [3], border tissue of Elschnig [1], and the scleral canal opening [4] can now be visualized. Overlay of optic disc clinical photographs with SD-OCT images has allowed clinicians to identify structures that correspond to common clinical landmarks, such as the clinical disc margin. New metrics such as the Bruch's membrane opening based minimum rim width (BMO-MRW) provide a more accurate measure of the retinal ganglion cell axons at the level of the ONH. This chapter reviews the properties, available scan patterns and tips on interpretation of the Spectralis OCT printouts (Heidelberg Engineering Inc., Heidelberg, Germany). Spectralis OCT uses an 870-nm wavelength super-luminescent diode laser as a light source and is capable of obtaining scans through a pupil size as small as 2.5 mm. The scanning speed of the first generation Spectralis OCT is 40,000 scans/s (85,000 scans/s in Spectralis OCT2). Scan depth is 1.9 mm with axial resolution of 3.87 μm and transverse resolution of 14 μm. Features of Spectralis OCT include automated anatomic positioning system (APS), and APS-linked unique scan patterns including ONH radial & circle scan (ONH-RC), posterior pole horizontal scan (PPoleH), and posterior pole vertical scan (PPoleV) (Fig. 6.1). These scan patterns facilitate analyses of the ONH, RNFL, posterior pole including measurement of individual retinal layers including ganglion cell layer (GCL) thickness.

A. Bayer
Department of Glaucoma, Dünyagöz Eye Hospital, Ankara, Turkey

© Springer International Publishing AG, part of Springer Nature 2018
A. Akman et al. (eds.), *Optical Coherence Tomography in Glaucoma*,
https://doi.org/10.1007/978-3-319-94905-5_6

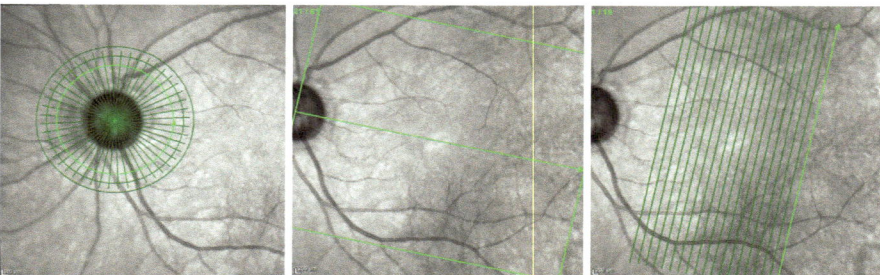

Fig. 6.1 Optic nerve head radial and circle scan (left), posterior pole horizontal scan (center), and posterior pole vertical scan (right) scan patterns of Spectralis optical coherence tomography instrument

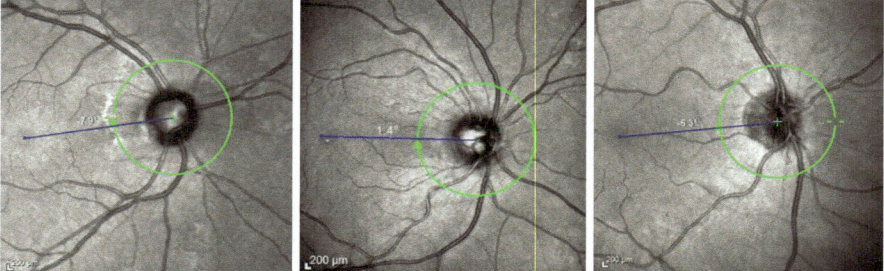

Fig. 6.2 Various examples of the varying angle between the foveal center and the BMO centroid relative to the horizontal axis defined on the fundus image. The mean angle of this axis is about −7°, i.e., the fovea is below the BMO centroid (left image). This angle can be positive (center) where the fovea is above the BMO centroid

6.2 The Automated Anatomic Positioning System

Currently available algorithms of OCT devices report regional data according to temporal, superior, nasal, and inferior sectors, which are established relative to the fixed horizontal and vertical axes of the current image, assuming that neuro-retinal rim width and area in a certain ONH sector refer to approximately the same anatomic location in all human eyes. As seen in clinical fundus images, in most individuals, the fovea is located below the level of the ONH (relative to the horizontal axis of the acquired image frame); the axis connecting the ONH or BMO centroid to foveal center (FoDi or FoBMO axis) deviates from horizontal meridian. A recent study of the angle between the FoBMO axis relative to the horizontal axis defined by the fundus image in 222 white patients with ocular hypertension or glaucoma showed that although the mean angle of this axis was −7° (the fovea being on average 7° below), the range varied from −17° to +6° (Fig. 6.2) [5]. OCT databases that do not correct for the FoBMO alignment have wider confidence intervals. Even a slight head tilt can shift the start/stop point of the TSNIT circle scan, adding alignment error to normative databases [6]. Test-retest variability is expected to be greater without alignment.

Fovea-to-Disc (FoDi) alignment function of the previous Spectralis OCT algorithm corrected for unwanted eye rotation. Two anatomically fixed landmarks relative to each other, center of the fovea and center of the ONH, define the coordinate system of the eye. FoDi technology ensured all circle scans start/stop at the same anatomical point, providing point-to-point accuracy between consecutive scans and eliminating alignment error in relation to the normative database.

The Glaucoma Module Premium Edition (GMPE) software of Spectralis OCT offers Automated APS which aligns follow-up scans with the baseline image according to FoBMO axis. As mentioned below, BMO is the outer anatomic boundary of the area where axons exit the eye and is used in preference to the FoDi axis. Since the anatomic path of the ganglion cell axon bundles between the fovea and the ONH is organized relative to the FoBMO axis, it is an anatomically consistent landmark for the regionalization of the ONH and retinal tissues [7, 8]. FoBMO alignment, therefore, ensures that all eyes are anatomically aligned correctly with the healthy control eyes (normative database), improving accuracy of measurements (Fig. 6.3). APS-based scan patterns are ONH radial scan for ONH analysis, ONH circle scanning for RNFL analysis, PPoleH scanning for thickness and asymmetry analyses of various retinal layers, and PPoleV for ganglion cell thickness analysis.

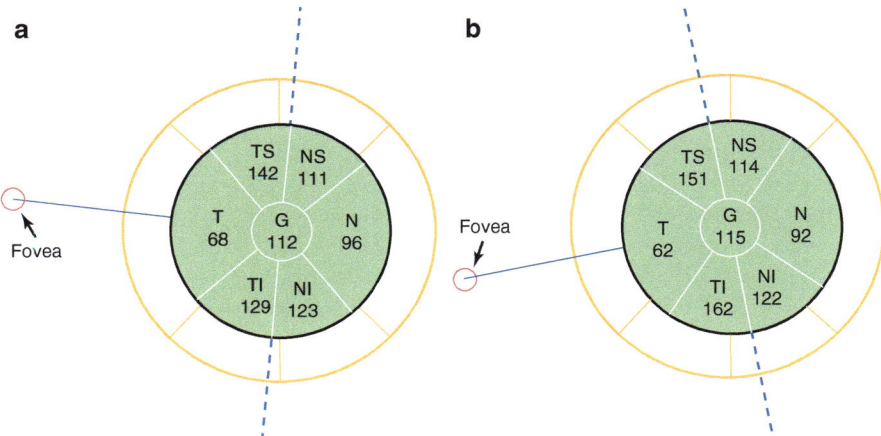

Fig. 6.3 If the correct anatomic orientation is ignored during acquisition of OCT scans, artificially large inter-subject differences in sectorial analyses are likely to occur. Blue line represents the Fovea to Bruch's membrane opening (FoBMO) axis of the individual eye. Two eyes with different anatomical positions of the fovea relative to the Bruch's membrane opening centroid are shown (**a** and **b**). Spectralis OCT scan orientation automatically is aligned along the eye's FoBMO axis. If the horizontal and vertical axes of the image frame are fixed (yellow grid), this would result in an orientation shift of the classification sectors relative to the normative database. When optic nerve head anatomy is not aligned with healthy control eyes, normal tissue may appear thin or thin tissue may appear normal leading to significant classification errors

6.3   Scan Properties of Spectralis OCT for Peripapillary Region

6.3.1   Standard 12 Degrees Scan Pattern

The original RNFL imaging algorithm of Spectralis OCT was based on a peripapillary circular scan 12° in diameter (which equates to a retinal diameter of 3.46 mm in eyes with average corneal curvature and axial length). It is automatically centered around the optic disc and 768 data points are analyzed (496 data points on the Z axis, 1.9 mm in depth). The temporal point where the FoDi or FoBMO axis crosses the measurement circle is designated as 0°; degrees are counted in a clockwise direction in the right eye and in counterclockwise direction in the left eye. The device also provides RNFL measurements in sectors consisting of temporal (316°-45°), temporal superior (46°-90°), nasal superior (91°-135°), nasal (136°-225°), nasal inferior (226°-270°), and temporal inferior (271°-315°) sectors. Measurements are compared to the normative database and displayed on the RNFL profile graph as well as quadrant and sectoral pie graphs. Normative database of the standard RNFL analysis (2009) included 218 eyes of healthy European subjects with ages between 20 and 87 years.

6.3.2   The Glaucoma Module Premium Edition

During RNFL analysis with GMPE software, three circle scans of 3.5, 4.1, and 4.7 mm are automatically centered around the BMO centroid and 768 data points are analyzed. The 3.5 mm RNFL circle scan is the default scan for analysis and is comparable to the standard 12° RNFL scan pattern. The two additional wider scans become important when the inner 3.5 mm circle is not interpretable due to confounding pathology such as peripapillary atrophy. In addition to the circular scans, the GMPE software performs 24 radial equidistant scans for ONH analysis (see below) (Fig. 6.4). RNFL thickness analysis is adjusted for BMO area and age on all three scans for a BMO area range of 1.0 –3.4 mm². Measurements are compared to the normative database and represented on the RNFL profile graph as well as quadrant and sectoral pie graphs. The current normative database of GMPE (2014) includes 246 eyes of healthy European subjects aged between 20 and 87 years.

6.4   Features of the Glaucoma Module Premium Edition Software for the Optic Nerve Head

6.4.1   The Optic Disc Margin

The optic disc margin or clinical disc margin is a clinical construct for the boundary that surrounds the neural tissue within the ONH. All quantitative measurements of the neuro-retinal rim with modern imaging techniques require the identification of

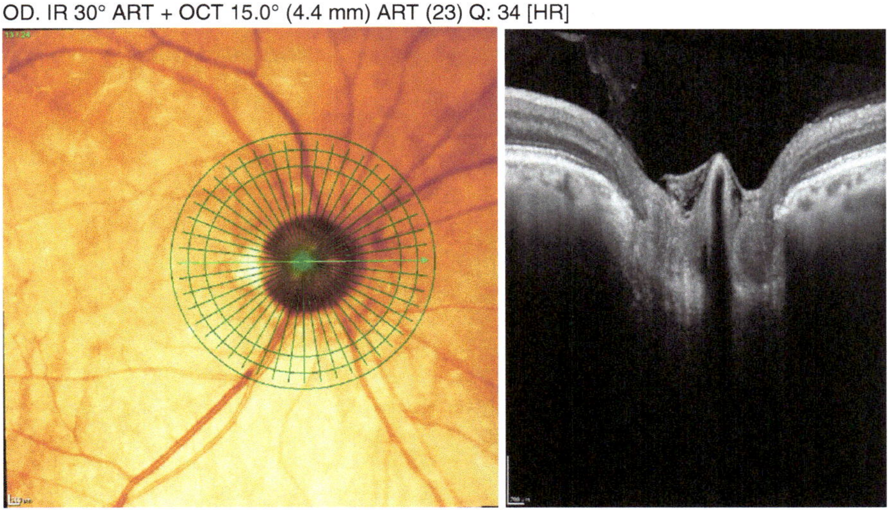

OD. IR 30° ART + OCT 15.0° (4.4 mm) ART (23) Q: 34 [HR]

Fig. 6.4 The Glaucoma Module Premium Edition software provides three circle scans (3.5, 4.1, 4.7 mm) for measuring the retinal nerve fiber layer and 24 radial scans for measurement of the Bruch's membrane opening-minimum rim width. The tomogram on the right shows the optic nerve head B-scan through the plane shown as an arrow on the fundus image

the disc margin. Traditionally, optic disc margin has been defined as the inner edge of the scleral rim and has been assumed to be a single and consistent anatomic structure around the ONH. Optic disc margin has been considered the true outer border of the neuro-retinal rim from which the width of the rim could be measured. However, what the clinician identifies as the disc margin in an individual eye is rarely a single structure. SD-OCT analysis of the ONH structures has revealed that the structures creating the appearance of the clinical disc margin vary according to configuration and relationship of the peripapillary tissues including the border tissue of Elschnig, sclera, and choroid and is highly variable within and between individual eyes. Histologic findings in monkey eyes and SD-OCT findings in human eyes have revealed that the clinical optic disc margin is rarely a single anatomic entity, nor are the structures that underlie it consistent in an individual eye [3, 9]. The structure corresponding to the optic disc margin at the 3 o'clock position may be different to that at the 9 o'clock position.

6.4.2   Bruch's Membrane Opening

The termination of Bruch's membrane around the ONH is defined as the BMO, which represents the opening through which all axons exit the eye. Axons cannot cross Bruch's membrane and must exit the eye beyond its edge [10]. The BMO defines the outermost edge of neural tissue at the level of the disc. While the BMO is consistently detected by SD-OCT imaging, it is rarely clinically visible in humans. The Bruch's membrane can extend beyond Elschnig border tissue (BT) or

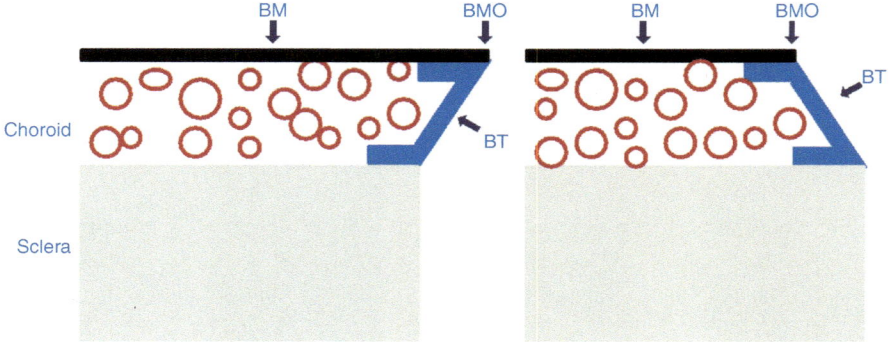

Fig. 6.5 Bruch's membrane configuration relative to the border tissue of Elschnig (BT). The BT configuration may be internally (left) or externally oblique (right). *BM* Bruch's membrane, *BMO* Bruch's membrane opening, *BT* Border tissue of Elschnig [3]

Fig. 6.6 Pseudo-color fundus image of a glaucoma patient demonstrates Bruch's membrane opening demarcation (red dots) based on automated segmentation by Spectralis OCT. Clinical disc margin is demarcated by green dashed curve. Note that the two do not overlap in most parts of the circumference of the optic nerve head

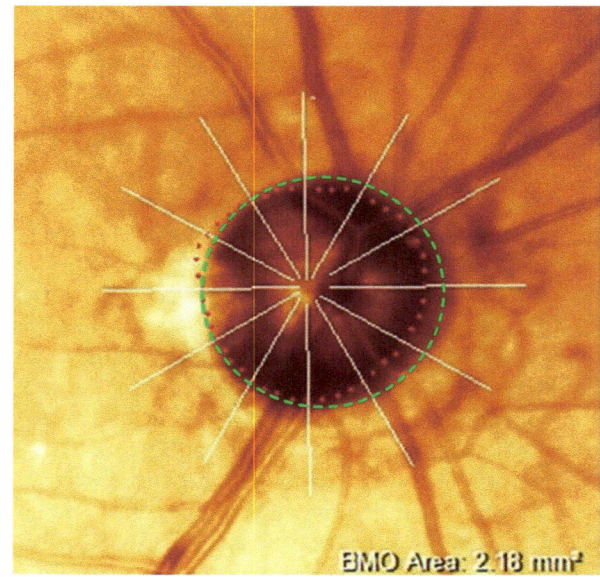

vice-versa (Fig. 6.5) creating various configurations around the ONH (Fig. 6.6) [3, 11].

The GMPE software automatically detects 48 BMO positions along 24 equidistant scan lines centered on the ONH centroid to determine the BMO-based disc margin (Figs. 6.1 and 6.4). BMO is a useful landmark in glaucoma given is its relative stability under a variety of conditions. The BMO remains unaltered despite large changes in intraocular pressure caused by glaucoma surgery [12].

Corneal curvature (CC) is an important factor to account for in order to obtain accurate measurements. The RNFL is thicker closer to the disc margin and thins out with increasing distance from the BMO. Therefore, the RNFL circle scan should be consistently placed for accurate assessment and comparison of RNFL measurements relative to the normative database. In an eye with flat cornea, the measurement circle falls closer to the BMO centroid and should be displaced away from the BMO centroid and vice versa. Therefore, before image acquisition, it is recommended to change the standard 7.7 mm corneal curvature value and enter the individual eye's mean corneal curvature. With the help of this CC value and the specific focus setting, the software is able to correct for image magnification or minification. Therefore, exact, diameters of the circle scans can be guaranteed.

6.4.3 The Neuro-Retinal Rim

The most anterior part of ONH contains the RGC axons, which make up the neuro-retinal rim. Figure 6.7 shows a B-scan displaying the structures of the ONH from the internal limiting membrane to the anterior lamina cribrosa. The neuro-retinal rim is separated from the vitreous by the inner limiting membrane (ILM) of Elschnig. ILM is an objective inner boundary of neuro-retinal rim tissue that is consistently

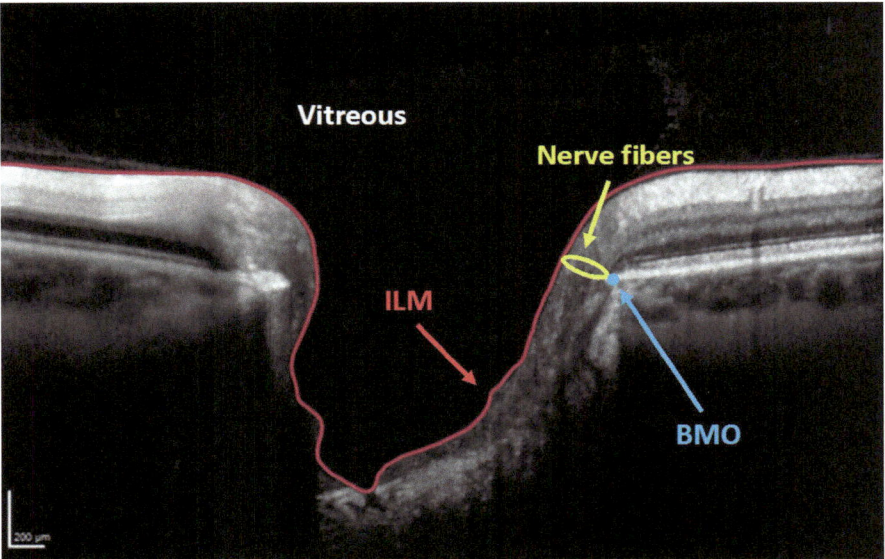

Fig. 6.7 The most anterior part of the optic nerve head contains the retinal ganglion cell axons, which make up the neuro-retinal rim. The neuro-retinal rim is separated from the vitreous by the internal limiting membrane. The Bruch's membrane opening represents the outer border of the rim tissue (nerve fibers), which is represented as a yellow ring. *BMO* Bruch's membrane opening, *ILM* internal limiting membrane

detected by SD-OCT. In order to avoid overestimation or underestimation, rim tissue must be measured in the correct geometric orientation. Ganglion cell axons may exit the eye almost parallel to the visual axis or even perpendicular to it. Significant errors in rim measurements can occur if the measurement plane is fixed.

Because of the varying orientation of the RGC axons upon their entry into the neural canal relative to the BMO, Povazay et al. and Chen and collaborators proposed that the minimum distance from BMO-RPE complex to the ILM represents the most accurate measurement of the axonal content in the neuro-retinal rim [13, 14]. The BMO is currently used as a reference by Spectralis OCT and the rim width is quantified as the minimum distance between the BMO and the internal limiting membrane. Chauhan and Burgoyne subsequently suggested using the end of the Bruch's membrane proper for this purpose and explored the difference between this measurement, termed BMO-minimum rim width (BMO-MRW) and conventional measurements, called horizontal rim width (BMO-HRW), and demonstrated the superiority of the BMO-MRW measurements (Fig. 6.8) [11, 15]. Strouthidis and associates showed the utility of BMO-MRW for detection of progressive ONH change in experimental primate glaucoma [9].

As mentioned above, the BMO-MRW analysis uses 48 equidistant data points, at which the BMO is identified and BMO-MRW calculated using an automated segmentation algorithm. The "BMO Overview" tab shows an overview of ONH anatomy at 12 equidistant locations around disc margin (Fig. 6.9) [16]. Clock hour anatomy is provided to the clinician for confirmation of automated segmentation, in addition to quantification of BMO-MRW to enhance clinical disc examination. Comparison to the normative database is then performed and results displayed as color-coded arrows. The neuro-retinal rim tissue is assessed perpendicular to the orientation of the axons and therefore, the varying trajectory of nerve fibers entering the ONH is taken into account at all points of measurement.

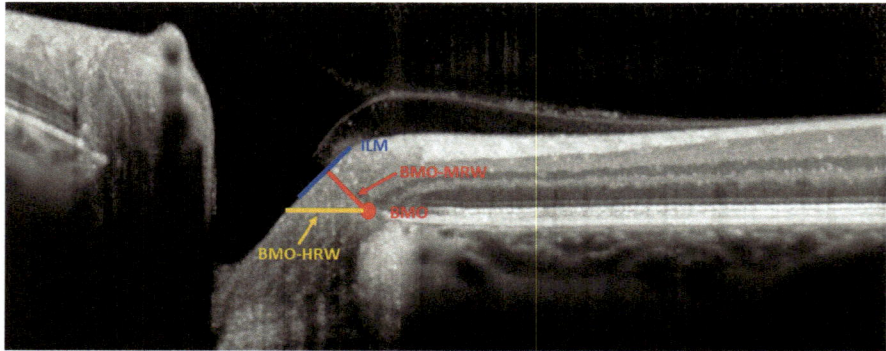

Fig. 6.8 The minimum distance from the Bruch's membrane opening to the internal limiting membrane represents the most accurate measurement of the neuro-retinal rim width. *BMO* Bruch's membrane opening, *BMO-MRW* Bruch's membrane opening-minimum rim width, *BMO-HRW* Bruch's membrane horizontal rim width, *ILM* internal limiting membrane

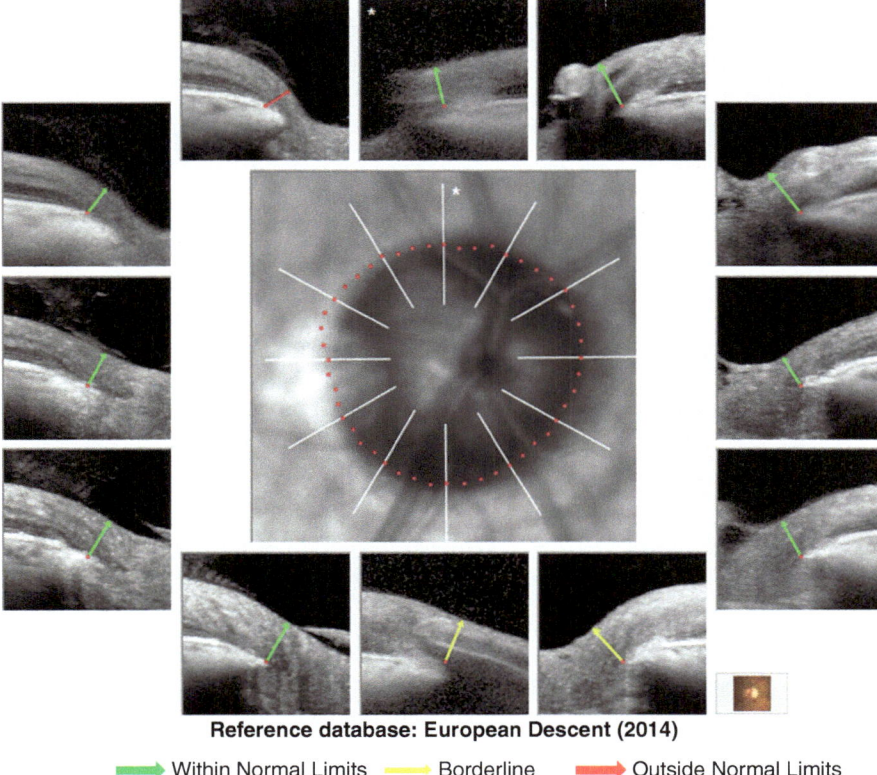

Reference database: European Descent (2014)

➡ Within Normal Limits   — Borderline   ➡ Outside Normal Limits

Fig. 6.9 Overview of the Bruch's membrane opening-minimum rim width (BMO-MRW) report of a patient with glaucomatous damage in the right eye. In the infrared image, the red dots represent Bruch's membrane opening delineated by the automated segmentation algorithm of Spectralis OCT at 48 equidistant points. The anatomic basis for BMO-MRW calculation at 12 equidistant locations around disc margin are also provided; classification of each location relative to a normative database is shown by color-coded arrows

The BMO segmentation should be confirmed after acquiring the ONH-RC scan. The BMO can sometimes be hidden by anatomical structures such as an overlying vessel; other times, it cannot be distinguished from neighboring structures due to the similar reflectivity. In such cases, changing the contrast scale from the standard settings of 12 to for example 15 may allow better visibility of the ONH structures. Detecting the wedge-shaped ending of the choroid may also be helpful in finding the BMO. It is well known that choriocapillaris does not exist without Bruch's membrane. Therefore, the BMO never ends before the choriocapillaris does, but it can extend further towards the ONH. The arrow representing the BMO-MRW should not cross retinal layers other than RNFL. There may be a jag in the height profile. This might indicate outlying BMO points or a wrong ILM segmentation.

In such a case, the segmentation of the OCT scan can be checked by placing the blue vertical lines onto the peak in the height profile. When it is not possible to detect the BMO point in one OCT scan, it is better to scroll through the neighboring scans till one BMO point has been identified clearly. After this, scan line should be dragged and dropped to the identified BMO point.

The BMO area affects the BMO-MRW profile. According to the ISNT rule, the thickness profile should show a slight double hump. In eyes with a small BMO area, the thickness profile graph is shifted upward (thicker) and for large BMO area, the thickness profile graph is shifted downward (thinner). Individual BMO-MRW height profile should be compared (black) with the BMO area- and age-adjusted normative database (green). Notches occur in case of rim thinning commonly matching RNFL defects. Since averaging can hide focal axonal defects in the classification chart, it is strongly recommended to review the height profile meticulously. The inferior and superior regions of the height profile should not be located below the nasal height profile; otherwise, the ISNT rule is clearly not respected.

6.5   The Posterior Pole Horizontal Algorithm (PPoleH)

The PPoleH scan is a volume scan of a $30° \times 25°$ area centered on the fovea. It consists of 61 horizontal B-scans aligned with the individual eye's FoBMO axis. The volume scan includes the total retinal thickness from the macula to the ONH across the posterior pole so that the complete path of the RGC axonal complex from the origin up to the entry point into the ONH can be assessed for macular RGCs (Fig. 6.10). Automated segmentation of the individual layers by the GMPE software allows evaluation of the thickness maps of the layers of interest in glaucoma (RNFL, GCL or IPL). The PPoleH scan covers the macular area corresponding to the majority of locations on the 24-2 visual field test for better structure and function correlation. The color scale of the posterior pole thickness map is finer than the standard retina thickness map and therefore, it is more sensitive for visualization of glaucomatous changes.

6.5.1   The Posterior Pole Asymmetry Analysis

The posterior pole asymmetry analysis is carried out by the software after a PPoleH scan. In the posterior pole asymmetry analysis tab, the posterior pole thickness map, the OCT raw scan for checking layer segmentation, and the posterior pole hemisphere asymmetry analysis are included.

The Posterior Pole Asymmetry Analysis combines mapping of the posterior pole retinal thickness with asymmetry analysis between the two eyes of the same individual and between the superior and inferior hemispheres of the same eye. Only the central $24° \times 24°$ of the macular volume scan is segmented and an 8×8 grid displaying retinal thickness on $3°$ superpixels is provided. Between-eye and superior-inferior thickness differences are also shown as a grayscale map where

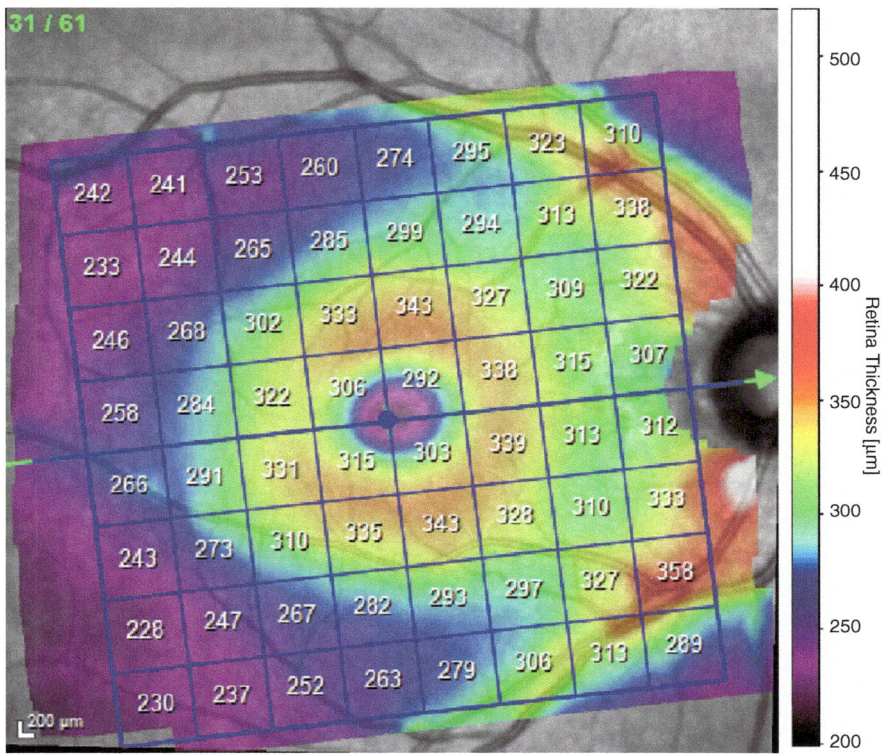

Fig. 6.10 Posterior pole horizontal scan of a healthy subject. The warmer colors on the thickness map represent thicker retina. The prominent thicker arcuate temporal-inferior and temporal-superior nerve fiber bundles appear red. The fovea as well as the peripheral retina appear purple or blue caused by physiologically thinner values

darker colors represent retinal thinning compared to the corresponding superpixel in either the fellow eye or the fellow vertical hemisphere. A difference of 30 μm results in a black superpixel indicating a significant difference. Three dark squares next to each other can indicate a defect (Fig. 6.11). Thickness differences along the nasal most superpixels are commonly caused by physiologically asymmetric distribution of the arteries and veins.

6.6   Posterior Pole Vertical Scan (PPoleV)

Pathologies of the outer retinal layers may affect the posterior pole thickness map. The PPoleV algorithm is an alternative macular volume scan. Nineteen vertical B-scans, encompassing a 30° × 15° scanning area, are carried out perpendicular to the FoBMO axis. These high resolution and noise-reduced scans allow for clear visualization of GCL and IPL layers after segmentation. Vertical scans provide more

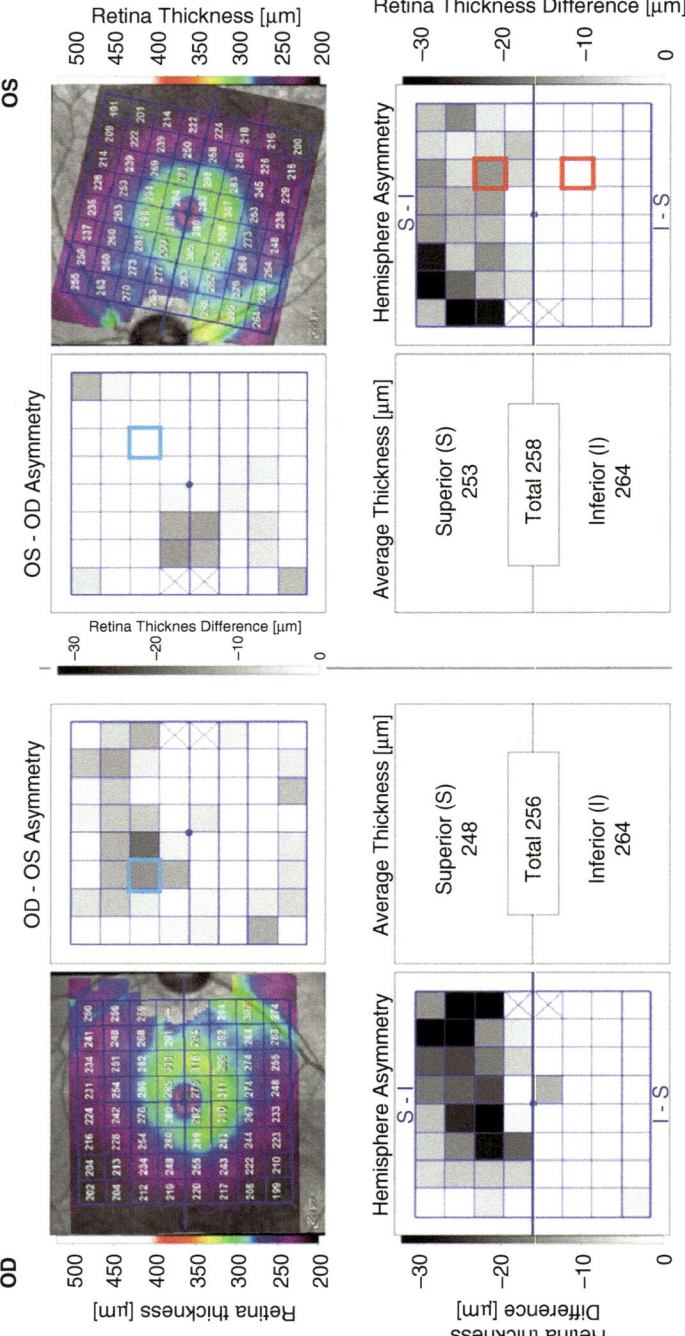

Fig. 6.11 Bilateral posterior pole asymmetry analysis of a patient with glaucoma. There is damage in both the superior and inferior nerve fibers in both eyes. This can be seen in the retinal thickness maps as thinning of the arcuate fibers both superiorly and inferiorly, and is more prominent superiorly in both eyes. In the hemisphere asymmetry charts, most of the squares in the superior hemisphere has colors with various tones of gray, representing thinning of the retina compared to the corresponding squares in the inferior hemisphere in both eyes. As an example, the red surrounded square in the upper hemisphere of the left eye shows a thickness of 269 microns, which is 14 microns thinner than the red surrounded corresponding square in the lower hemisphere. In the OD-OS asymmetry chart the blue surrounded square in the right eye shows a thickness of 254 microns, which is 15 microns thinner than the corresponding location in the left eye. This square has a gray color, representing thinning of the retina compared to the white colored corresponding square in the left eye

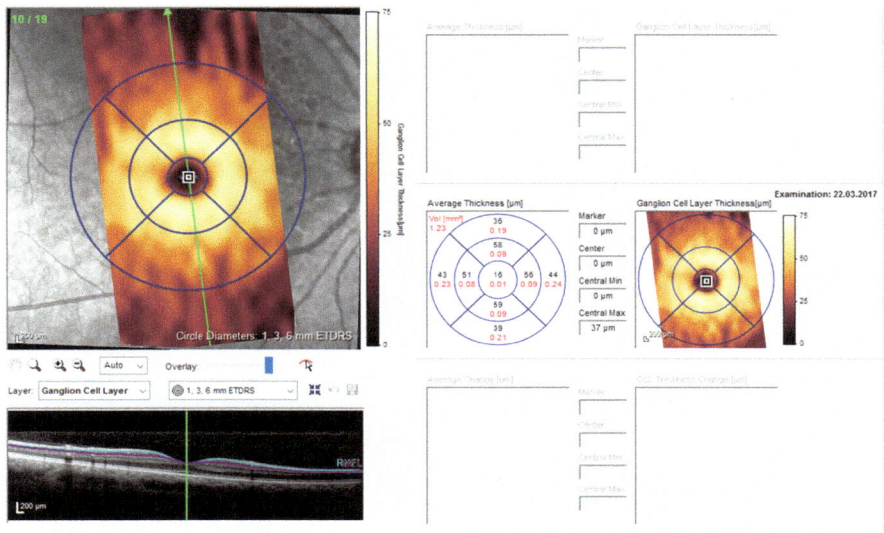

Fig. 6.12 Heat map of the ganglion cell layer of a healthy eye obtained following posterior pole vertical analysis and segmentation. Average thickness and volume measurements are provided on an ETDRS grid

sensitive symmetry analysis of superior vs. inferior macular layers on each individual B-scan and major horizontal vasculature does not create shadowing. Specifically, the GCL thickness is symmetrical between the superior and inferior macular hemispheres compared to the temporal and nasal hemispheres; The vertical asymmetry in GCL across the horizontal meridian was reported to be the most sensitive biomarker for detection of various stages of glaucoma including the preperimetric stage [17, 18].

After the PPoleV analysis and manual or automated segmentation, GCL thickness is provided as a color map on a circular grid. This thickness map can be displayed as a standard heat map (Glow Scale) (Fig. 6.12) or color map (Color Scale). Lack of a continuum of colors in the color map may lead to misleading of thickness values as some borderline values may fall in one color spectrum vs. another. Since heat maps offer a more continuous spectrum of color-scales, the standard heat map is preferred. Ganglion cell layer thickness maps and average thickness values are provided in a ETDRS grid format.

6.7 Interpretation of the Printouts

6.7.1 The Standard RNFL Single Exam Report

See Fig. 6.13.

1. **Patient and Test Information**: Displays general patient information including patient name, patient ID, diagnosis, date of birth, examination date and gender.

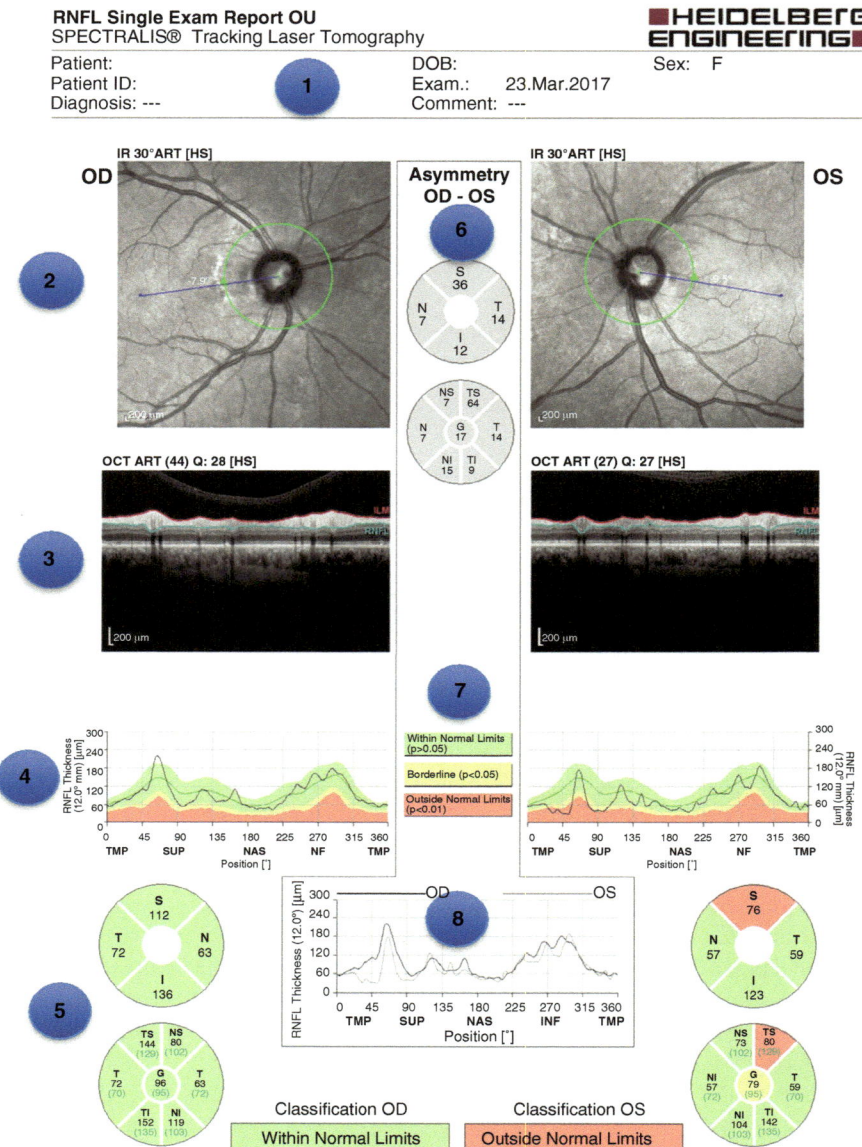

Fig. 6.13 The standard RNFL single exam report of a patient with a glaucomatous superior RNFL defect in the left eye. This eye is classified as outside normal limits. The right eye is classified as within normal limits

The examiner should verify the name and date of birth of the patient, as the results are compared to age-matched data from the normative database.

2. **Fundus Image Information**: The infrared reflectance (IR) image is an image of the fundus where the peripapillary circular scan is delineated. This image should be checked for even illumination, as well as proper location of circular scan, and fovea to disc alignment (or FoDi) axis. Abnormalities such as myelinated nerve fibers, peripapillary atrophy, and vitreous opacities should be excluded. The string above each fundus image notes the settings used for that image. In this example:

   (a) "IR" is imaging modality.
   (b) "30°" is the field of view.
   (c) "ART" indicates that the automatic real-time function was active during image capture.
   (d) "[HR]" is the resolution setting (High Speed/High Resolution).

3. **RNFL Profile Image:** RNFL profile (raw image) should be checked for abnormalities of the vitreo-retinal interface as well as the segmentation errors.

   The string above each OCT image notes the settings used for that image. In this example:

   (a) "ART" indicates that the automatic real-time function was active during image capture.
   (b) "(44)" is the number of averaged frames, i.e., the number of times the circular scan was repeated.
   (c) "Q:28" is the Quality score on a scale of 1–40. Values of <20 are considered poor quality image.
   (d) "[HR]" is the resolution setting (High Speed/High Resolution).

4. **RNFL Thickness Profile:** The black line indicates the thickness values of the patient's scan around the optic disc starting from 9 o'clock in the temporal quadrant (3 o'clock in the left eye) and going through the superior, nasal, inferior quadrants to end in the temporal quadrant (TSNIT). Background colors indicate normative data ranges (see Classification Colors). The dark green line plots the average thickness values from the normative database. Thickness profile should be characterized by distinctive humps along the temporal superior and temporal inferior sectors and values should fall within the range of normal limits for all sectors.

5. **Classification Chart:** The RNFL thickness is averaged and compared to the normative database in four quadrants and six sectors (temporal, temporal superior, nasal superior, nasal, nasal inferior, temporal inferior), as well as globally. This chart shows the average RNFL thickness (in microns) for each sector of each eye. Global (G) average is shown in the center. Sector colors indicate classification compared to the normative database. The black numbers represent the

average RNFL thickness in each sector. The numbers in parentheses (green) are the expected normal values, adjusted for age. The classification bar displays the classification of the worst sector in the pie graph.

6. **The Asymmetry Chart:** Displays the difference (in microns) between the thickness of corresponding quadrants (top) or sectors (bottom) of the right and left eye. If the RNFL thickness is similar in the two eyes, the value will be close to zero.
7. **Classification Colors**: Indicate comparison against the normative database. Green color represents "Within Normal Limits" values, i.e., measurements within the 95% prediction limits for normality ($p > 0.05$). Yellow represents "Borderline", with values outside the 95% but within 99% prediction interval of the normal distribution ($0.01 < p < 0.05$). Red color represents "Outside Normal Limits", with RNFL thickness measurements less than 99% of the healthy population ($p < 0.01$).
8. **Combined RNFL Profile:** Provides plots the RNFL thickness graph of both eyes. If the correlation between the two eyes is good, the lines on the graph will be very similar.

6.7.2 The RNFL Single Exam Report of the Glaucoma Module Premium Edition Software

GMPE's RNFL single exam report is similar to the standard report with a few differences. As mentioned above, the GMPE software performs three circle scans (3.5, 4.1, 4.7 mm in diameter). All scans are aligned with the individual eye's FoBMO axis. Since the normative database is different than the standard report and takes the BMO area into consideration, the classification chart has some differences from the standard report that are summarized below (Fig. 6.14).

1. **Fundus Image Information**: Interpretation of the IR fundus image is similar to that of standard report. In the GMPE report, although the default setting of circular scan is 3.5 mm, it is possible to see the results of the other two circular scans 4.1 and 4.7 mm in dimeter. The setting of the current circular scan is shown in bold. The circle scan diameter and BMO area is presented in the right lower section of the fundus image.
2. **Classification Chart:** RNFL thickness is analyzed and classified in four quadrants, Garway-Heath sectors and globally. The two charts show average RNFL thickness (in microns) for each sector and quadrant. Global (G) average is shown in the center of the former. Sector or quadrant color indicates classification based on the normative database of the GMPE. The black numbers represent the average RNFL thickness values in each sector. The numbers in parentheses shows the ranking of the RNFL thickness in percentile within the normative database.

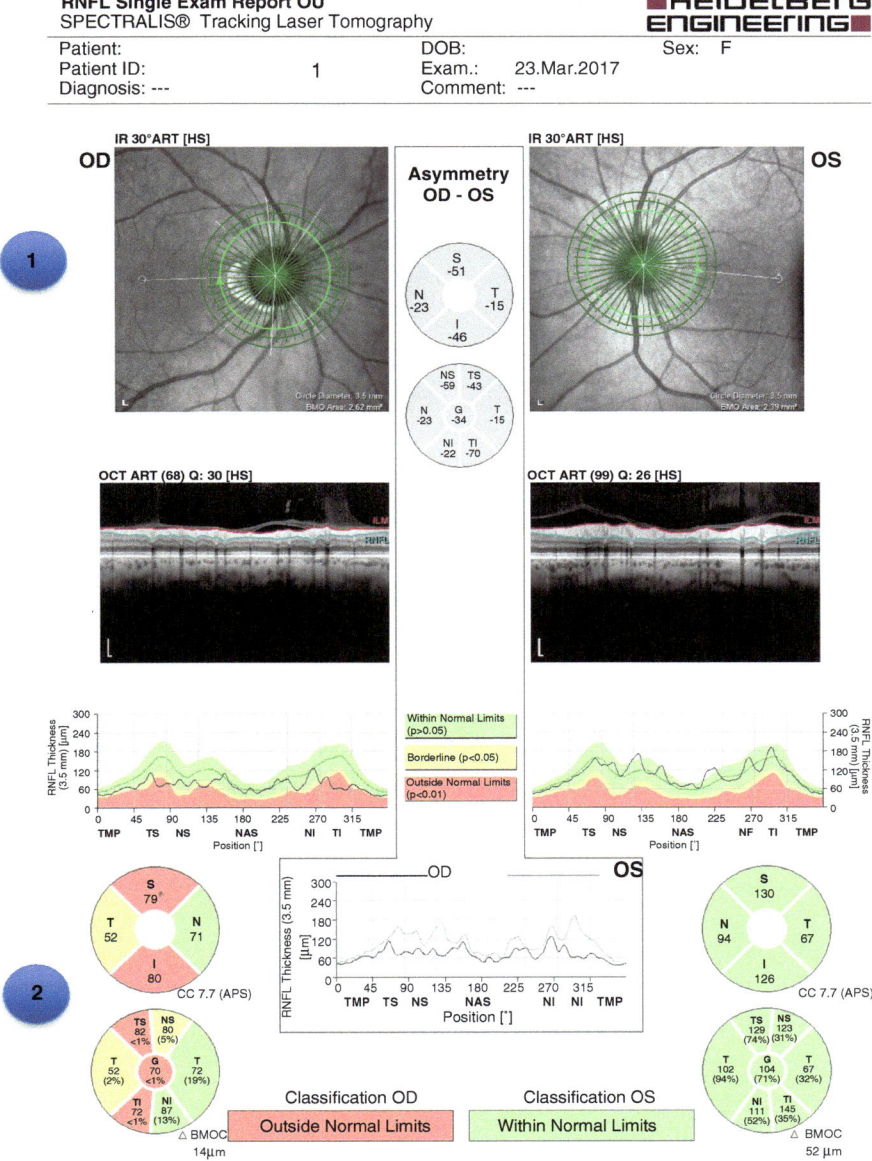

Fig. 6.14 Glaucoma Module Premium Edition software RNFL single exam report of a patient with glaucomatous superior, temporal and inferior RNFL defects in the right eye on the 3.5 mm circle scan. This eye is classified as outside normal limits. The left eye is classified to be within normal limits

Classification colors are similar to that of the standard RNFL report. The classification bar in the bottom displays the classification of the worst sector in the pie graph. CC represents corneal curvature, and Δ BMOC shows the distance between the BMO and the optic disc centroids.

6.7.3 The Minimum Rim Width Analysis Report of the Glaucoma Module Premium Edition Software

See Fig. 6.15.

1. **Patient and Test Information**: Displays general patient information such as patient name, patient ID, diagnosis, date of birth, examination date and gender. The name and date of birth of the patient need to be verified as the results are compared to age-matched data from the normative database.
2. **BMO Overview Tab**: Shows an overview of ONH anatomy at 12 equidistant locations around the BMO. The BMO area is displayed on the bottom left of the central IR image (1.96 mm^2 in the right eye and 1.98 mm^2 in the left eye) and the BMO is marked in red. Arrows show the anatomic structures that form the basis for measurement of the MRW at each location. The color of the arrows flags the classification of the MRW based on the normative database. ILM is represented in red.

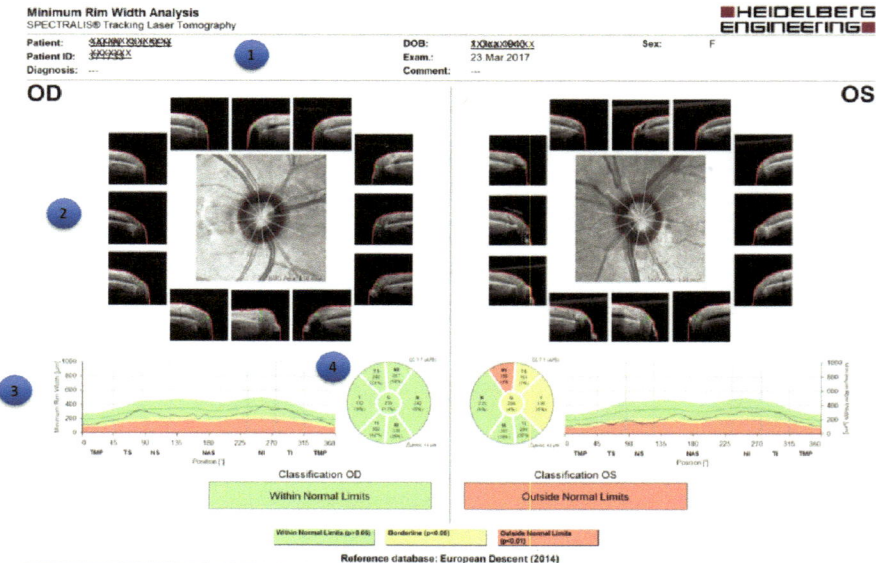

Fig. 6.15 Glaucoma Module Premium Edition software minimum rim width analysis report of the patient in Fig. 6.13 with superior and temporal glaucomatous rim thinning in the left eye. This eye is classified as outside normal limits. Right eye is classified as within normal limits

3. **BMO-MRW Height Profile (TSNIT Graph):** The measured BMO-MRW is provided in color codes and in microns along the optic disc circumference starting from 0°, which is the point located temporally at the junction of the FoBMO axis and BMO. The black curve indicates the thickness values of the patient's scan. Age and BMO area adjusted MRW of normal eyes is also represented in the height profile as a green curve. The height profile should show a slight double hump according to the ISNT rule. In a case with glaucoma, the MRW profile does not show a temporal inferior and temporal superior hump and the ISNT rule is not fulfilled. Notches in the temporal inferior or temporal superior height profile correspond to focal neuroretinal rim loss or nerve fiber bundle defects.

4. **Classification Chart:** The measured average BMO-MRW thickness in microns, corresponding percentiles of the normal distribution adjusted for age and the BMO area of the individual eye are shown for each individual Garway-Heath sector (T, TS, NS, N, NI, TI) and globally. The black numbers represent the average MRW thickness values in each sector. The numbers in parentheses shows the percentile of the MRW thickness value of that sector. Classification colors are similar to that of the standard RNFL report. The overall classification bar below the Garway-Heath sector map reflects results of the thinnest sector. Classification colors are similar to the previous reports. CC represents corneal curvature, and Δ BMOC shows the distance between the BMO and the optic disc centroids.

6.7.4   The Posterior Pole Asymmetry Analysis Report

See Fig. 6.16.

1. **Patient and Test Information**: Displays general patient information as patient name, patient ID, diagnosis, date of birth, examination date and gender.

2. **Posterior Pole Thickness Map:** In each $3° \times 3°$ superpixel on the 8×8 grid, the average retinal thickness within the superpixel is displayed. The warmer (the redder) the color of the thickness map, the thicker the measured retinal area. The compressed color scale on the right side of the map is used to localize even the smallest differences in retinal thickness between adjacent areas.

3. **Inter-Ocular Asymmetry Map:** The retinal thickness at 64 superpixels in one eye is compared to the corresponding thickness measurements in the fellow eye. Superpixels with shades of gray demonstrate reduced thickness compared to the corresponding superpixels in the fellow eye. The intensity of the gray scale reflects the magnitude of differences between corresponding superpixels of the eyes.

4. **Hemisphere Asymmetry Map:** The average retinal thickness in superpixels in one hemisphere is compared to the corresponding superpixels in the opposite hemisphere. Superpixels displaying various shades of gray in one hemisphere have reduced thickness compared to those on the corresponding hemisphere. The intensity of the gray color is a function of the amount of difference between corresponding superpixels of the two hemispheres (black: ≥ 30 μm difference).

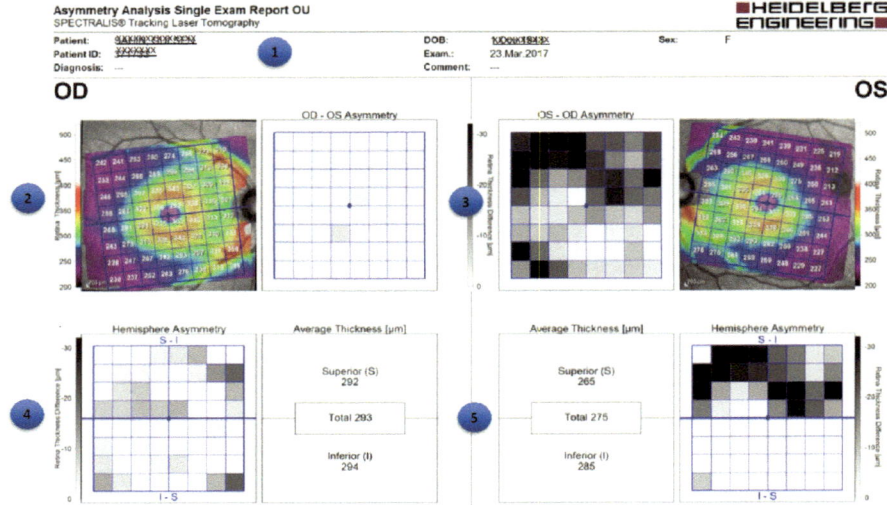

Fig. 6.16 The Posterior Pole Asymmetry analysis of the patient in Figs. 6.13 and 6.15. The prominent arcuate temporal-inferior and temporal-superior nerve fiber bundles appear red in the right eye. In the left eye, there is glaucomatous damage in the superior quadrant, which can be seen in the retinal thickness map as thinning of the arcuate fibers superiorly. In the hemisphere asymmetry chart of the left eye, most of the superpixels in the superior hemisphere are flagged various shades of gray, representing thinning of the retina compared to the corresponding superpixels in the inferior hemifield. In the OS-OD asymmetry chart (3), most of the superpixels are flagged with various shades of gray, depicting retinal thinning in the left eye compared to the right eye

5. **Average Thickness Chart:** The averaged retinal thickness of the central $24° \times 24°$ area is provided in addition to the superior and inferior hemisphere thickness measurements.

6.8   Key Points

- Poor signal strength leads to a faint image resulting in the software being unable to accurately identify the boundaries of the retinal layers. The technician needs to ensure that the patient blinks just before image acquisition or instill artificial tears to improve the image quality.
- The eye typically has five micro-saccades per second. Unless there is image tracking, motion artifact is very likely even with the most cooperative patient. That is why a decrease in image acquisition time improves image quality.
- Accurate acquisition of the image without cutoff at the edges and with good centration of the optic nerve or the fovea is very important for an acceptable test.
- After confirming that all the requirements have been met, the physician must rule out the presence of coexisting pathology that may confound the results and therefore, the interpretation. The most common offenders include vitreous

traction on the RNFL and epiretinal membranes in the peripapillary and macular region.

- The physician should confirm that the auto-segmentation function of the software has correctly identified the layers it is trying to measure.
- The clinician needs to determine if the patient's ocular condition merits comparison to a normative database. For example, high myopes are not included in OCT normative databases, and therefore, their measurements typically read as abnormal.
- It is very important for the clinician to have ready access to the raw images acquired before looking at the interpretation provided in the report.

References

1. Strouthidis NG, Grimm J, Williams GA, Cull GA, Wilson DJ, Burgoyne CF. A comparison of optic nerve head morphology viewed by spectral domain optical coherence tomography and by serial histology. Invest Ophthalmol Vis Sci. 2010;51:1464–74.
2. Lee EJ, Kim TW, Weinreb RN, Park KH, Kim SH, Kim DM. Visualization of the lamina cribrosa using enhanced depth imaging spectral-domain optical coherence tomography. Am J Ophthalmol. 2011;152:87–95e81.
3. Reis AS, Sharpe GP, Yang H, Nicolela MT, Burgoyne CF, Chauhan BC. Optic disc margin anatomy in patients with glaucoma and normal controls with spectral domain optical coherence tomography. Ophthalmology. 2012a;119:738–47.
4. Strouthidis NG, Yang H, Reynaud JF, Grimm JL, Gardiner SK, Fortune B, Burgoyne CF. Comparison of clinical and spectral domain optical coherence tomography optic disc margin anatomy. Invest Ophthalmol Vis Sci. 2009;50:4709–18.
5. He L, Ren R, Yang H, Hardin C, Reyes L, Reynaud J, Gardiner SK, Fortune B, Demirel S, Burgoyne CF. Anatomic vs acquired image frame discordance in spectral domain optical coherence tomography minimum rim measurements. PLoS One. 2014;9:e92225. [PubMed: 24643069]
6. Valverde-Megías A, Martinez-de-la-Casa JM, Serrador-García M, Larrosa JM, García-Feijoó J. Clinical relevance of foveal location on retinal nerve fiber layer thickness using the new FoDi software in spectralis optical coherence tomography. Invest Ophthalmol Vis Sci. 2013;54:5771–6.
7. Jansonius NM, Nevalainen J, Selig B, Zangwill LM, Sample PA, et al. A mathematical description of nerve fiber bundle trajectories and their variability in the human retina. Vis Res. 2009;49:2157–63.
8. Hood DC, Raza AS, de Moraes CG, Liebmann JM, Ritch R. Glaucomatous damage of the macula. Prog Retin Eye Res. 2013;32:1–21.
9. Strouthidis NG, Fortune B, Yang H, Sigal IA, Burgoyne CF. Longitudinal change detected by spectral domain optical coherence tomography in the optic nerve head and peripapillary retina in experimental glaucoma. Invest Ophthalmol Vis Sci. 2011;52:1206–19.
10. Chauhan BC, Burgoyne FC. From clinical examination of the optic disc to clinical assessment of the optic nerve head: a paradigm change. Am J Ophthalmol. 2013;156:218–27.
11. Reis AS, O'Leary N, Yang H, Sharpe GP, Nicolela MT, Burgoyne CF, Chauhan BC. Influence of clinically invisible, but optical coherence tomography detected, optic disc margin anatomy on neuroretinal rim evaluation. Invest Ophthalmol Vis Sci. 2012b;53:1852–60.
12. Reis AS, O'Leary N, Stanfield MJ, Shuba LM, Nicolela MT, Chauhan BC. Laminar displacement and prelaminar tissue thickness change after glaucoma surgery imaged with optical coherence tomography. Invest Ophthalmol Vis Sci. 2012d;53:5819–26.

13. Chen TC. Spectral domain optical coherence tomography in glaucoma: qualitative and quantitative analysis of the optic nerve head and retinal nerve fiber layer (an AOS thesis). Trans Am Ophthalmol Soc. 2009;107:254–81.
14. Povazay B, Hofer B, Hermann B, et al. Minimum distance mapping using three-dimensional optical coherence tomography for glaucoma diagnosis. J Biomed Opt. 2007;12:041204.
15. Chauhan BC, O'Leary N, Almobarak FA, Reis AS, Yang H, Sharpe GP, Hutchison DM, Nicolela MT, Burgoyne CF. Enhanced detection of open-angle glaucoma with an anatomically accurate optical coherence tomography-derived neuroretinal rim parameter. Ophthalmology. 2013;120:535–43.
16. Danthurebandara VM, Sharpe GP, Hutchinson DM, Dennis J, Nicolela MT, McKendrick AM, Turpin A, Chauhan BC. Enhanced structure-function relationship in glaucoma with an anatomically and geometrically accurate neuroretinal rim measurement. Invest Ophthalmol Vis Sci. 2011;56:98–105.
17. Nakano N, Hangai M, Nakanishi H, Mori S, Nukada M, Kotera Y, Ikeda HO, Nakamura H, Nonaka A, Yoshimura N. Macular ganglion cell layer imaging in preperimetric glaucoma with speckle noise-reduced spectral domain optical coherence tomography. Ophthalmology. 2011;118:2414–26.
18. Yamada H, Hangai M, Nakano N, Takayama K, Kimura Y, Miyake M, Akagi T, Ikeda HO, Noma H, Yoshimura N. Asymmetry analysis of macular inner retinal layers for glaucoma diagnosis. Am J Ophthalmol. 2014;158:1318–29.

Chapter 7
Examples of Optical Coherence Tomography Findings in Glaucoma Eyes with Varying Stages of Severity

Ahmet Akman

7.1 Early (Pre-perimetric) Glaucoma

Seventy-year-old male glaucoma suspect referred for glaucoma evaluation. The BCVA was 20/20 OU. The anterior segment exam was normal with grade one nuclear sclerosis in both eyes. The posterior segment exam was normal OU. Intraocular pressures (IOPs) were 32 mmHg OD and 26 mmHg OS without treatment (Figs. 7.1, 7.2, 7.3, 7.4, 7.5, and 7.6).

A. Akman
Department of Ophthalmology, School of Medicine, Başkent University, Ankara, Turkey

© Springer International Publishing AG, part of Springer Nature 2018
A. Akman et al. (eds.), *Optical Coherence Tomography in Glaucoma*,
https://doi.org/10.1007/978-3-319-94905-5_7

78   A. Akman

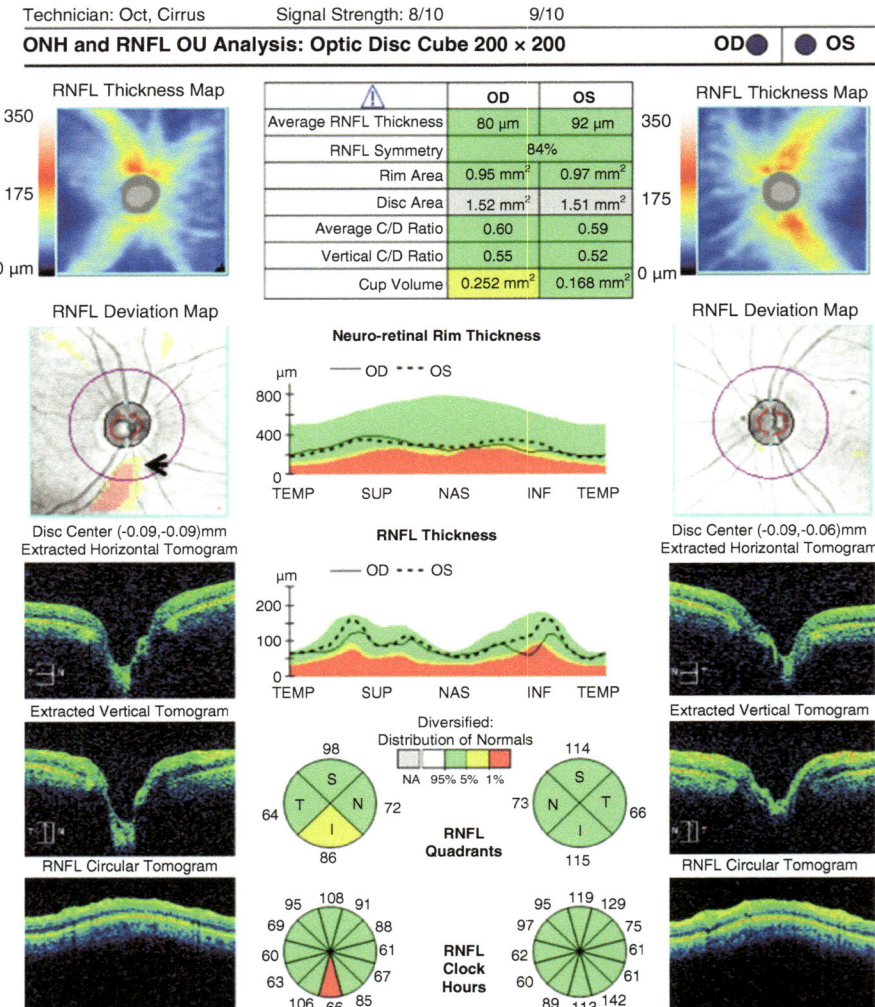

Fig. 7.1 (Cirrus HD-OCT) This is a good quality OCT scan with SS value of 8 OD and 9 OS; there are no artifacts or anatomical variations. The RNFL thickness map shows that the inferior RNFL bundle is thinner than the superior bundle in the right eye and compared with the inferior bundle of the left eye (see TSNIT curves). Although the average RNFL thickness measurements are still in the normal range in both eyes, there is an inferior RNFL defect on the RNFL deviation map (black arrowhead). The TSNIT plot and clock hour graphs also demonstrate this defect at the 6 o'clock position. The only abnormal finding among ONH parameters is the cup volume in the right eye, which is borderline abnormal

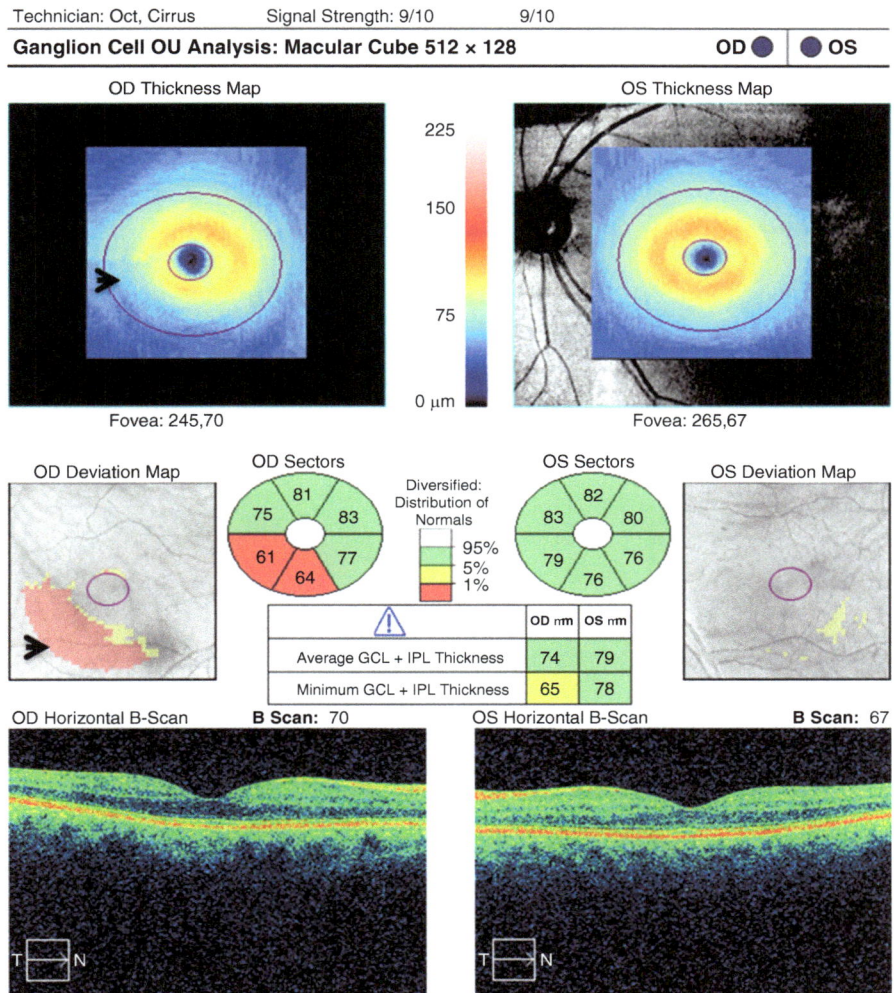

Fig. 7.2 (Cirrus HD-OCT) Macular Ganglion Cell Analysis also shows a local abnormal area in the inferior temporal part of the macula in the right eye (black arrowheads), which corresponds to the inferior RNFL defect on the optic disc cube. The inferotemporal and inferior sectors are also abnormal at <1% level and the minimum GCL + IPL thickness is borderline abnormal despite the average GCL + IPL being in the normal range. The right eye with corresponding defects in the peripapillary area and the macula can be classified as early glaucomatous damage as the 30-2 visual field is within normal limits (see below)

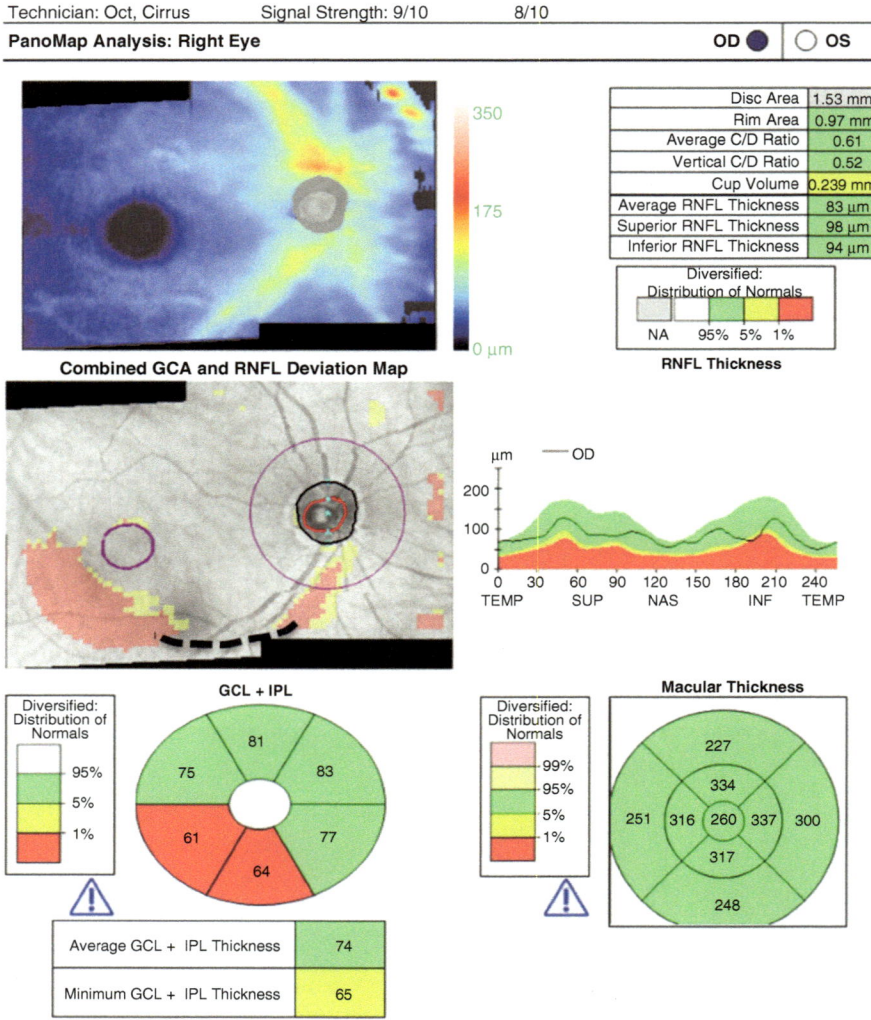

Technician: Oct, Cirrus   Signal Strength: 9/10   8/10

PanoMap Analysis: Right Eye   OD ●   ○ OS

Fig. 7.3 (Cirrus HD-OCT) The Panomap analysis shows the peripapillary and macular thinning in a single printout. The area of inferior RNFL thinning appears to be continuous with the region demonstrating macular GCL + IPL thinning, but part of the defect is outside the scan cubes so a gap seems to exist between the peripapillary and macular components of the defect in this printout (black dashed line)

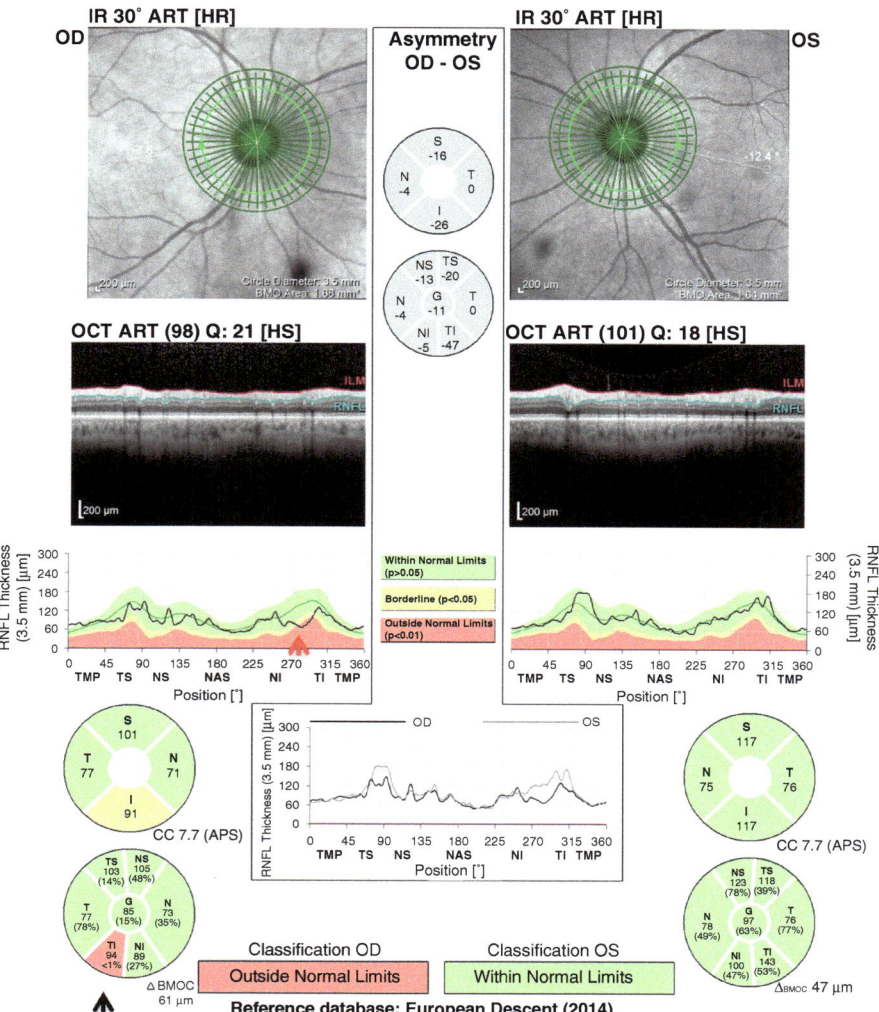

Fig. 7.4 (Spectralis GMPE module) The Spectralis OCT also demonstrates the RNFL defect in the right eye consistent with the Cirrus HD-OCT. The Garway–Heath sectors locate the defect in the inferior temporal quadrant (black arrowhead). The TSNIT graph also shows the defect at around 270–300 degrees (red arrowhead)

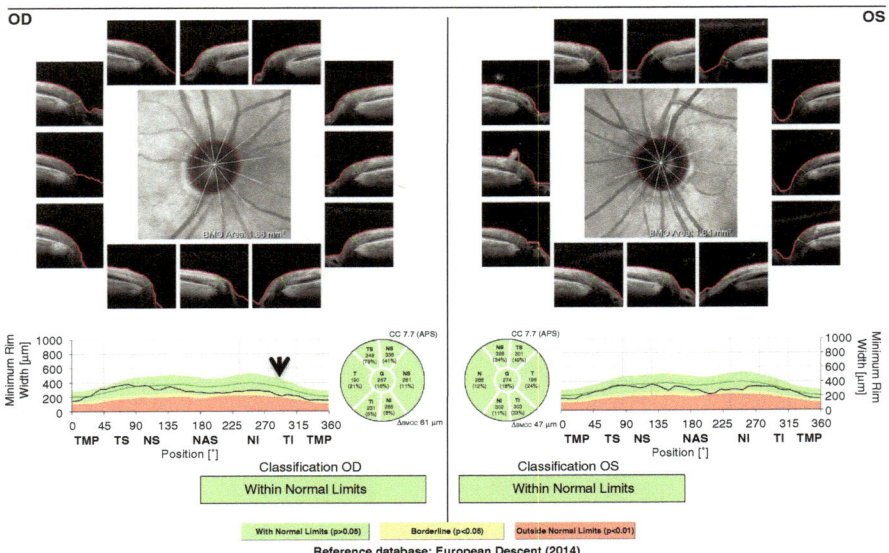

Fig. 7.5 (Spectralis GMPE module) The Minimum Rim Width analysis demonstrates ONH topography. GMPE analysis is more detailed than the Cirrus HD-OCT ONH findings and although the MRW parameter is borderline in the temporal inferior (TI) quadrant of the right eye in the TSNIT graph (black arrowhead), the TI quadrant of the classification chart is still in green range as it is a very early and localized defect

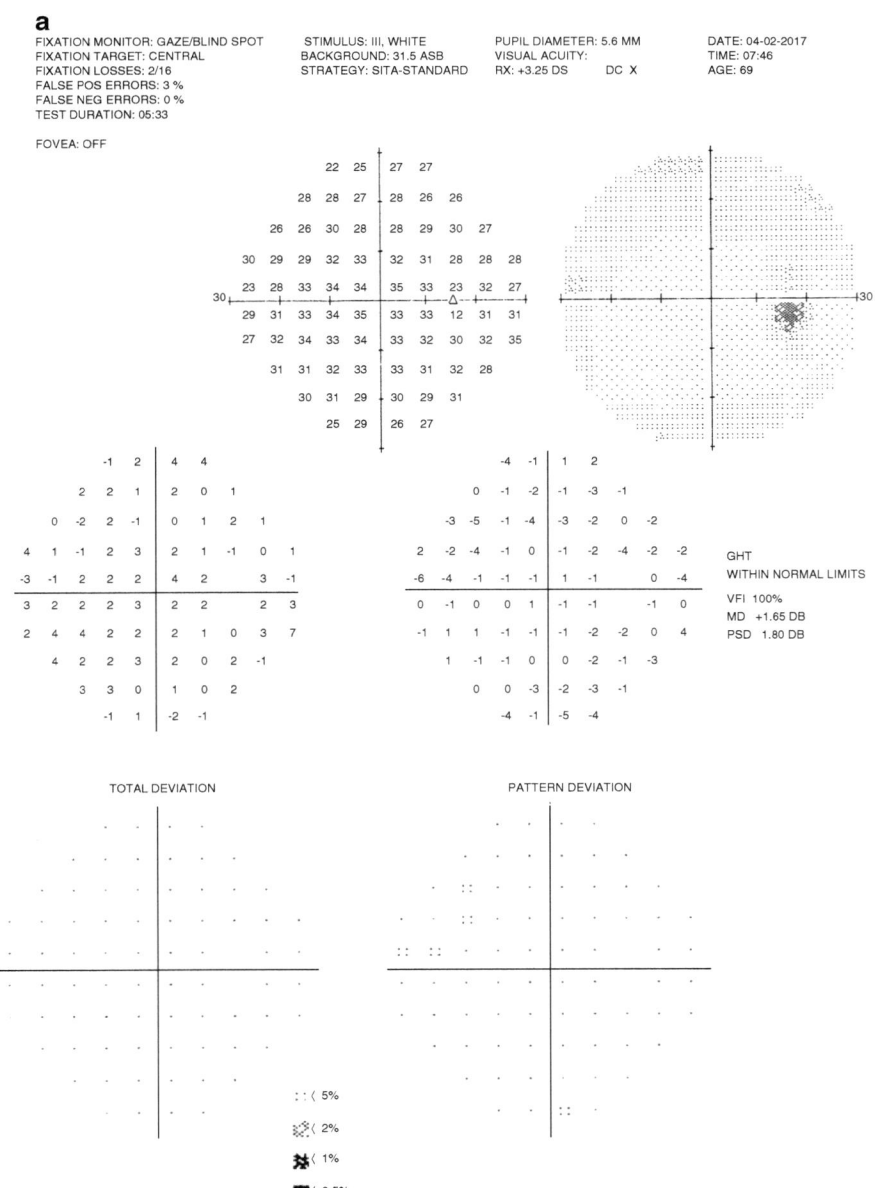

Fig. 7.6 (**a** and **b**) The Humphrey visual field tests are classified as within normal limits in both eyes

b

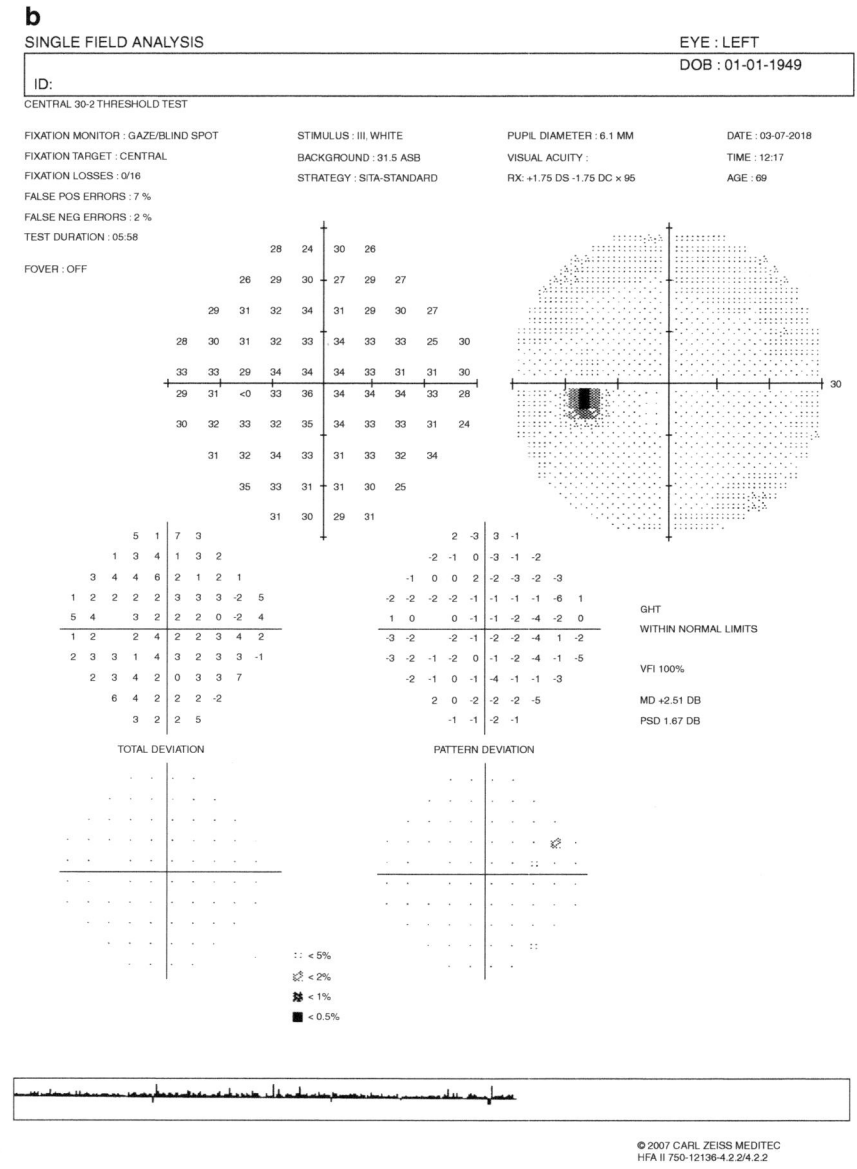

Fig. 7.6 (continued)

Conclusion: This case represents an example of early glaucomatous damage, which can be classified as pre-perimetric glaucoma as there is no functional damage on visual field (VF) testing. The retinal nerve fiber layer (RNFL) defect was demonstrated by two different OCT systems; however, both devices failed to show optic nerve head (ONH) topographic damage. Given the high IOP (32 mmHg) and presence of early glaucomatous defects in OCT tests, starting anti-glaucomatous treatment at this stage is a viable option to prevent further damage in the right eye.

7.2   Moderate Glaucoma

Seventy-one-year old male with newly diagnosed exfoliative glaucoma, who had IOP measurements of 22 and 38 mmHg in the right and left eyes, respectively. The anterior segment exam revealed exfoliative material at the pupillary margin and on the anterior lens capsule in both eyes. BCVA was 20/20 OU (Figs. 7.7, 7.8, 7.9, 7.10, 7.11, 7.12, and 7.13).

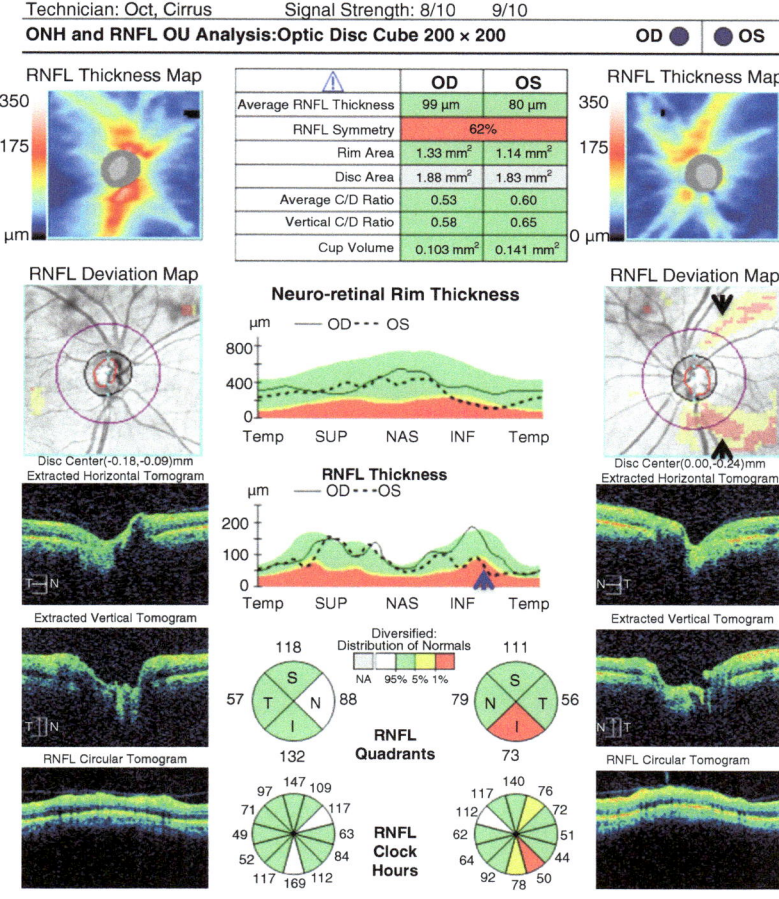

Fig. 7.7 (Cirrus HD-OCT) Good quality scan with high signal strength (9/10) OU. In the key parameters plot, average RNFL thickness is within normal limits in both eyes although the left eye average RNFL value is 19 μm thinner than that of the right eye. This difference resulted in the RNFL symmetry box being flagged in red. The RNFL thickness map of the left eye shows some RNFL loss and the RNFL deviation map, which compares the patient's RNFL measurements to the normative database, reveals definitive inferior RNFL loss and a possible superior RNFL defect (black arrowheads). The TSNIT graph demonstrates the inferior RNFL defect in the left eye (blue arrowhead). The superior RNFL defect could be a real defect, but it can also be shifted RNFL artifact, which will be discussed in the Chap. 8. Quadrant and clock hour pie graphs confirm the inferior RNFL defect. Although the cup/disc ratios are still in the green zone (see the key parameters table), the neuro-retinal rim area TSNIT graph demonstrates neuro-retinal rim loss in the inferior quadrant

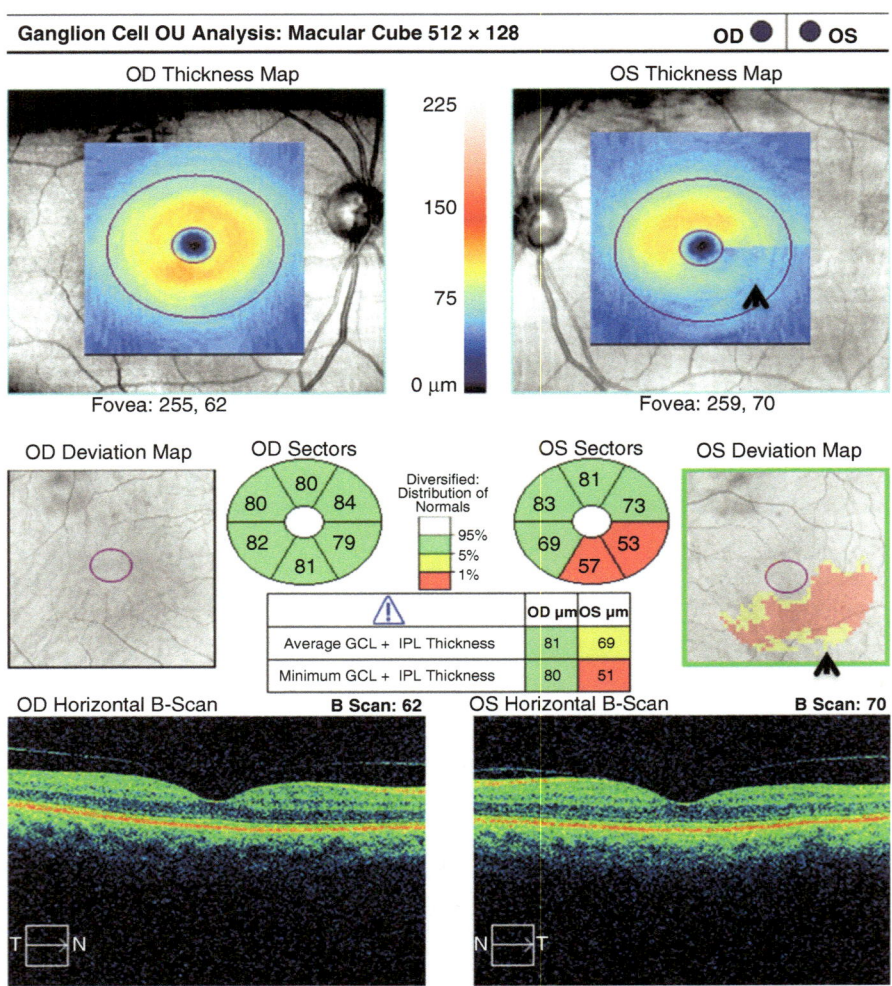

Fig. 7.8 (Cirrus-HD OCT) Ganglion Cell Analysis shows normal GCL + IPL thickness in the right eye; a large area of GCL + IPL damage is evident in the inferior and temporal regions of the left macula confirmed by abnormal inferior and inferotemporal sectors and average GCL + IPL thickness (black arrowheads). The superior half of the GCL + IPL thickness map is within normal limits

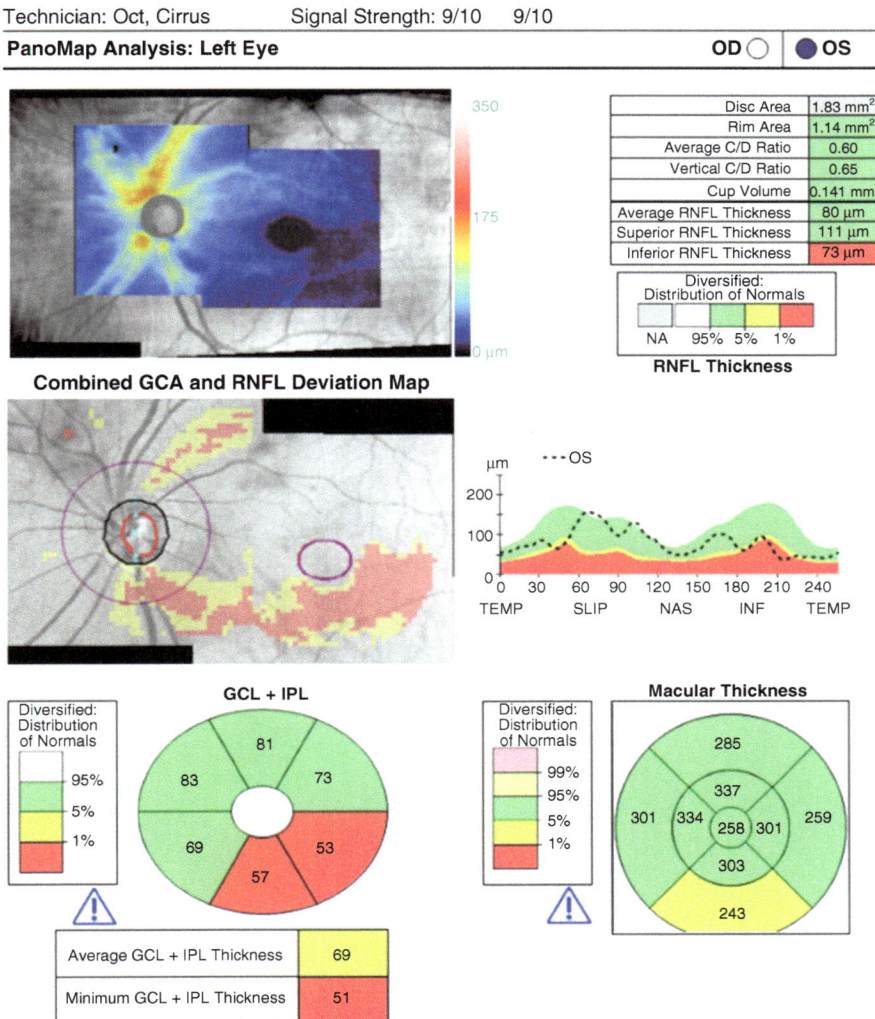

Fig. 7.9 (Cirrus-HD OCT) Panomap report of the left eye demonstrates the peripapillary RNFL loss and macular ganglion cell loss in wide-field format

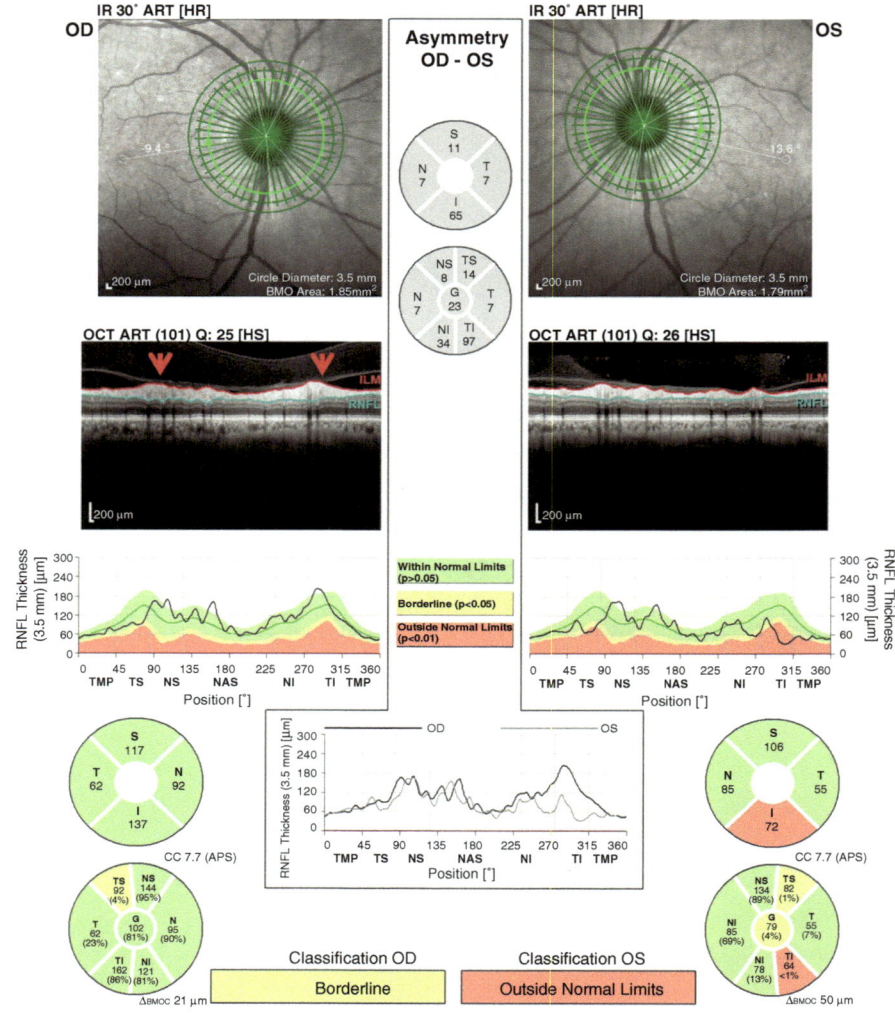

Fig. 7.10 (Spectralis, GMPE module) Spectralis OCT demonstrates the RNFL loss in the inferior quadrant and in the inferotemporal sector of the left eye. The borderline RNFL finding in the superior temporal sectors of both eyes could be the result of shifted RNFL peaks as the TSNIT graphs show that the RNFL peaks in superior quadrants are not that thin and do not fit the configuration expected from the normative database. Another important point on this OCT printout is the possibility of vitreoretinal traction around the optic nerve head. Vitreous adhesions to the RNFL can be observed in an extended area on the raw OCT image of the right eye. The superior-nasal-inferior adhesions (red arrowheads) could be the reason for the thick RNFL values of the right eye on the TSNIT graph. The vitreous/RNFL adhesion and possible traction could hide RNFL loss and may lead to a green disease artifact, which will be discussed in the Chap. 8

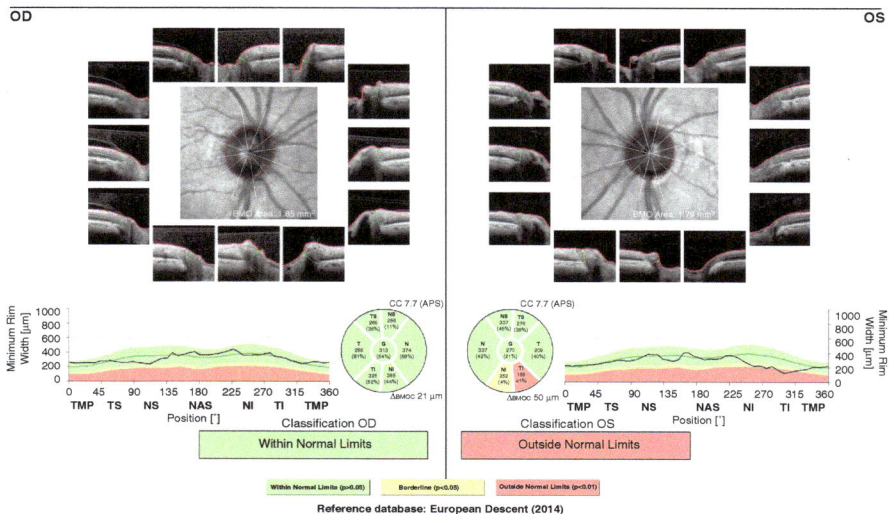

Fig. 7.11 (Spectralis GMPE module) The Minimum Rim Width analysis demonstrates inferior rim loss in the left eye consistent with the neuro-retinal rim changes observed on Cirrus HD-OCT printout

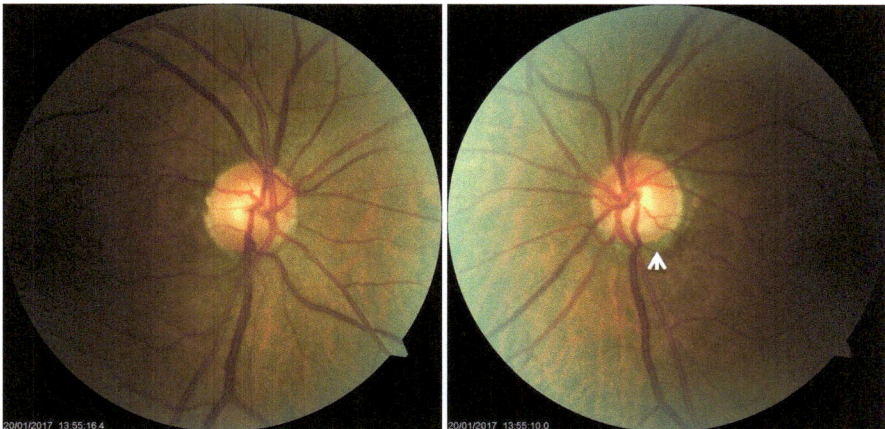

Fig. 7.12 Inferior notching at the left optic nerve head is evident on the disc photographs (white arrowhead)

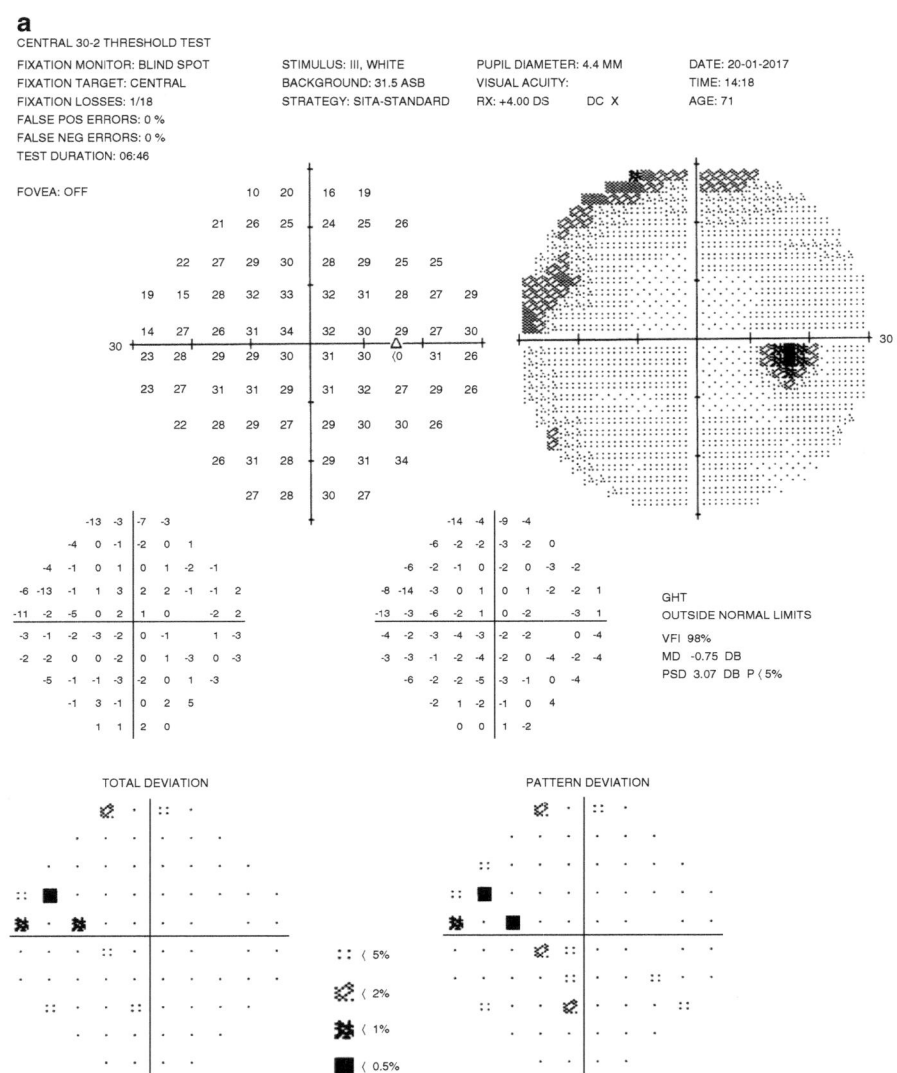

Fig. 7.13 (**a**) Humphrey visual field of the right eye may be classified as outside normal limits because of an early nasal step. (**b**) Visual field of the left eye shows a dense arcuate defect in the superior hemifield, which is compatible with the inferior RNFL defect. The visual field findings suggest a moderate level of damage

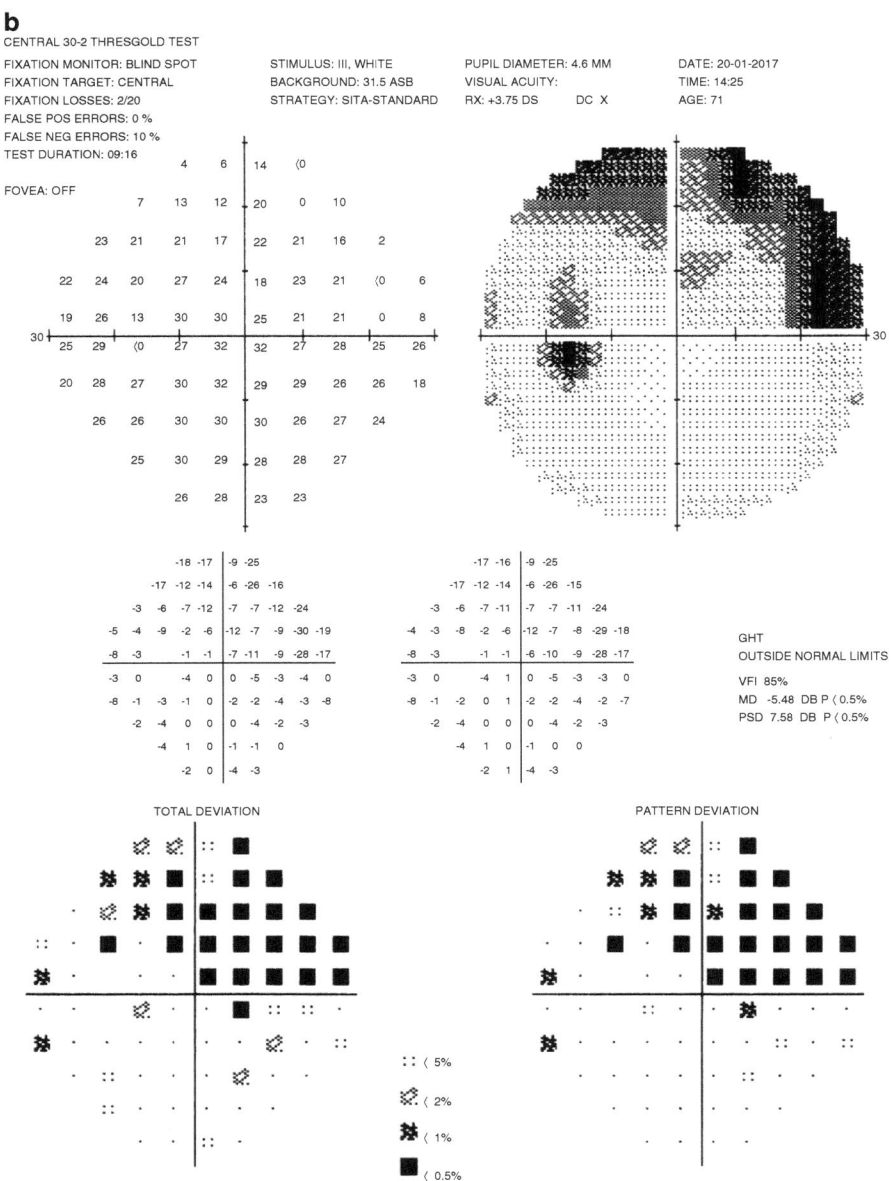

Fig. 7.13 (continued)

Conclusion: This case represents a patient with a moderate degree of glaucomatous damage. Both the structural test (OCT) and functional test (VF) show corresponding damage in the left eye. Also, two different OCT devices show similar RNFL loss patterns and neuro-retinal rim damage at the same location. In eyes with moderate damage, both structural and functional tests are important in diagnosing the disease and monitoring the progression. The right eye of the patient must also be followed closely as there is a possibility of green disease.

7.3 Advanced Glaucoma

Sixty-eight-year old female, diagnosed with bilateral primary open angle glaucoma seven years ago. The right eye underwent two trabeculectomies and the left eye had one trabeculectomy in the last five years. On the last examination, IOP was 16 mmHg in the right eye and 14 mmHg in the left eye (Figs. 7.14, 7.15, 7.16, 7.17, 7.18, 7.19, 7.20, and 7.21).

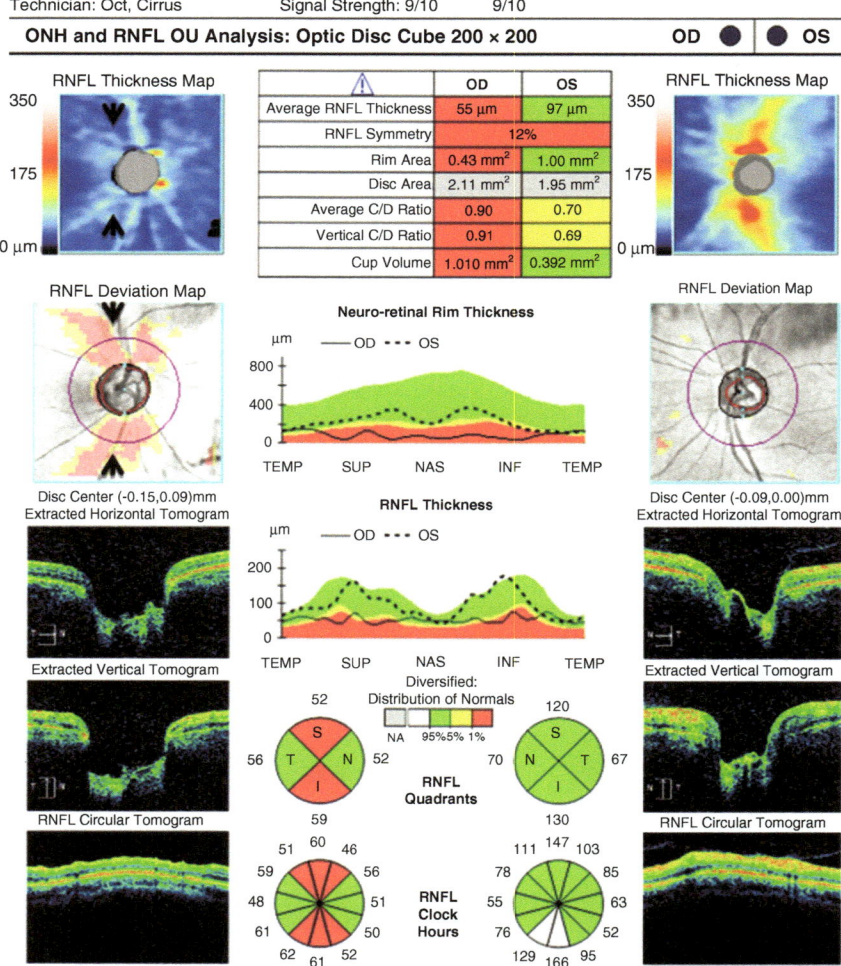

Fig. 7.14 (Cirrus-HD OCT) Scan quality is excellent (9/10) in both eyes. In the key parameters table, all RNFL and ONH parameters of the right eye are outside normal limits. The RNFL thickness map of the right eye shows advanced RNFL loss and the RNFL deviation map, which compares the patient's RNFL to the normative database, reveals nearly total RNFL loss (black arrowheads). The TSNIT graph demonstrates advanced RNFL loss in the right eye in all quadrants. Quadrant and clock hour pie graphs also confirm the advanced RNFL loss evident on the TSNIT graph. Neuro-retinal rim area TSNIT graph also demonstrates advanced neuro-retinal rim loss in all quadrants

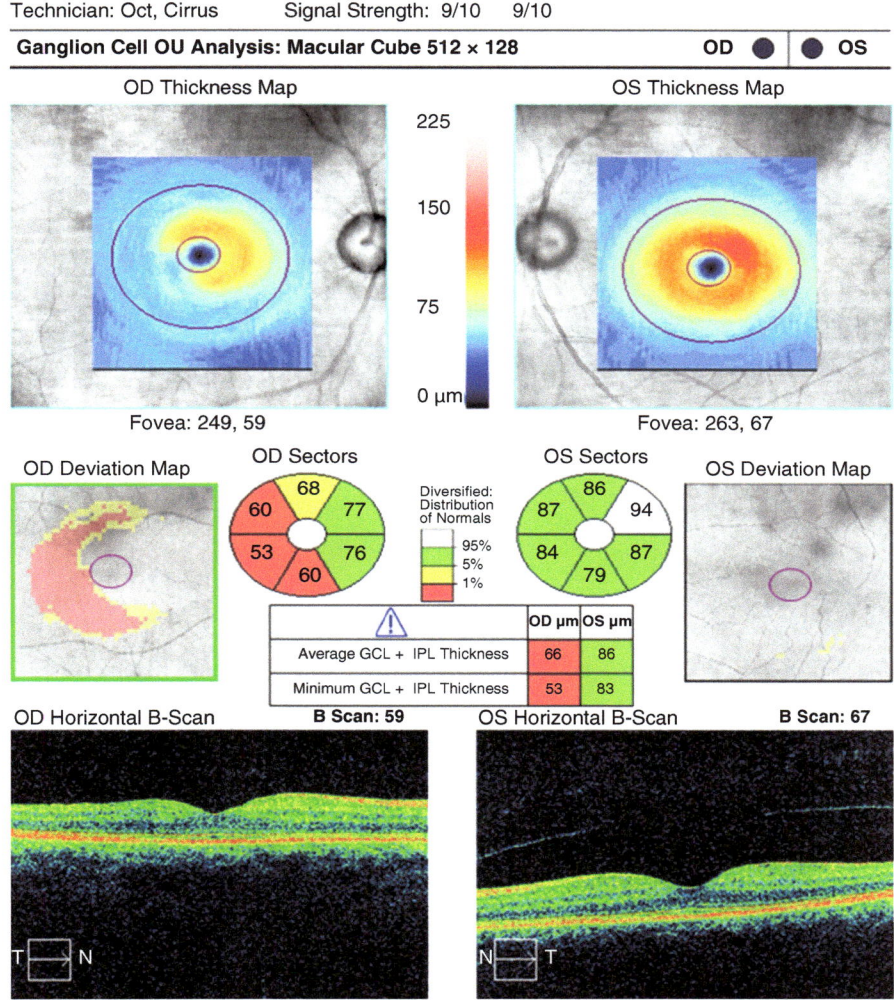

Fig. 7.15 (Cirrus-HD OCT) Ganglion Cell Analysis shows severely depressed GCL + IPL thickness in the superior and inferior temporal regions of the right eye. The left eye seems within normal limits

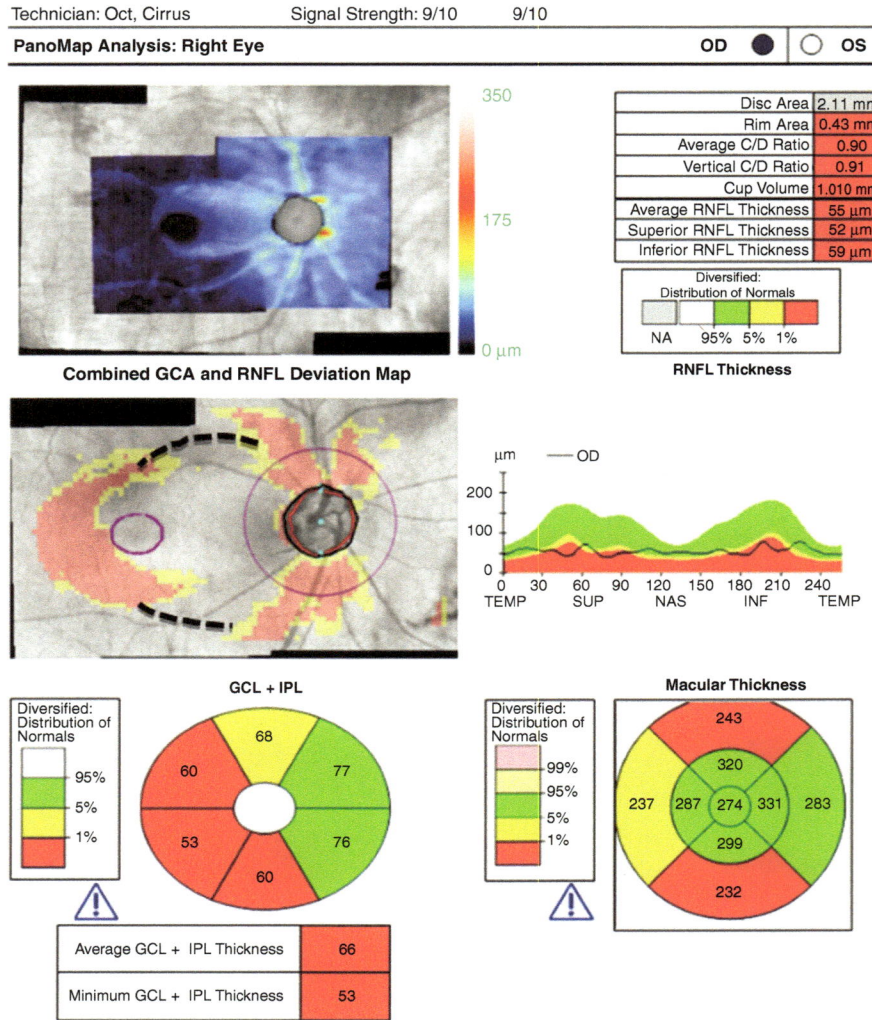

Fig. 7.16 (Cirrus-HD OCT) Panomap report of the right eye demonstrates severe RNFL loss around the disc and ganglion cell loss in the macula. OCT uses only the elliptical annulus for comparing the GCL + IPL thickness to the normative database and comparison data for areas outside this annulus are not provided and such regions are not flagged on the GCL + IPL map leading to discontinuity in the RNFL and macular defects (dashed black lines)

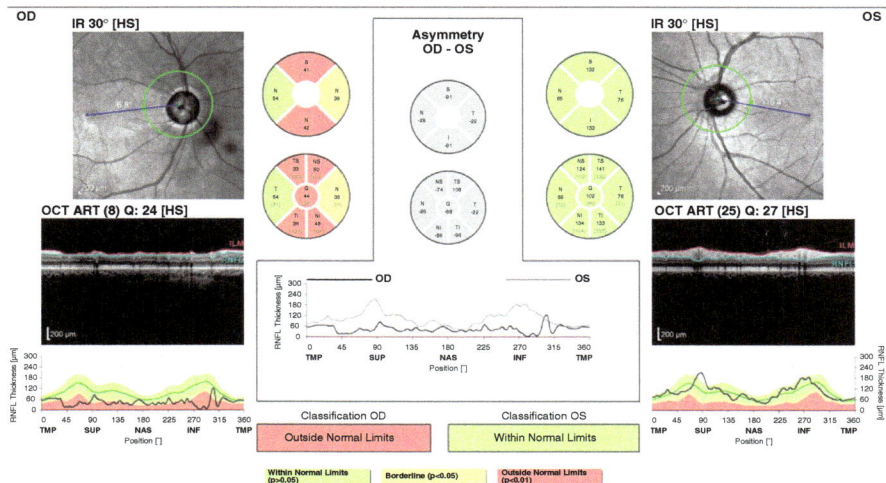

Fig. 7.17 (Spectralis OCT) The advanced RNFL loss is evident in the right eye. The RNFL TSNIT graph also shows RNFL loss in all quadrants. There is a segmentation error in the inferior quadrant of the right eye which leads to zero micron RNFL thickness between 280° and 300° in the TSNIT plot

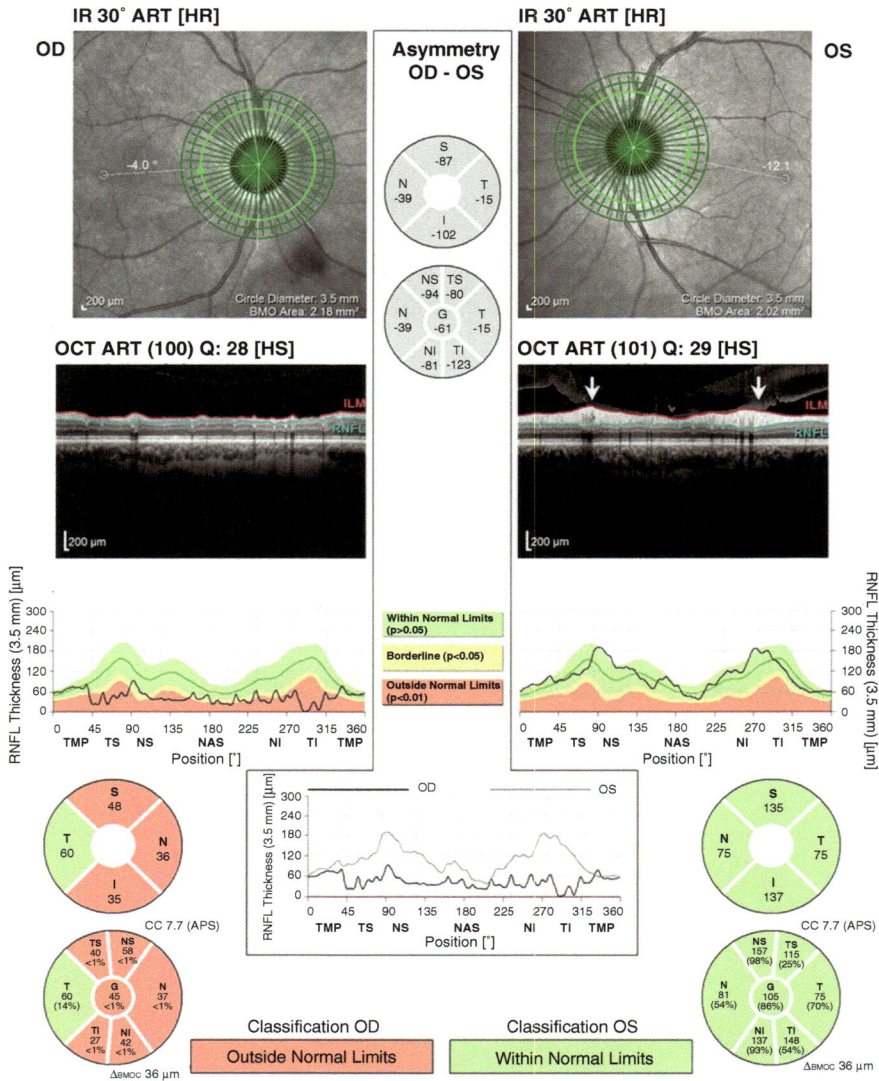

Fig. 7.18 (Spectralis, GMPE module) Spectralis OCT report with the newer GMPE module also demonstrates RNFL loss in the superior, nasal and inferior quadrants of the right eye. Vitreous/RNFL adhesions can be observed on the raw OCT image of the left eye. These superior-nasal-inferior adhesions (the area between white arrowheads) could explain the thick RNFL measurements of the left eye on the TSNIT graph. These adhesions could hide RNFL loss and may lead to a green disease artifact

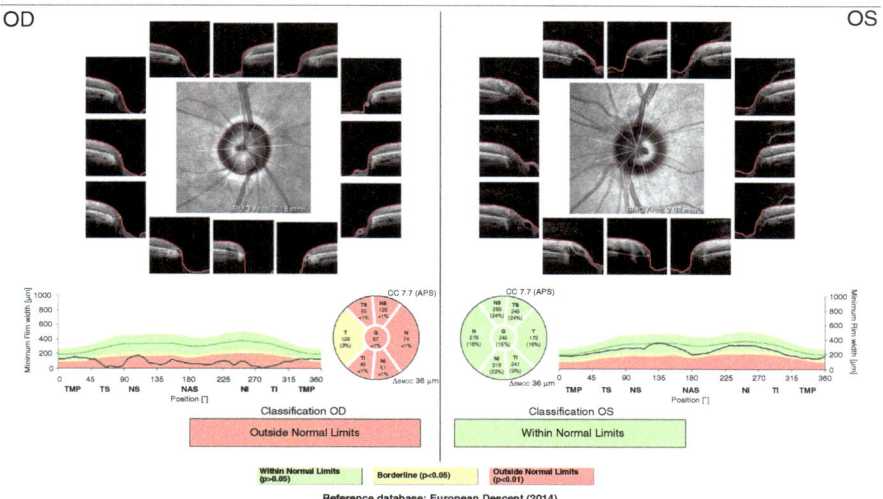

Fig. 7.19 (Spectralis, GMPE module) The Minimum Rim Width analysis demonstrates loss of neuro-retinal rim in all sectors of the right eye

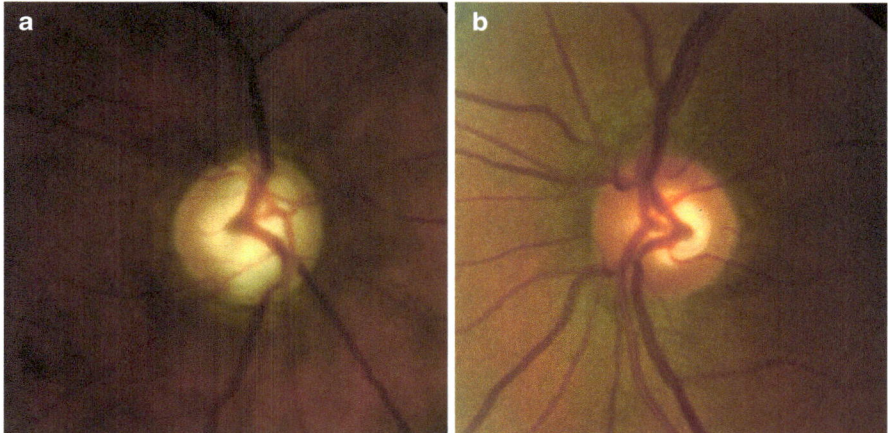

Fig. 7.20 (**a**) Advanced glaucomatous damage of the right optic nerve head can be seen. (**b**) Left optic nerve head is normal

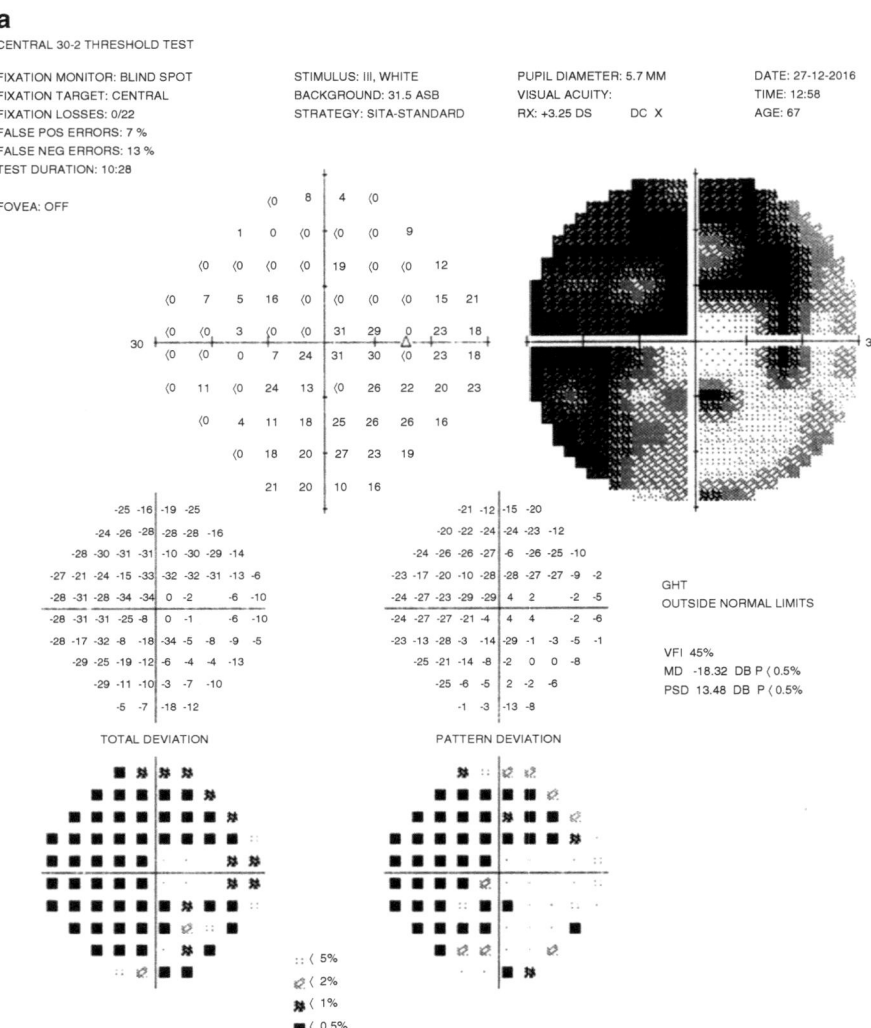

Fig. 7.21 (**a**) Visual field exam of the right eye shows advanced glaucomatous damage, which is consistent with the OCT findings in this eye. (**b**) The visual field of the left eye is essentially within normal limits

b

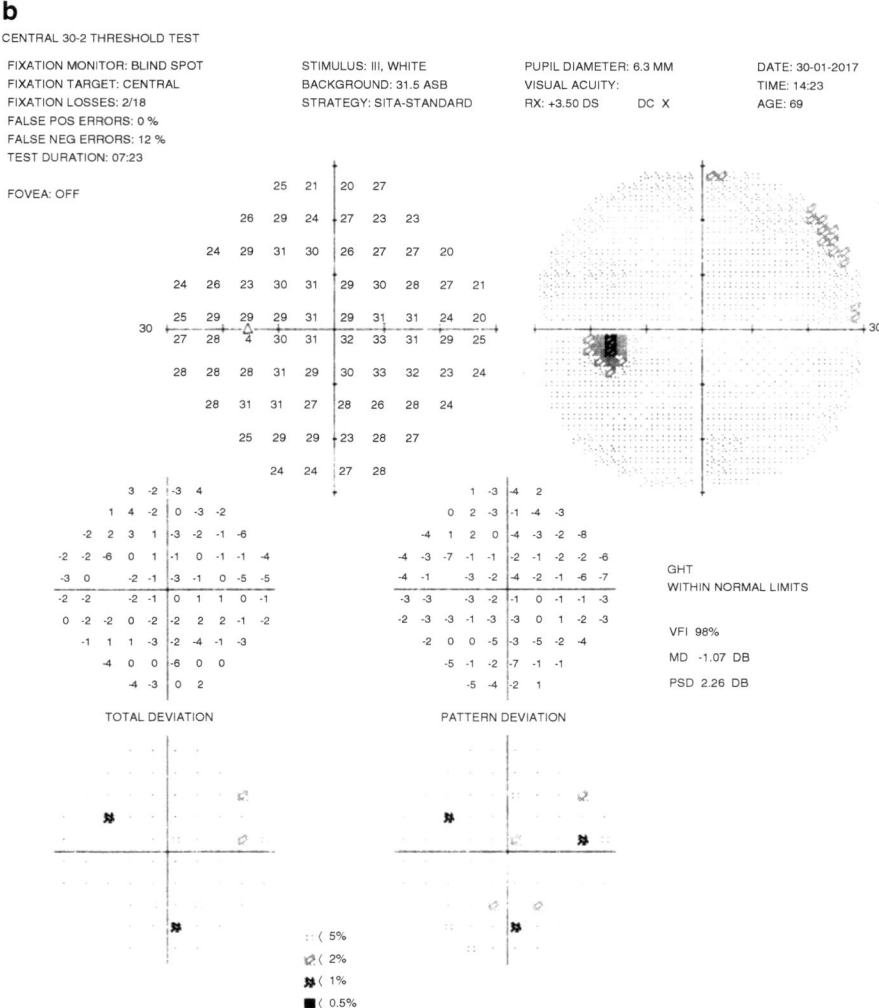

CENTRAL 30-2 THRESHOLD TEST

FIXATION MONITOR: BLIND SPOT   STIMULUS: III, WHITE   PUPIL DIAMETER: 6.3 MM   DATE: 30-01-2017
FIXATION TARGET: CENTRAL   BACKGROUND: 31.5 ASB   VISUAL ACUITY: TIME: 14:23
FIXATION LOSSES: 2/18   STRATEGY: SITA-STANDARD   RX: +3.50 DS   DC X   AGE: 69
FALSE POS ERRORS: 0 %
FALSE NEG ERRORS: 12 %
TEST DURATION: 07:23

FOVEA: OFF

GHT
WITHIN NORMAL LIMITS

VFI 98%

MD -1.07 DB

PSD 2.26 DB

TOTAL DEVIATION   PATTERN DEVIATION

:: (5%
 (2%
 (1%
■ (0.5%

Fig. 7.21 (continued)

Conclusion: The RNFL- and ONH-based OCT parameters demonstrate advanced glaucomatous damage in the right eye. Neuro-retinal rim loss in all quadrants is evident on the optic disc photographs and the VF shows advanced glaucomatous damage. Beyond this stage of the disease, the peripapillary RNFL thickness measurements become less important for monitoring the disease as further deterioration is likely difficult to detect due to the floor effect (see Sect. 8.2.1). Macular thickness outcomes frequently reach their measurement floor later than the peripapillary RNFL and hence, GCL + IPL thickness may still be used for monitoring the disease at this stage. Also, functional tests become more important for follow-up at the advanced stage of the disease.

Chapter 8
Artifacts and Anatomical Variations in Optical Coherence Tomography

Ahmet Akman

8.1 Introduction

Optical coherence tomography (OCT) is currently the most important imaging tool for early diagnosis of glaucoma and is widely used by ophthalmologists worldwide in daily practice [1–3]. Ophthalmologists are now basing their treatment plans on OCT results in early glaucoma patients or glaucoma suspects. As with any new technology, it takes time for the users to understand the potential limitations and pitfalls. By understanding these limitations and interpreting OCT results with proper education, clinicians can diagnose very early glaucoma and monitor progression of the disease with great confidence that was never possible before.

In order to interpret an OCT printout correctly, the clinician must not limit him- or herself to the summary report of the OCT instrument, which depends on the normative database of the manufacturer and may contain artifacts. Clinicians should evaluate the whole printout including the en-face images, TSNIT profiles, individual tomograms and need to understand how the data is analyzed by the software. In addition, s/he must have good knowledge of common artifacts [4–7]. This is the only way to differentiate what is a real defect and what is an artifact or anatomical variation. It is the clinician's responsibility to make this differentiation in order to benefit from this powerful technology and optimally implement the results in patient care.

One of the most common errors by less experienced ophthalmologists is interpreting the normative database comparisons without evaluating the results for each patient individually. A potential undesirable consequence is that many patients who do not have glaucoma are diagnosed, followed and treated as a result of an abnormal OCT scan. In addition to the side effects of the glaucoma medications, a false positive diagnosis for a potentially blinding disease can be a psychological burden for a

A. Akman
Department of Ophthalmology, School of Medicine, Başkent University, Ankara, Turkey

© Springer International Publishing AG, part of Springer Nature 2018
A. Akman et al. (eds.), *Optical Coherence Tomography in Glaucoma*,
https://doi.org/10.1007/978-3-319-94905-5_8

patient for many years. This chapter is devoted to the most common artifacts and anatomical variations that can lead to diagnostic errors in OCT.

8.2 Causes or Mechanisms of OCT Artifacts

8.2.1 Floor Effect

In contrast to early and moderate glaucoma, OCT becomes less useful in the follow-up of advanced stages of glaucoma. At this stage of the disease, progressive thinning of retinal nerve fiber layer (RNFL) stops due to the presence of glial cells and retinal vasculature [4, 5]. In other words, no more structural progression can be demonstrated with OCT after this stage of the disease and functional tests like visual field (VF) examination supersede OCT for monitoring glaucoma.

The current segmentation algorithms almost never measure RNFL thickness less than 30 μm [4]. Even in blind eyes with total cupping and complete loss of RNFL, OCT will measure RNFL thickness values of 30 μm or more. If a scan shows RNFL thickness values <30 μm, the interpreter must carefully re-evaluate this scan for artifacts or image quality issues.

8.2.2 Red and Green Diseases

Red and green are the main colors for the OCT platforms to indicate that the results are within normal limits (within the 5–95% prediction interval) or abnormal (less than 1% prediction interval) when compared with the normative database. *Red disease* is a false positive diagnosis where the software mistakenly identifies an eye abnormal although there is no glaucomatous damage [4, 8]. *Green disease* is the opposite, i.e., although there is some glaucomatous damage, the software is unable to identify it [9]. Clinicians should not assume that every time there are red regions on the OCT report, there must be damage and that everything is normal when an OCT report is all green so that a false diagnosis of glaucoma is not made or early glaucoma missed.

In addition to the device related artifacts, the interpreter should keep in mind that the red and green colors in OCT evaluations depend on the normative database of the manufacturer, which commonly includes 300–500 patients. Depending on the manufacturer, these normative databases may not include patients with high refractive errors, children or eyes from diverse races or correct for such variations.

8.3   Common Artifacts and Anatomical Variations in OCT

The artifacts causing red or green disease in OCT can be classified as follows:

1. Imaging artifacts
2. Patient-related artifacts

8.3.1   Imaging Artifacts

8.3.1.1   Poor Image Quality

A good quality scan is indispensable for a reliable OCT result. All OCT devices use quality control systems for image quality. Cirrus HD-OCT displays a parameter called signal strength. The Cirrus HD-OCT manufacturer recommends that scans with a signal strength less than 6 should be repeated. However, in some patients, media opacities, dry eyes or inability to fixate properly may prevent a good quality scan. Poor OCT lens cleaning, older devices, poor centration and an inexperienced operator can also result in lower quality scans. In addition, some scans can still have artifacts that prevent reliable interpretation of the results, although the signal strength is higher than 6.

The importance of scan quality in RNFL measurements has been demonstrated in many published articles in the past. A poor scan quality leads to thinner RNFL measurements [10–12].

Case 1: Image Quality—Cataract

OCT printout of a 44-year-old woman with bilateral uveitic glaucoma and posterior subcapsular cataracts (Fig. 8.1). Her vision was 20/60 OU, the intraocular pressure (IOP) was 18 mmHg OD and 16 mmHg OS on medical treatment.

104   A. Akman

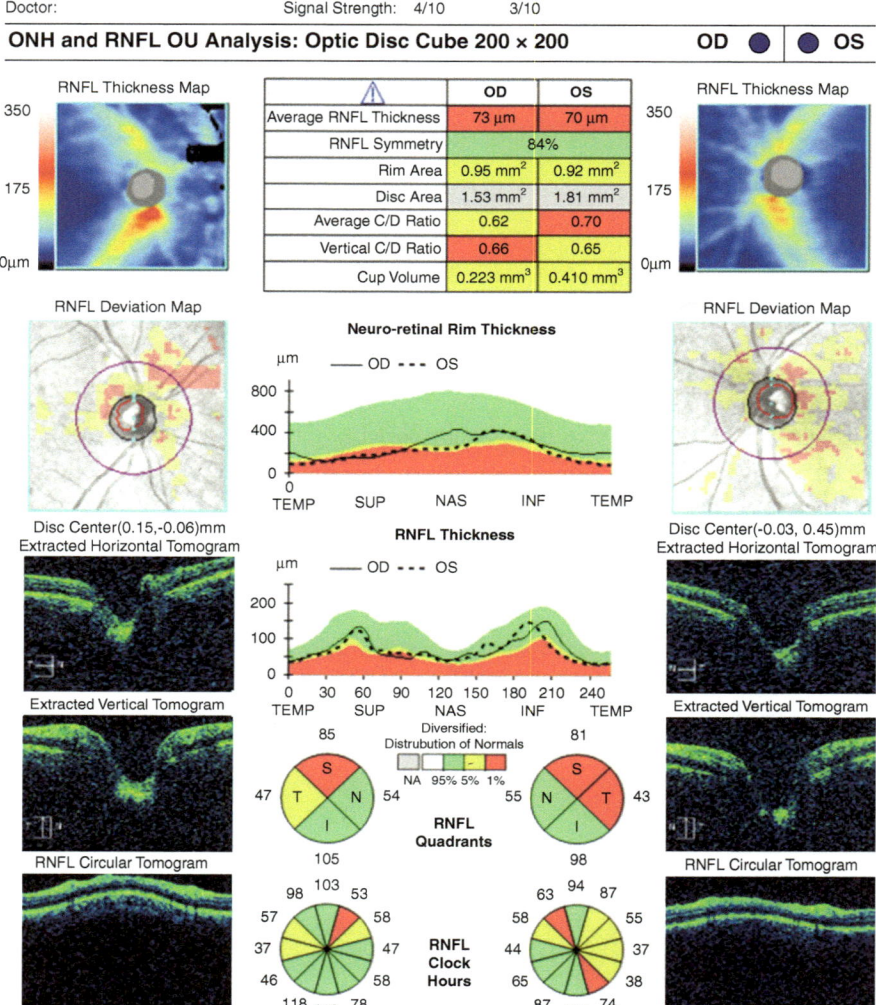

Fig. 8.1 (Cirrus HD-OCT) This is a very poor-quality OCT scan with signal strength (SS) values of 4 OD and 3 OS. The patient's cataract prevented a good quality scan and the RNFL thickness map shows areas that are not scanned at all (black areas on the RNFL thickness map). The unscanned area is outside the calculation circle. In the remaining areas, the RNFL thickness is out of normal limits with an average RNFL thickness value of the 73 μm in the right eye and 70 μm in the left eye. The TSNIT profile, quadrant and clock hour graphs also show widespread thinning although the two eyes are very symmetric, a clue that this generalized thinning is likely caused by poor image quality

Rescan of the Same Patient One-Year Later After Cataract Surgery (Fig. 8.2)

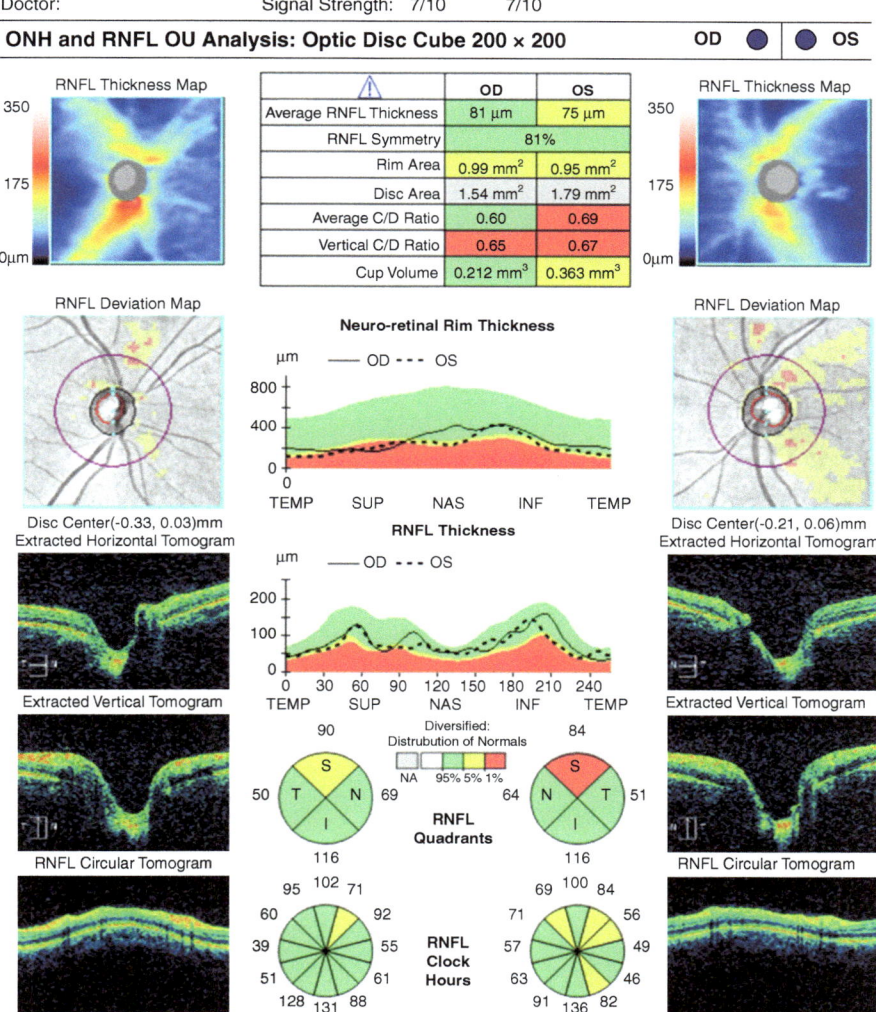

Fig. 8.2 Cirrus HD-OCT of the same patient after bilateral cataract surgery. Now the SS is 7 in both eyes and RNFL thickness maps are free of artifacts. The average RNFL thickness values increased to 81 μm and 75 μm in the right and left eyes respectively. The TSNIT profile, quadrant and clock hour graphs show less damage after cataract removal

Conclusion: Cataracts are one of the most common causes of low-quality scans. Low-quality scans generally show thinner RNFL values with a lot of artifacts. These low-quality scans should not be used for decision making unless an artifact free scan with good SS and is obtained.

Case 2: Image Quality—OCT Device Related

A 24-year-old female, juvenile glaucoma suspect, IOP 20 mmHg OU without any medication. Her vision was 20/20 OU, anterior and posterior segment examinations were normal. Possible RNFL defect is present in the left eye with normal visual fields (Fig. 8.3).

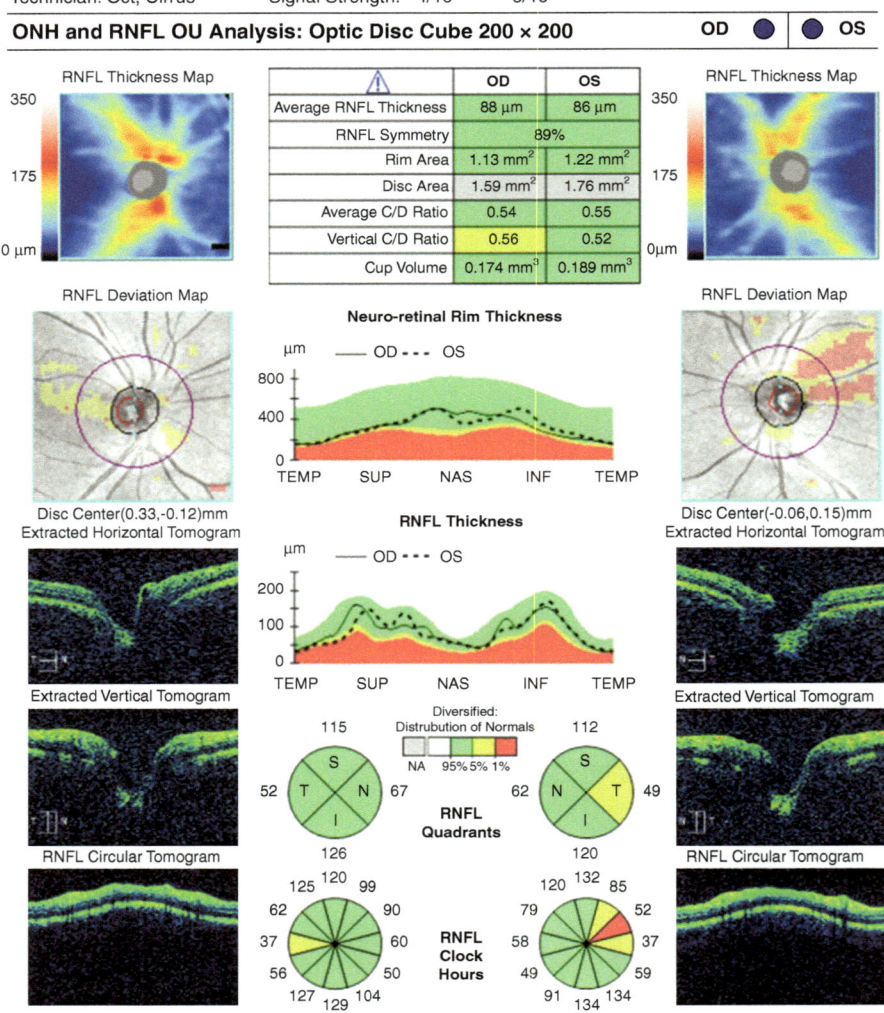

Fig. 8.3 (Cirrus-HD OCT) OCT scan shows possible wedge-shaped RNFL defect on the superior temporal quadrant of the left eye. Average RNFL thickness is 88 μm, in the right eye and 86 μm in the left eye. In addition, the TSNIT profile, RNFL quadrant and clock hour graphs are abnormal in the left eye. The important point is low SS (4 and 5) values in both eyes. These values are below manufacturer's recommendations. This is a young patient without ocular pathology like media opacities. Low SS must either be related to device malfunction, poor patient cooperation or poor scanning technique of the technician. The scan needs to be repeated

The SS was still low on repeat scans on the same day. A device malfunction was suspected. The manufacturer inspected the OCT device, replaced the light source (superluminescent light emitting diode), calibrated the spectrometer and cleaned the optics.

Rescan of the Patient One-Year Later (Fig. 8.4)

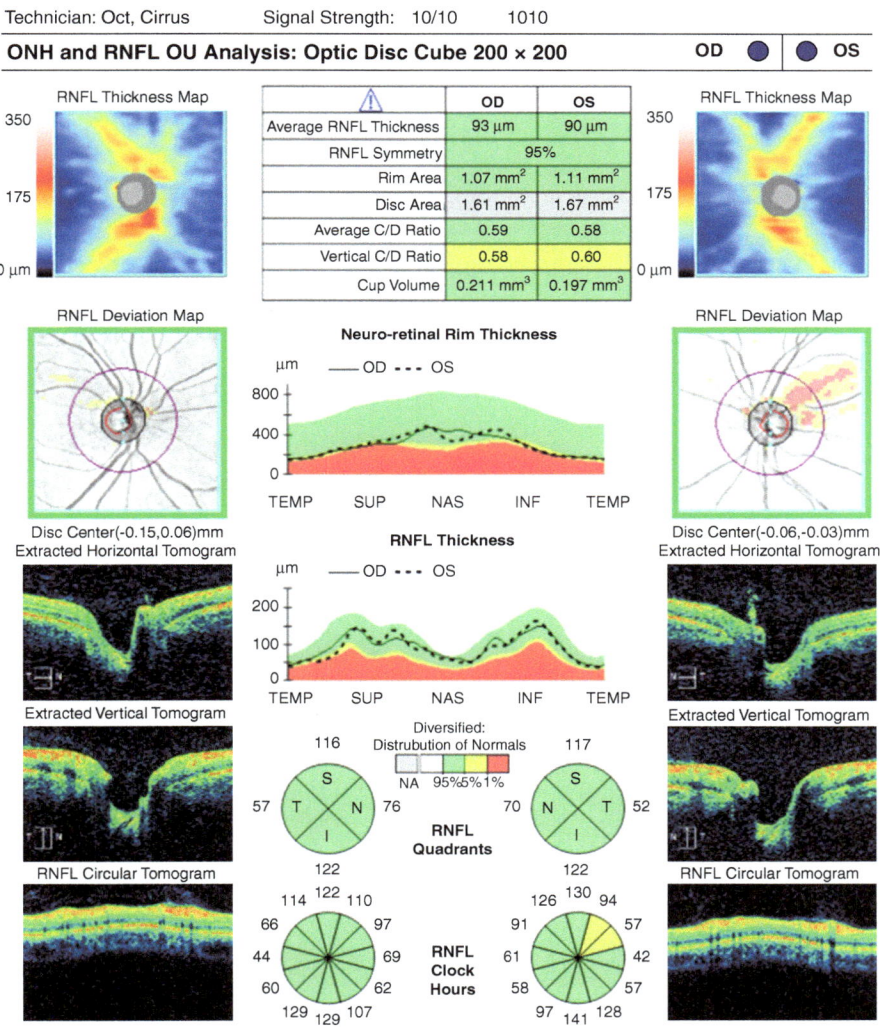

Fig. 8.4 (Cirrus-HD OCT) The patient was scanned again a year later, a high-quality scan was obtained with SS values of 10 in both eyes. Average RNFL thickness has increased to 93 μm in the right eye and 90 μm in the left eye. In addition, TSNIT profile, RNFL quadrant and clock hour graphs are better with this high-quality scan in the left eye. There is still an area of borderline RNFL thinning when compared to the normative database in the left eye (possibly a red disease artifact caused by the shifted RNFL variation, which will be described in the following pages)

Conclusion: Lower quality scans should not be used for decision-making. Low-quality scans generally show thinner RNFL values. If it is not possible to obtain a good quality scan, particularly in young patients without cataract or ocular pathology, check the device and contact the manufacturer for possible malfunction.

Case 3: Image Quality—Poor Quality Image Acquisition Related to Cataract, Ocular Surface Disease and Poor OCT Device Performance

OCT printout of a 70-year-old male with pseudo-exfoliation glaucoma, ocular surface disease and grade two nuclear sclerosis (Fig. 8.5). His BCVA was 20/40 OD and 20/80 OS, IOP was 18 mmHg OD and 17 mmHg OS with topical travoprost and timolol combination.

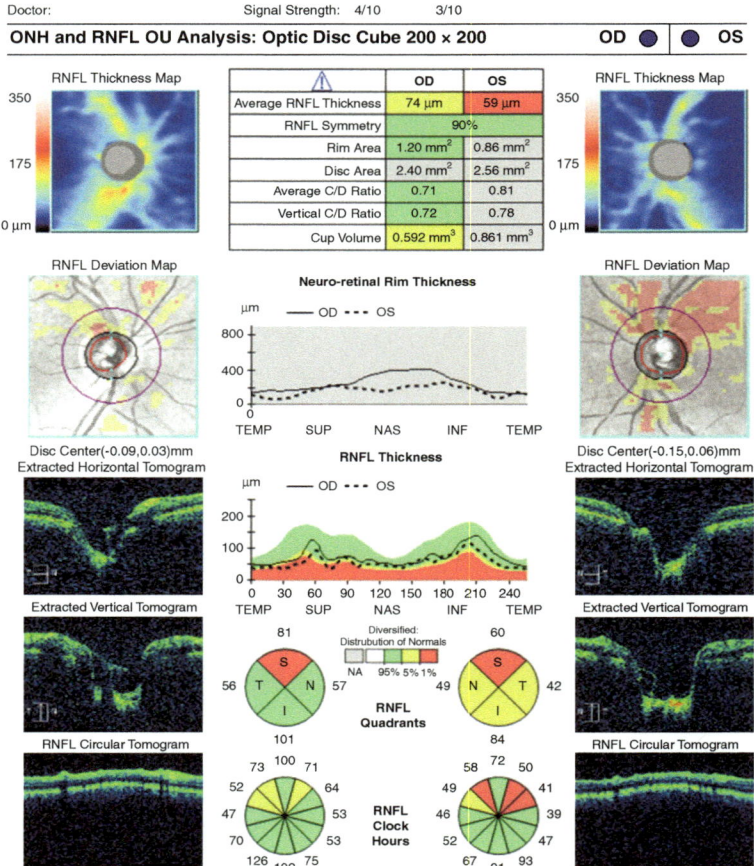

Fig. 8.5 (Cirrus-HD OCT) Poor quality OCT scan of a pseudo-exfoliation glaucoma patient, possibly due to nuclear cataract, poor performance of the OCT device and ocular surface problems of the patient. The Rescans also resulted in similar SS. This OCT scan with SS of 3 and 4, shows early damage in the right eye and advanced damage in the left eye. Average RNFL thickness is 74 μm and 59 μm in the right and left eye, respectively. This scan has very poor SS and should not be used for decision-making

Rescan of the Patient Two-Years Later (Figs. 8.6 and 8.7)

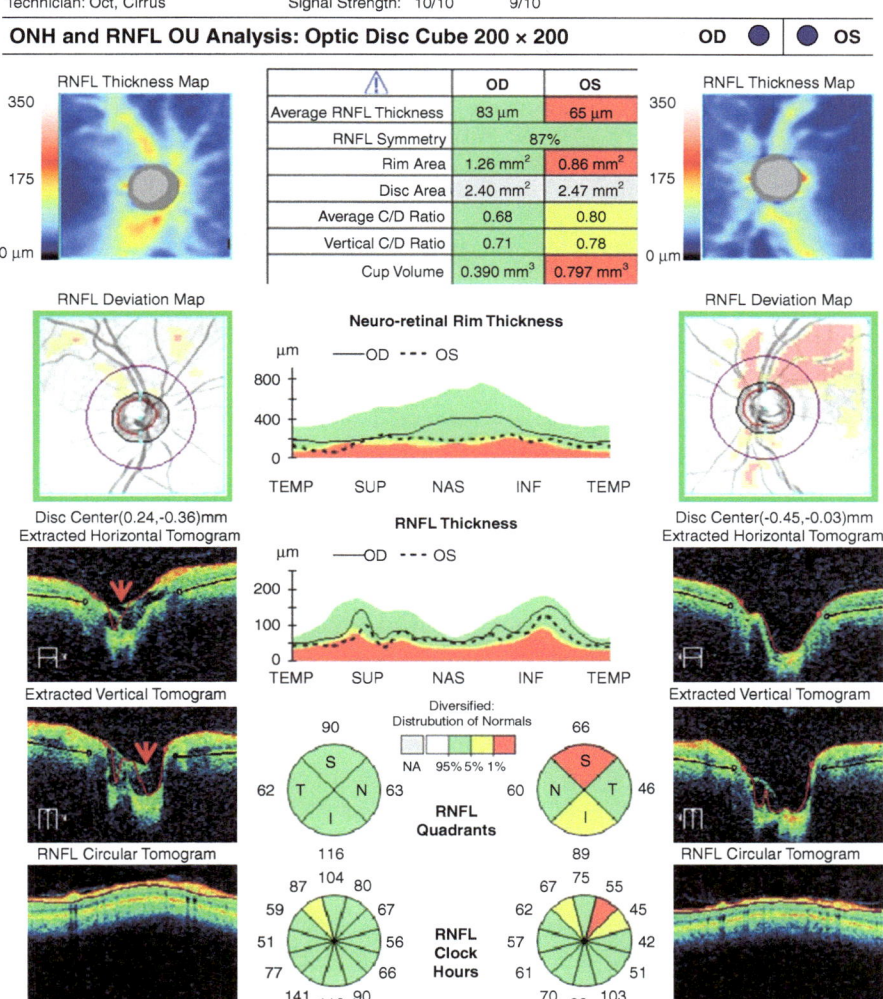

Fig. 8.6 (Cirrus-HD OCT) OCT scan of the same patient 2 years later with a new Cirrus OCT device, after cataract surgery and treatment of the ocular surface disease. The SS is 10 OD and 9 OS. The RNFL defect in the right eye is not present anymore and the left eye has only a superior bundle defect, which is also evident as rim thinning on the fundus photograph (see Fig. 8.7b, white arrowhead). Average RNFL thickness has increased to 83 μm in the right eye and to 65 μm in the left eye. This case is a good example of the relation of the SS and RNFL thickness measurements and defects. Another interesting point in this scan is the remnants of the fetal hyaloid artery (Bergmeister papilla) in the right eye, which prevents correct segmentation of the optic nerve head (red arrowheads). This can be seen in the fundus photograph of the right eye (see Fig. 8.7a, black arrowhead)

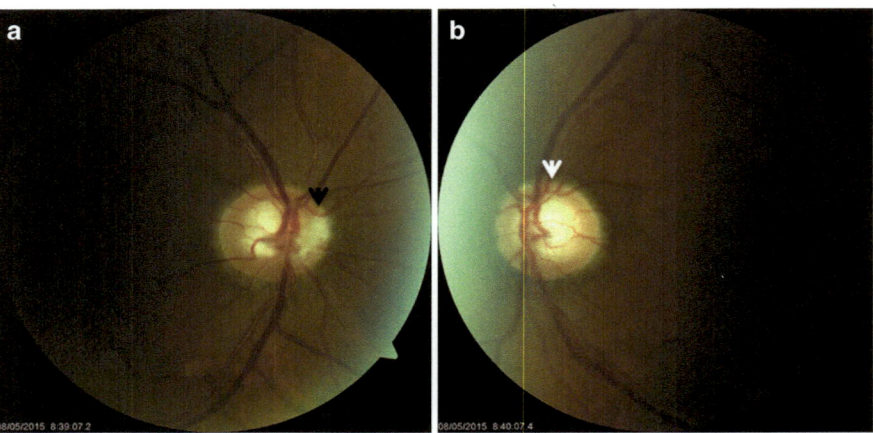

Fig. 8.7 (**a**) Fundus photograph of the right eye showing remnants of the fetal hyaloid artery (Bergmeister papilla) (black arrowhead) (**b**) Fundus photograph of the left eye showing neuroretinal rim thinning in the superior quadrant (white arrowhead)

Conclusion: In addition to patient and technician related problems causing artifacts, as an OCT device gets older, the power of the superluminescent light emiting diode decays over time and the optics become dirty. The result is poor quality scans in almost all patients but, especially in patients with early cataracts or dry eyes. In this patient, a device problem in addition to early cataract resulted in a very poor scan quality, which caused thinner RNFL measurements and artifacts. The second scan was performed 2 years later with a new Cirrus HD-OCT device and after bilateral cataract surgery. The second scan has perfect scan quality resulting in thicker RNFL measurements and artifact free scans that are compatible with the rim loss seen in the fundus photograph. The fetal hyaloid artery remnant that is present on the right optic nerve head is also another interesting feature of this scan.

Case 4: Image Quality—Motion Artifact

OCT scans of a 27-year-old female glaucoma suspect (Figs. 8.8, 8.9 and 8.10). BCVA 20/20 OU, IOP was 21 mmHg OD and 23 mmHg OS without any treatment. Anterior and posterior segment exams were unremarkable.

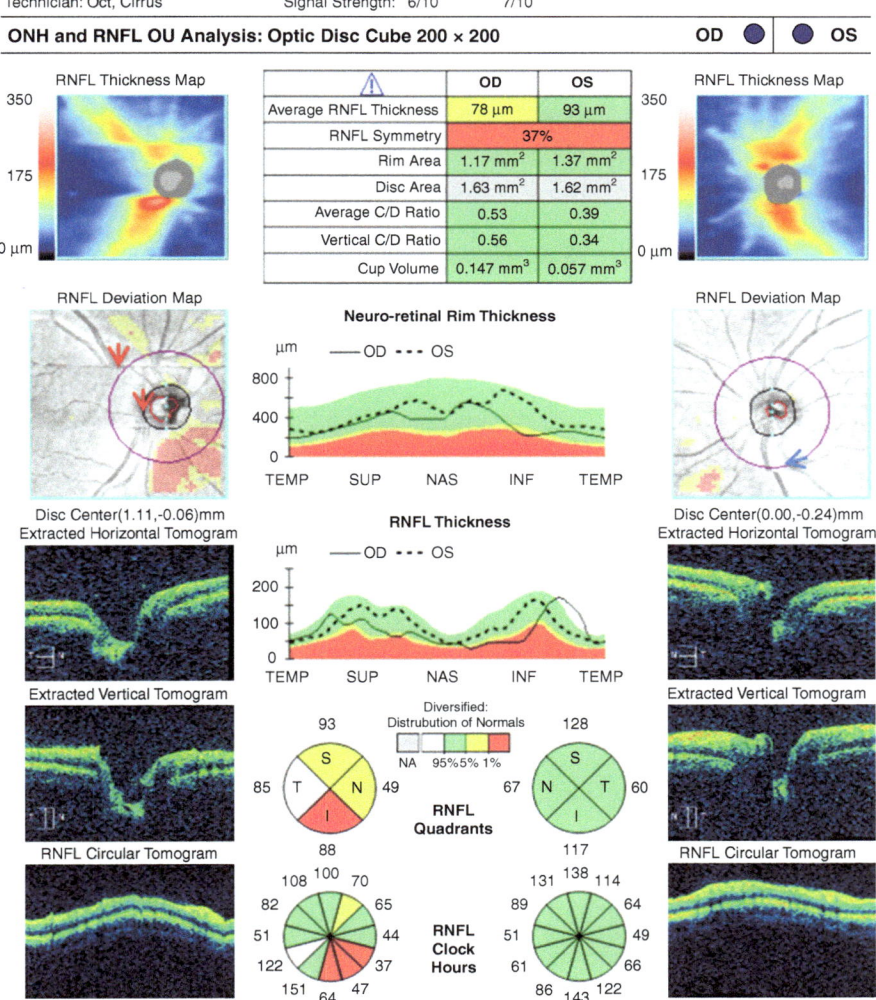

Fig. 8.8 (Cirrus-HD OCT) Although SS is acceptable (>= 6 OU), RNFL Deviation map of the right eye shows significant movement artifacts (note the broken course of the vessels, red arrowheads), RNFL Deviation Map of the left eye, also demonstrates movement artifacts (blue arrowhead). Average RNFL thickness is 78 μm in the right eye and 93 μm in the left eye. In addition, the TSNIT profile, RNFL quadrant and clock hour graphs of the right eye are abnormal. See next page for the results of the repeat scan

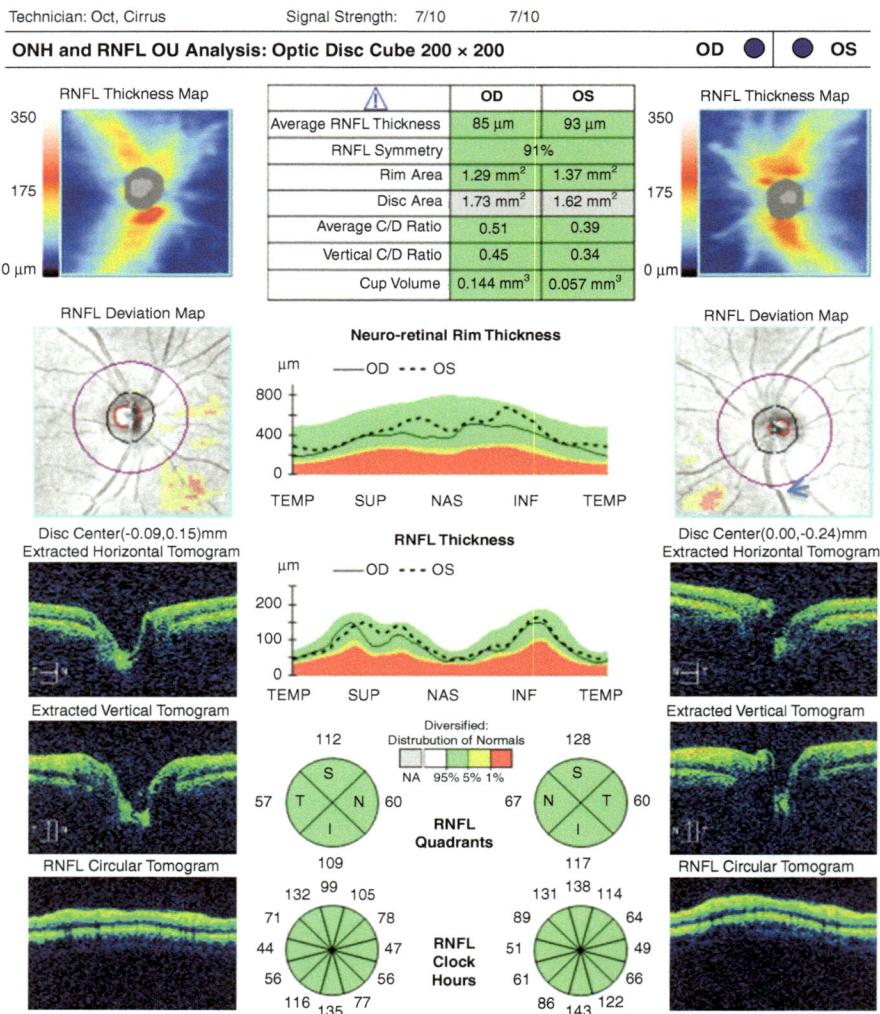

Fig. 8.9 (Cirrus-HD OCT) Rescan of the same patient, same day, now SS = 7 OU, no movement artifact in the right eye. Left eye still shows a motion artifact (blue arrowhead). Average RNFL increased to 85 μm in the right eye. The TSNIT profile, RNFL quadrant and clock hour graphs are all in the normal range for the right eye. Also see next page

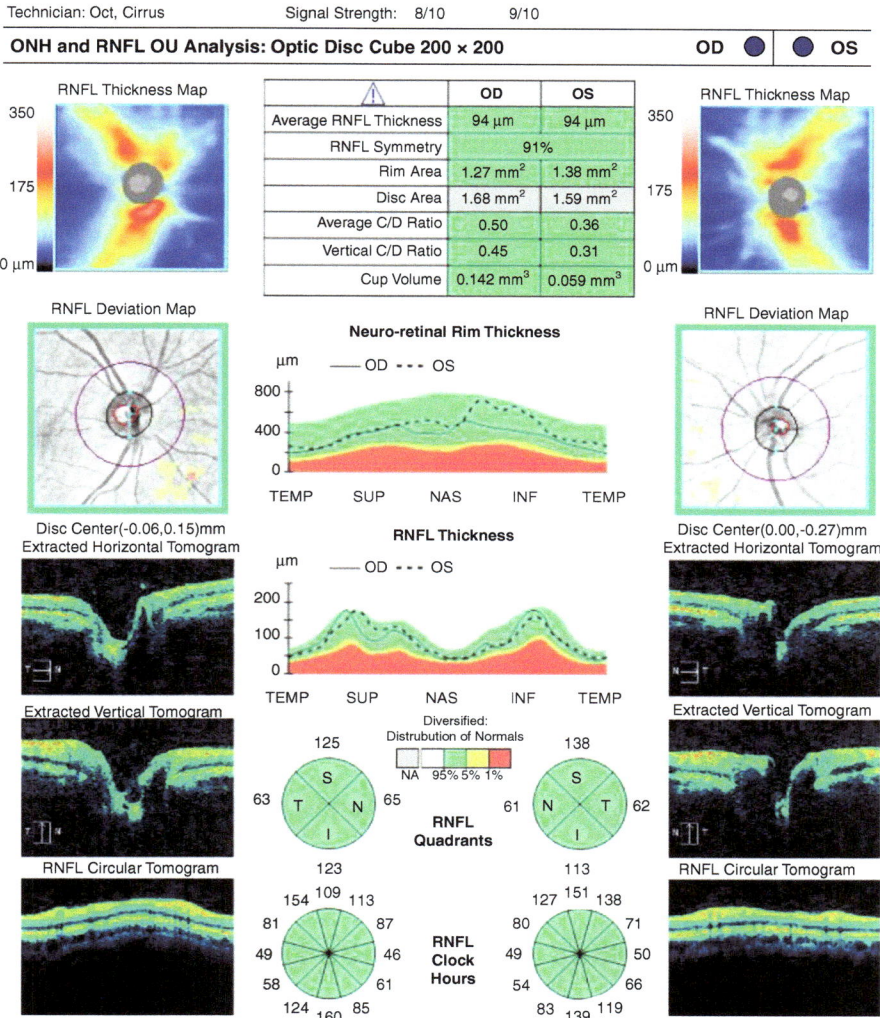

Fig. 8.10 (Cirrus-HD OCT) Rescan of the same patient, 8 months later. No eye movement artifact is present and SS is 8 OD and 9 OS. Average RNFL thickness has increased to 94 μm in both eyes with better SS

Conclusion: The reviewer should check the en-face OCT image in RNFL deviation map and RNFL thickness map in addition to SS values in order to identify artifacts that can affect the results. In some cases, the OCT scan with a high SS can still have significant imaging artifacts. With a repeat scan free of the artifacts, all the presumed RNFL defects disappeared and average RNFL thickness values increased in this patient.

Case 5: Image Quality—Motion Artifact and Poor Centration

OCT scan of a 49-year-old male with presbyopia complaints and unremarkable ocular exam. His IOP was 16 mmHg OD and 17 mmHg OS. He has a family history of glaucoma. OCT scan was obtained during this routine eye exam (Fig. 8.11).

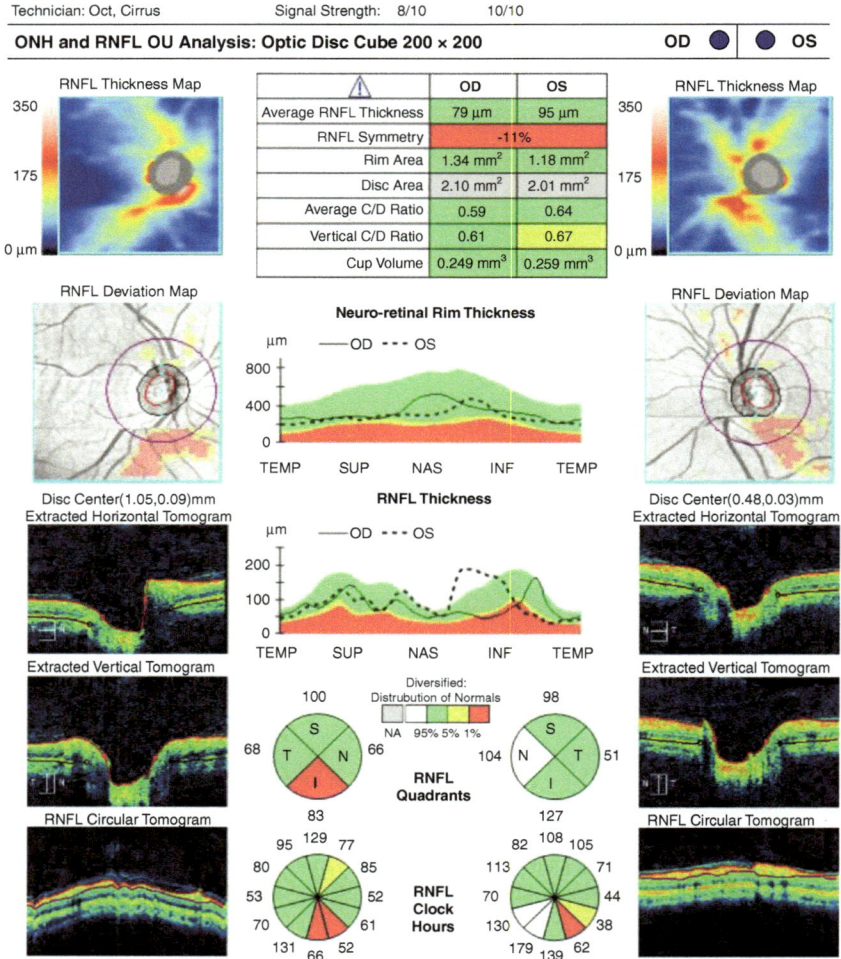

Fig. 8.11 (Cirrus-HD OCT) A very good quality OCT scan based on the SS (8 and 10 respectively). OCT looks abnormal with significant RNFL defects nearly in all maps. A careful evaluation of the RNFL deviation map shows poor centration of the disc and motion artifacts. Although the SS is perfect, the motion artifacts resulting from the eye movements of the patient and inability of the technician to center the optic nerve head during the scan resulted in a poor-quality scan. An experienced technician must be able to identify these types of artifacts and rescan the patient

Rescan of the Patient Three Months Later (Fig. 8.12)

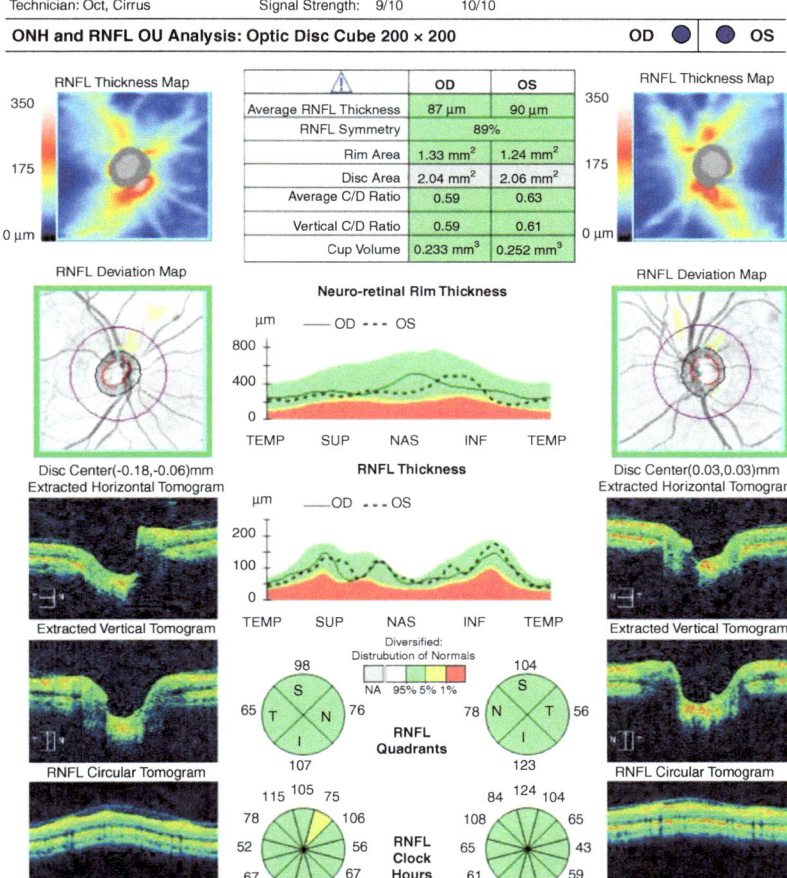

Fig. 8.12 (Cirrus-HD OCT) Rescan of the patient with proper fixation and centration resulted in a normal OCT report

Conclusion: As it is evident in this case and the previous case, a scan even with a perfect SS does not always guarantee an artifact free OCT report. In addition to the SS values, all other parts of the report must be evaluated for detecting various sources of artifacts.

8.3.1.2   Segmentation Errors

All OCT devices use segmentation algorithms or layer seeking algorithms to measure the thickness of the target retinal layers. If the software is unable to determine the layers correctly, segmentation errors will be present and RNFL thickness could be measured as zero with large areas of abnormal thickness flagged as red areas.

One needs to consider the floor effect in this kind of scan, as the RNFL thickness almost never falls under 30 μm on OCT scans. RNFL thickness < 30 μm is almost always due to segmentation or imaging errors.

Case 6: Segmentation Error—High Myopia and Tilted Disc

OCT scan of a 69-year-old male with high myopia, tilted disc, peripapillary atrophy and open angle glaucoma (Fig. 8.13). BCVA of the patient was 20/40 with −10.5 D correction in the right eye and 20/30 with −8.0 D correction in the left eye.

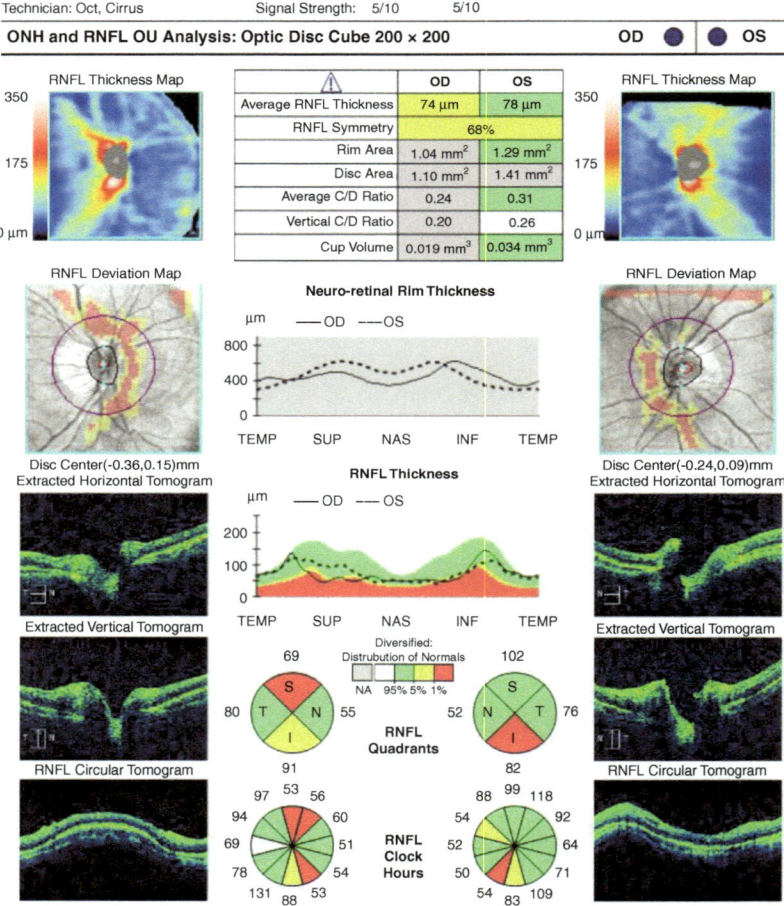

Fig. 8.13 (Cirrus-HD OCT) A poor quality OCT scan with SS = 5 OU, likely due to high myopia. RNFL analysis shows significant RNFL loss mostly in the nasal areas in both eyes. This is typically caused by the more temporal location of the blood vessels causing temporal displacement of the RNFL peaks and showing as thinning of the nasal and inferonasal regions. A magnification effect could also partially contribute to this pattern as the measurements are in general farther out than assumed in an average eye in such myopic eyes

Rescan of the Patient Two Years Later (Figs. 8.14 and 8.15)

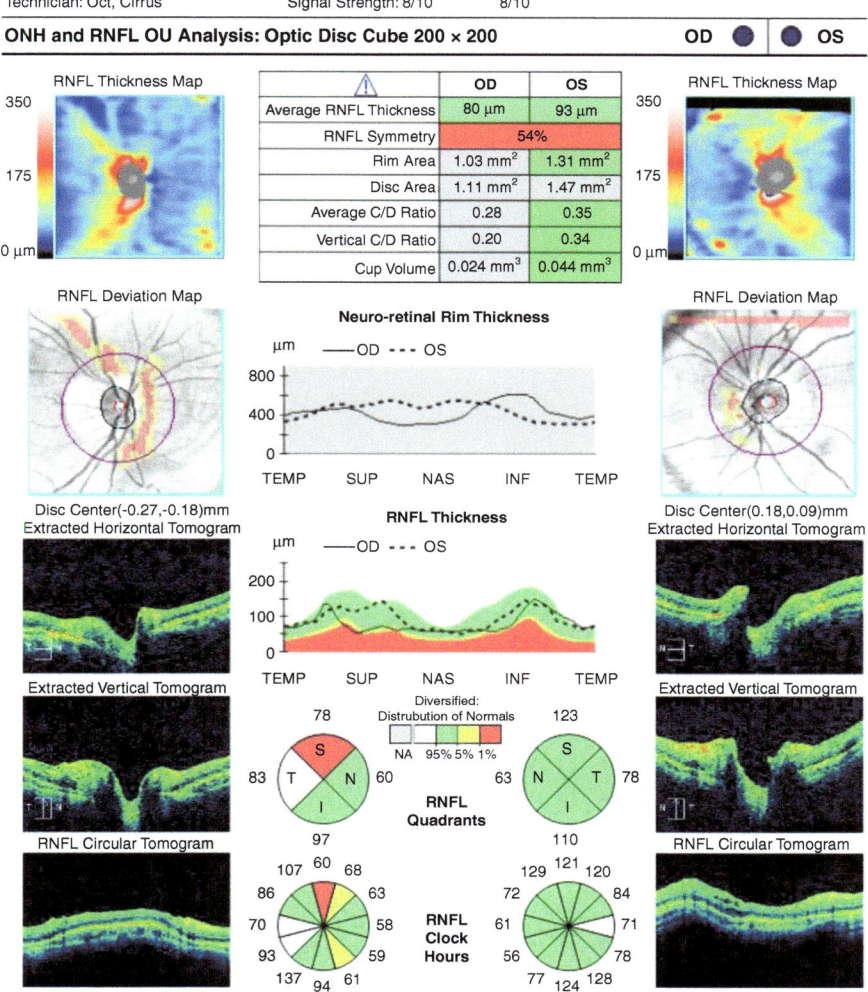

Fig. 8.14 (Cirrus-HD OCT) Rescan of the same patient 2 years later. A better quality (SS = 8, OU) scan was obtained and RNFL defects were less significant in the left eye but the unusual pattern RNFL defect in the right eye is still present. The patient was scanned again with Spectralis OCT, see the results on the next page

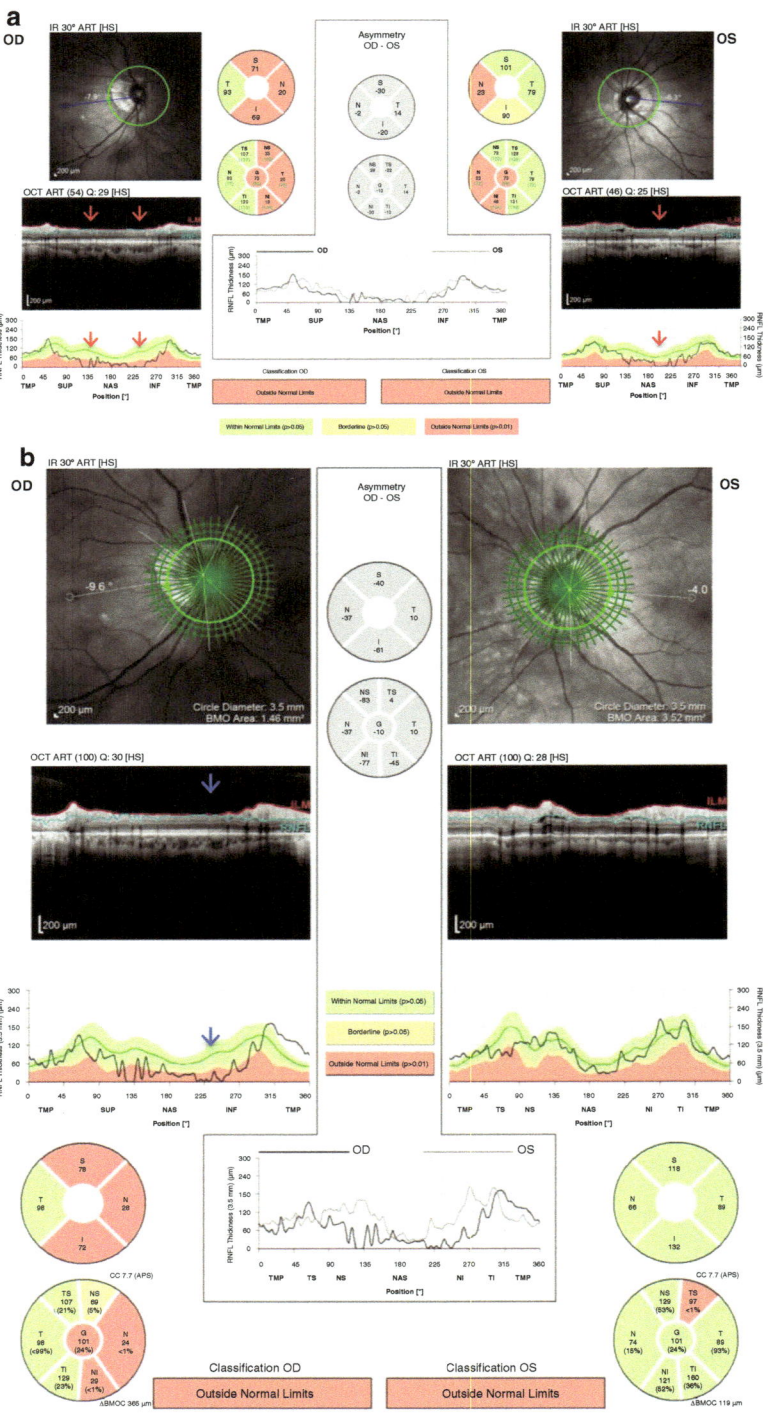

Reference database: European Descent (2014)

Conclusion: High myopia, tilted discs, peripapillary atrophy and myelinated nerve fibers make segmentation very difficult for the layer seeking algorithms of OCT devices. This case is a good example in which segmentation problems were observed with two different OCT platforms. OCT results in these kinds of eyes must be interpreted cautiously as these artifacts can also affect the progression analysis capabilities of the devices.

Case 7: Segmentation Problem—Myelinated Retinal Nerve Fibers

OCT scan of a 32-year-old ocular hypertensive male with myelinated retinal nerve fibers in the left eye (Figs. 8.16, 8.17, 8.18 and 8.19).

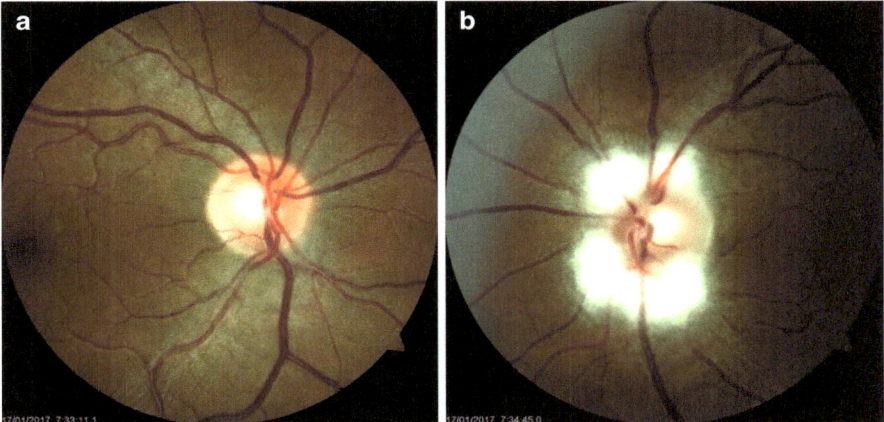

Fig. 8.16 (**a, b**) Fundus photographs of the patient showing myelinated retinal nerve fibers in the left eye

Fig. 8.15 (Spectralis OCT) (**a**) Standard report of the Spectralis OCT, there are segmentation issues in both eyes due to the peripapillary atrophy (red arrowheads). In some areas of the calculation ring, the RNFL thickness is zero, which is not possible due to the floor effect. (**b**) GMPE module report of the Spectralis OCT. Although segmentation is better in the left eye, it is still not possible in the right eye (blue arrows). As Spectralis OCT shows the segmentation lines on the TSNIT OCT image, one can see the areas in which the segmentation is not correct (blue arrowheads)

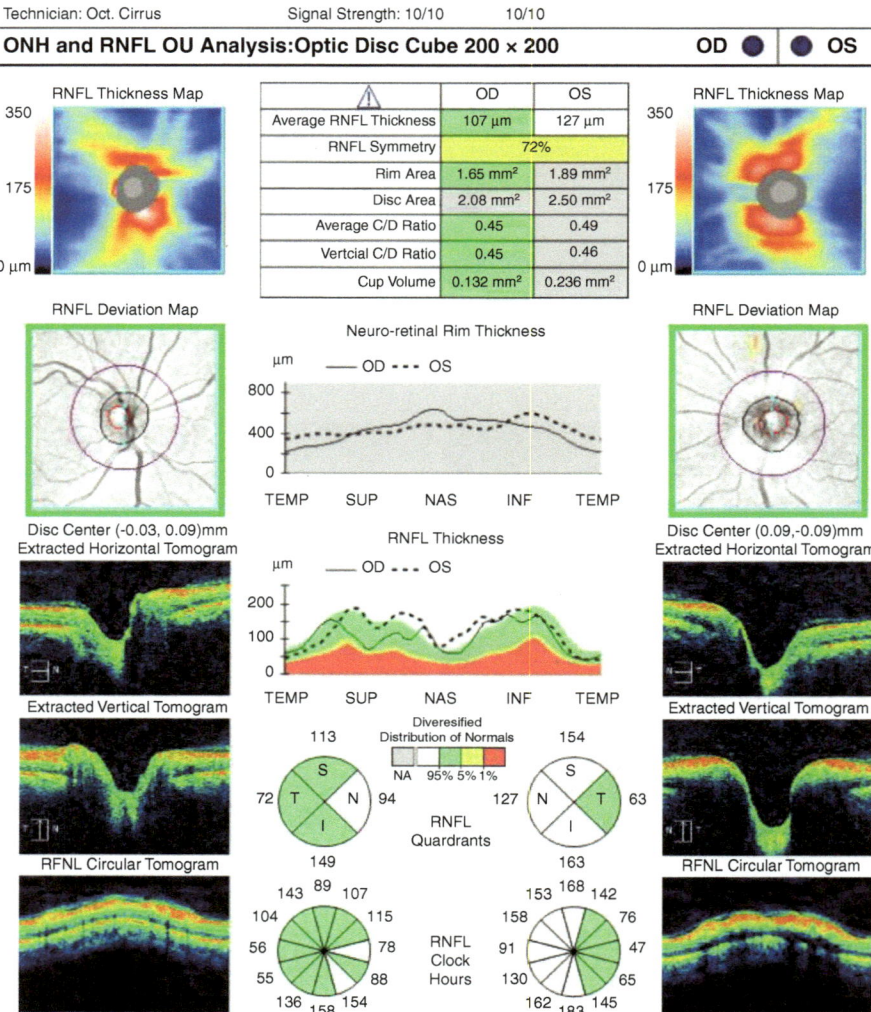

Fig. 8.17 (Cirrus-HD OCT) Myelinated nerve fibers are quite common. The thick myelinated nerve fibers may hide the RNFL loss in glaucoma and it is one of the reasons for green disease. In this patient, although he does not have RNFL loss, being ocular hypertensive makes him a potential candidate for future damage. Monitoring the RNFL with OCT will not be a good option for diagnosis and follow-up in such eyes. The Spectralis OCT images below show the same pattern

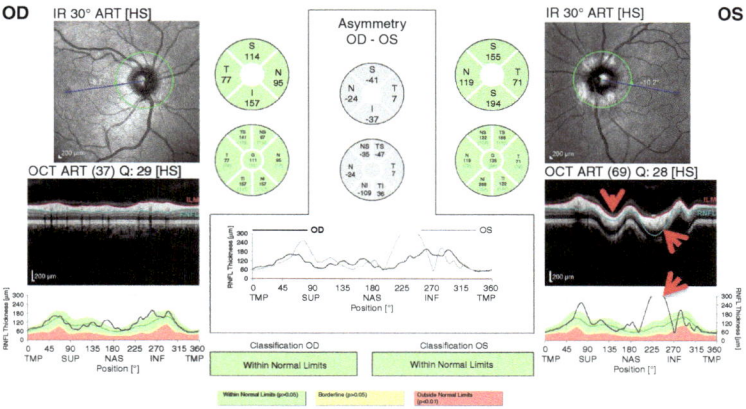

Fig. 8.18 (Spectralis OCT) Similar to Cirrus HD-OCT, Spectralis OCT shows a thick RNFL in the right eye and very thick RNFL in the left eye (red arrowheads) with segmentation problems

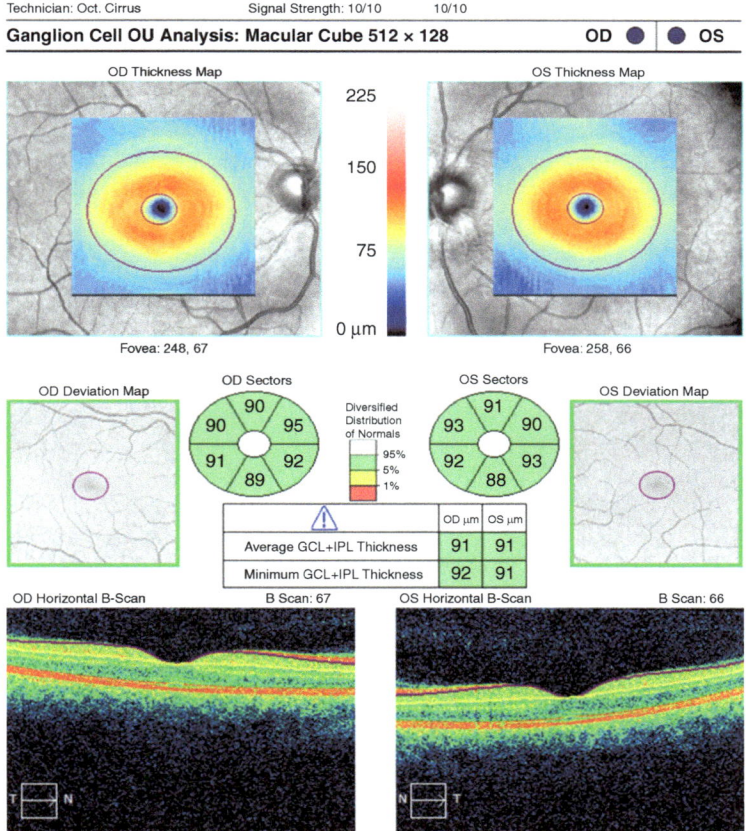

Fig. 8.19 (Cirrus HD-OCT) Macular Ganglion Cell Analysis of the patient with myelinated retinal nerve fibers. Macular scans are helpful for diagnosis and follow-up of glaucoma in eyes with RNFL segmentation problems in the peripapillary area

Conclusion: Segmentation errors can either cause red disease in myopic, tilted discs or can cause green diseases in eyes with myelinated retinal nerve fibers. OCT must be reviewed carefully in these eyes.

8.3.2 Patient Related Artifacts

These are the most confusing artifacts for the ophthalmologists. It is very common to see a young patient with a good quality OCT scan as a part of a routine eye exam many red areas on the printout. These patients are either diagnosed as early glaucoma or referred for glaucoma evaluation. In either case, the end result is a young individual suspected or diagnosed with a potentially blinding disease that requires lifelong treatment. This could lead to enormous psychological burden to the patient and the family. To prevent this kind of a false diagnosis, every ophthalmologist must able to differentiate the common anatomical variations that can lead to red disease on OCT.

8.3.2.1 Split Bundle or Shifted RNFL Peaks

In most individuals, the superior and inferior poles of the ONH receive the largest number of axons of the retinal ganglion cells (the RNFL) as two thick bundles of axons. This configuration is the basis for the color-coded normative database comparisons of TSNIT profiles. In some patients, however, the superior, inferior or both bundles may be split and can enter the optic nerve as two distinct bundles. This phenomenon was first described on the scanning laser polarimetry (GDx) reports [13]. Split nerve fiber layer configuration of RNFL was later confirmed in a histopathologic study and the authors concluded that split RNFL is a common anatomical variant rather than an imaging artifact [14]. With the widespread use of OCT, this variation has been more commonly observed masquerading as a local RNFL defect. This finding is one of the most common reasons for red disease in younger patients with good quality OCT scans.

Shifted RNFL peaks is another anatomical variant as the RNFL thickness is in the normal range but the RNFL configuration does not fit the expected configuration of TSNIT profiles on OCT normative database. In other words, patient's TSNIT profile is completely normal but the position of the two humps does not fit the predicted location on the normative database because of differences in topography of the bundle location.

Both of these two configurations, as being normal variants, should be distinguished from real RNFL loss.

Case 8: Split RNFL

Forty-six-year-old female referred for possible RNFL defect on OCT (Figs. 8.20, 8.21 and 8.22). BCVA was 20/20 OU and IOP is 16 mmHg OU without any treatment. Anterior and posterior segment exam were unremarkable.

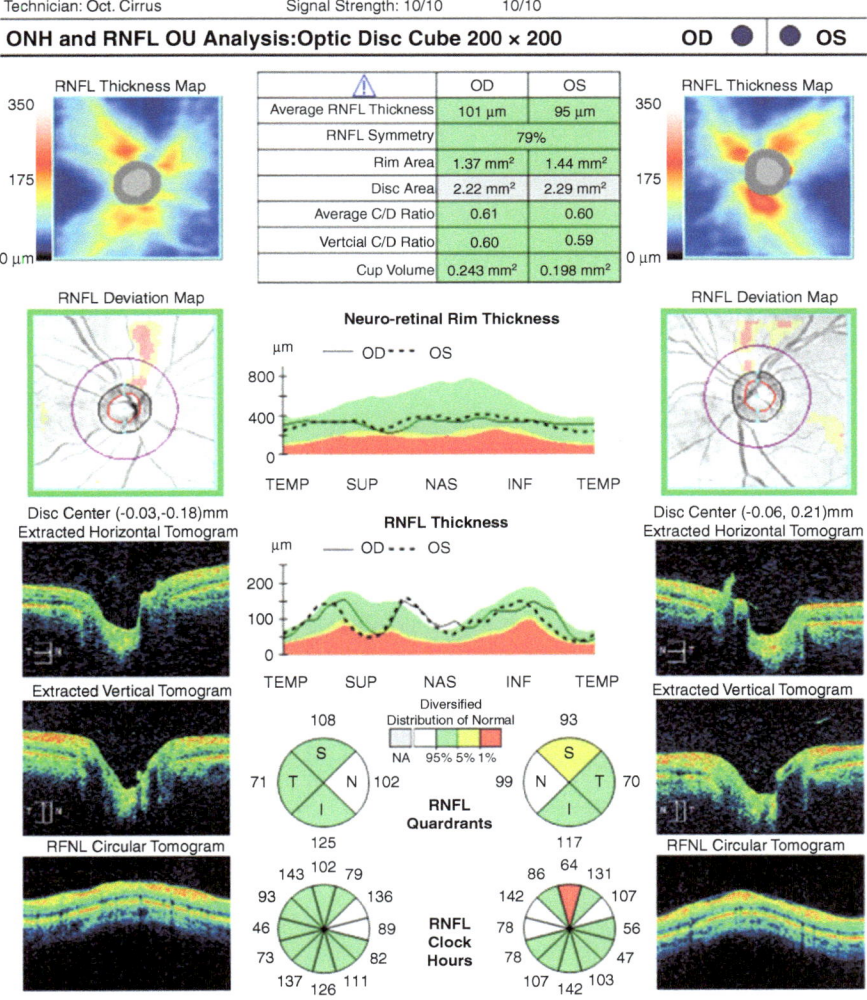

Fig. 8.20 (Cirrus HD-OCT) The patient has typical split nerve configuration at the superior RNFL bundle in both eyes; one can see that on the TSNIT profile there are two prominent RNFL humps with a marked depression in between. RNFL thickness map shows healthy RNFL bundles in the split configuration, and average RNFL thickness values are normal nearly in all quadrants. Two prominent humps with a marked depression in between within the superior or inferior quadrant are typical for the split RNFL configuration, which is observed more frequently in the superior quadrant

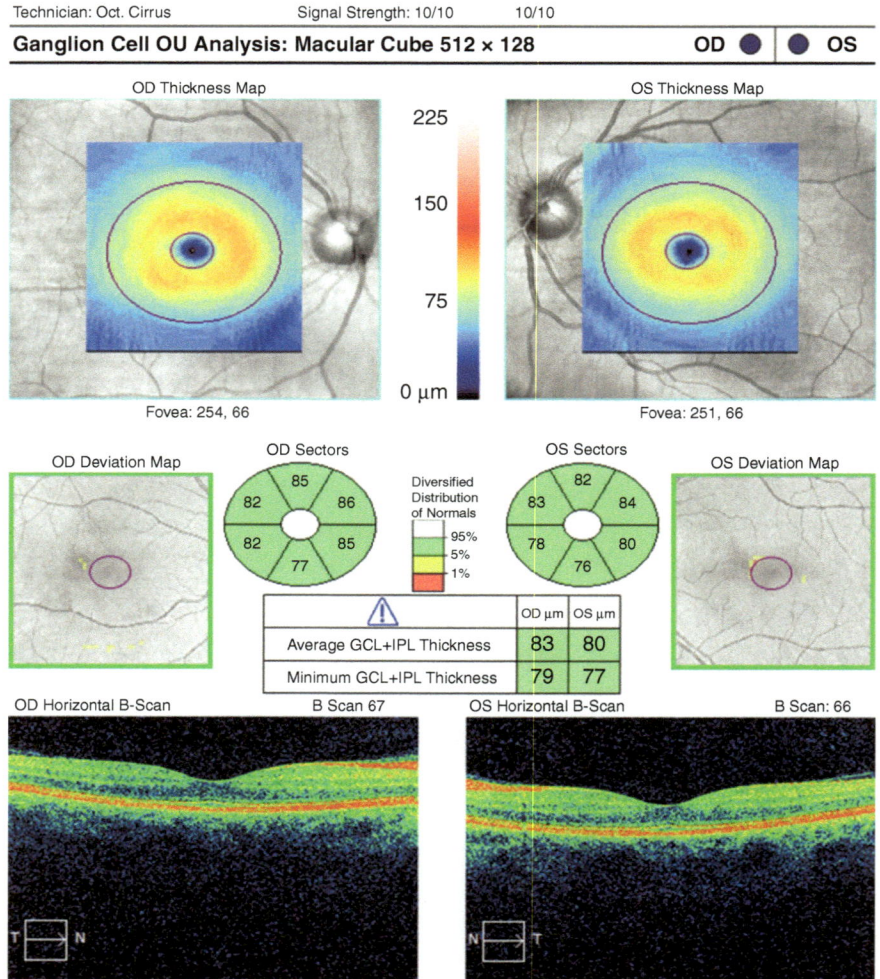

Fig. 8.21 (Cirrus HD-OCT) Ganglion Cell Analysis of the same patient is completely normal

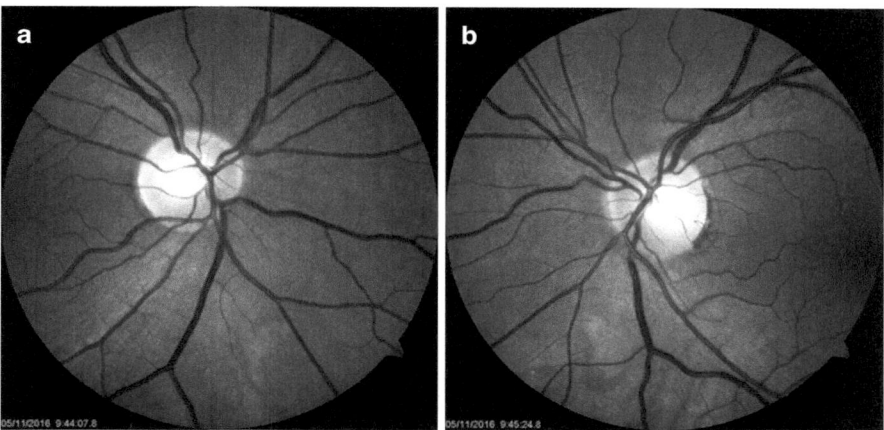

Fig. 8.22 (**a, b**) Red free disc photos of the patient. Careful examination of the photos shows areas of RNFL thinning (split bundle configuration) in the superior quadrant

Conclusion: Split RNFL configuration is one of the common artifacts that can lead to red disease. A careful evaluation of the RNFL TSNIT profiles, lack of ONH parameter abnormalities, normal macular Ganglion Cell Analysis and typical split RNFL images on the RNFL thickness maps are important clues for correct diagnosis.

Case 9: Split RNFL Bundle

OCT scan of a 27-year-old female patient referred for possible RNFL loss (Fig. 8.23). Her UCVA was 20/20 OU, IOP was 16 mmHg OU, anterior and posterior segment exams were unremarkable.

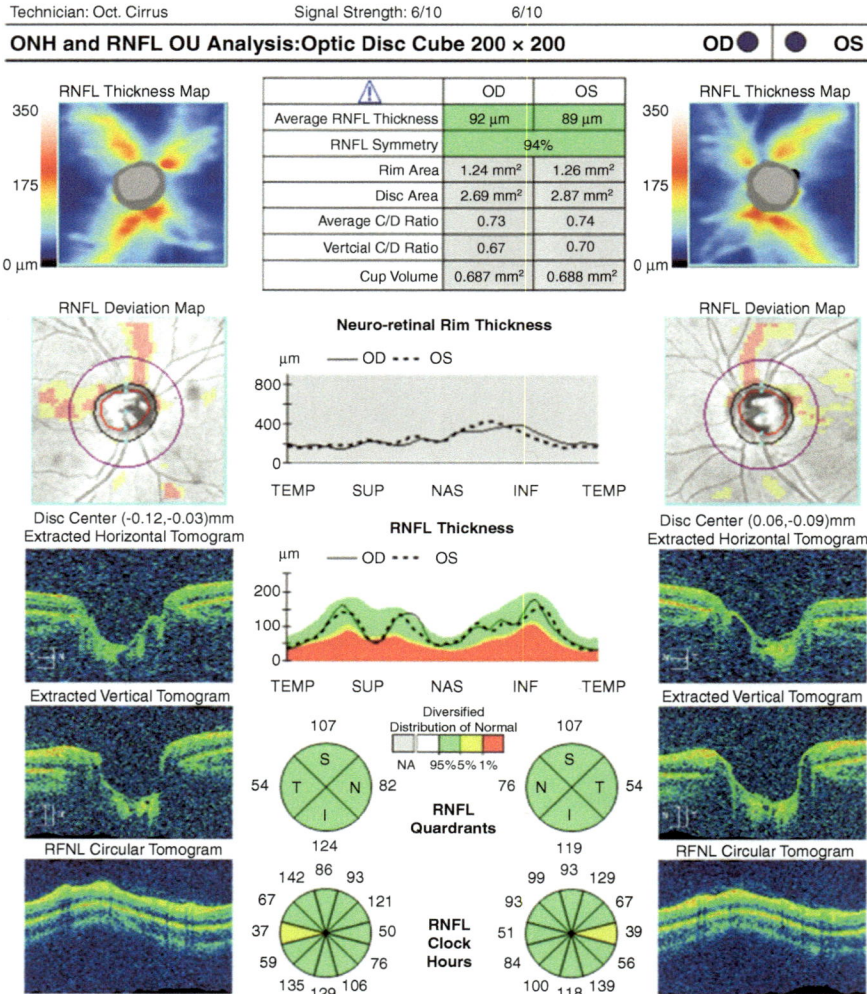

Fig. 8.23 (Cirrus HD-OCT) Scans with borderline quality OU (SS = 6). Another example of split RNFL configuration in the superior RNFL bundle in both eyes. RNFL thickness map shows good RNFL thickness in two superior bundles, RNFL deviation map shows a defect between two bundles when compared to the normative database. TSNIT profiles demonstrate two prominent RNFL peaks for both eyes superiorly, although the RNFL thickness is low between the two peaks; this should be considered a normal anatomic variant with two thick RNFL bundles separated with an area of thinner RNFL

Conclusion: TSNIT profile evaluation is very important to differentiate the split RNFL configuration.

Case 10: Shifted RNFL Peaks

Forty-four-year-old male glaucoma suspect referred for work-up (Fig. 8.24). His BCVA was 20/20 OU. IOPs were 20 mmHg OD and 19 mmHg OS without treatment. Anterior and posterior segment exams are normal.

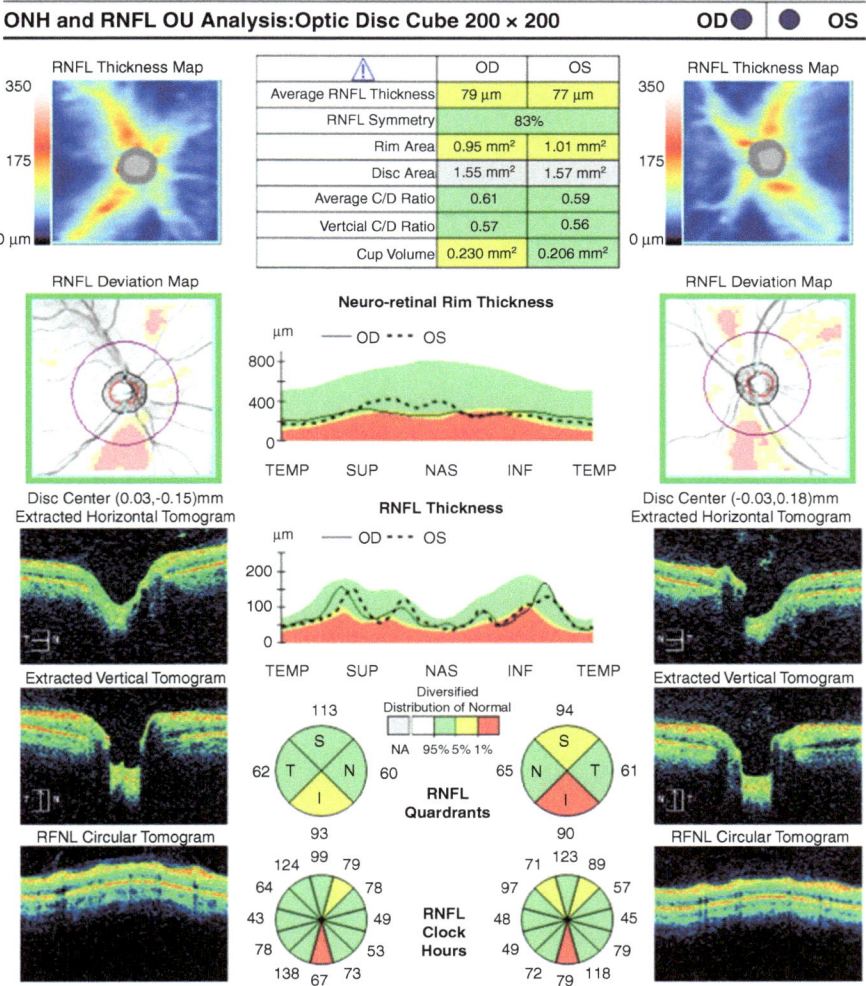

Fig. 8.24 (Cirrus HD-OCT) This OCT report shows RNFL defects OU and the average RNFL thickness values were classified as borderline by the normative database in both eyes. Inferior RNFL thickness in both eyes and superior RNFL thickness in the left eye are out of normal limits. After careful evaluation of the TSNIT profiles, one can notice that the graphs representing RNFL thickness values look normal with a double-hump pattern but they do not fit to the green areas, the typical topography expected in the average normative database. The inferior RNFL peaks are shifted to temporal side

If the RNFL thickness peaks were not shifted to the temporal area, the RNFL thickness lines would fit to the normative database values (Figs. 8.25, 8.26 and 8.27).

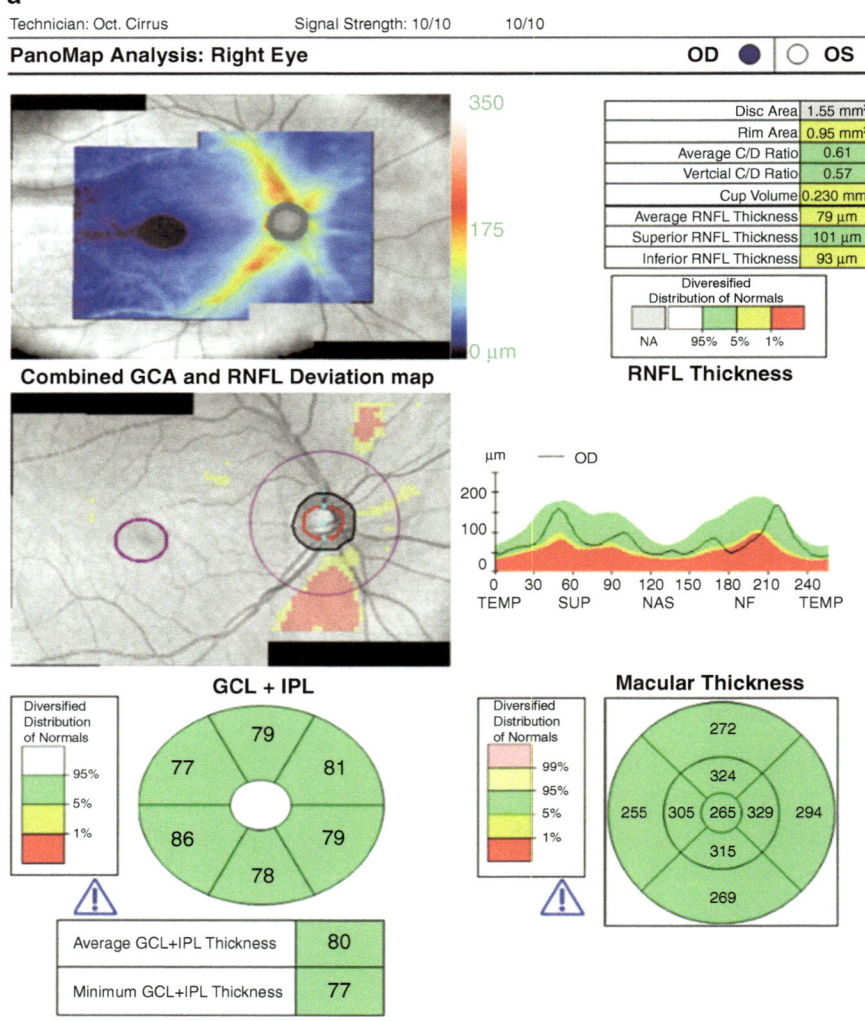

Fig. 8.25 (**a**, **b**) (Cirrus HD-OCT) Panomap reports of both eyes show the artifacts related to the temporal shift of the inferior and nasal shift of the superior RNFL bundles

b

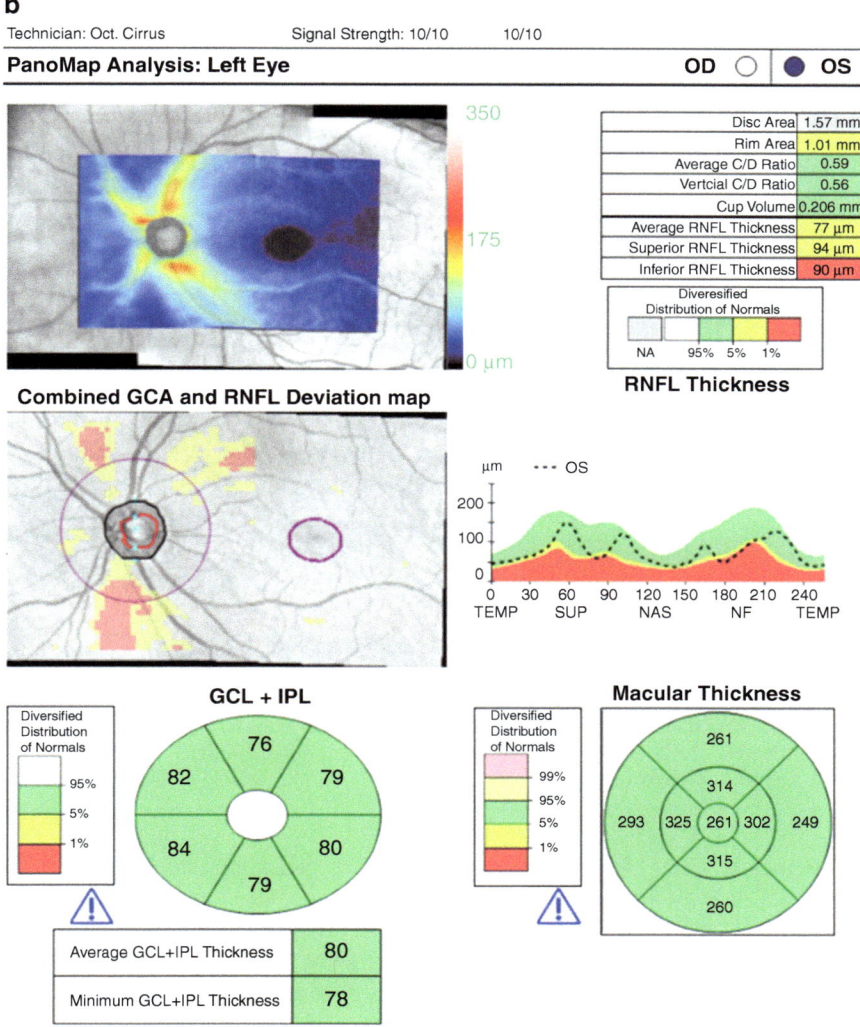

Technician: Oct. Cirrus   Signal Strength: 10/10   10/10

PanoMap Analysis: Left Eye   OD ○ | ● OS

Disc Area	1.57 mm²
Rim Area	1.01 mm²
Average C/D Ratio	0.59
Vertcial C/D Ratio	0.56
Cup Volume	0.206 mm²
Average RNFL Thickness	77 µm
Superior RNFL Thickness	94 µm
Inferior RNFL Thickness	90 µm

Diveresified Distribution of Normals

| NA | 95% | 5% | 1% |

RNFL Thickness

Combined GCA and RNFL Deviation map

µm   --- OS

200
100
0

0   30   60   90   120   150   180   210   240
TEMP   SUP   NAS   NF   TEMP

GCL + IPL

Diversified Distribution of Normals

95%
5%
1%

76
82   79
84   80
79

| Average GCL+IPL Thickness | 80 |
| Minimum GCL+IPL Thickness | 78 |

Macular Thickness

Diversified Distribution of Normals

99%
95%
5%
1%

261
314
293 325 261 302 249
315
260

Fig. 8.25 (continued)

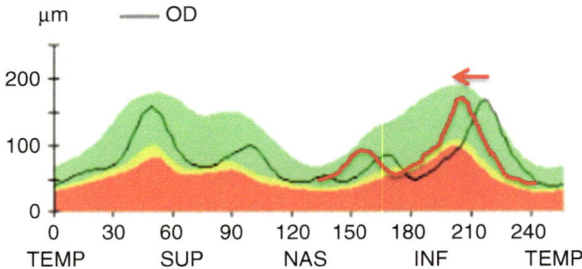

Fig. 8.26 TSNIT graphs of case 10. In the right eye, the superior RNFL bundle fits the green regions, i.e., is within normal statistical range; on the other hand, the inferior bundle is located more temporally but it has a normal thickness. If the RNFL TSNIT profile can be displaced to the nasal side artificially (red line), the new RNFL thickness line would fit to the green area

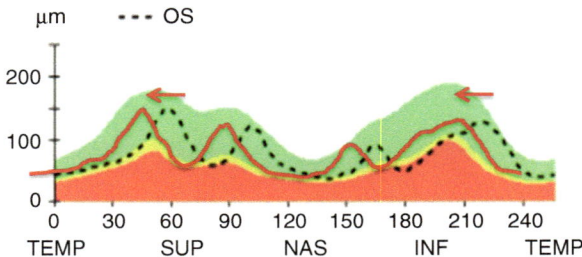

Fig. 8.27 For the left eye, both the inferior and superior bundles seem to displaced and again moving the RNFL TSNIT profile to the left (red line) results in a good fit to the normative database normal (green) region

Conclusion: Hong et al. showed that the RNFL peaks may deviate in normal individuals leading to red diseases artifacts [15]. They studied eyes of 269 Korean volunteers and concluded that in subjects with increased distance between the foveola and optic disc center, myopia and increased axial length, RNFL bundles tend to shift to temporal side [15]. Hood et al. found that the locations of peak RNFL thicknesses in TSNIT profiles largely correlate with the angles of major retinal vessels [16]. This case demonstrates the importance of evaluating the TSNIT profiles in order to avoid a diagnosis of red disease in eyes with unusual RNFL bundle patterns.

Case 11: Shifted RNFL Peaks

OCT scans of a 21-year-old male with myopia (Figs. 8.28, 8.29, 8.30, 8.31 and 8.32). His BCVA was 20/20 with −1.0D correction OU, IOPs were 17 mmHg and visual fields were normal. The anterior and posterior segments were normal except for signs of allergic conjuncitivitis.

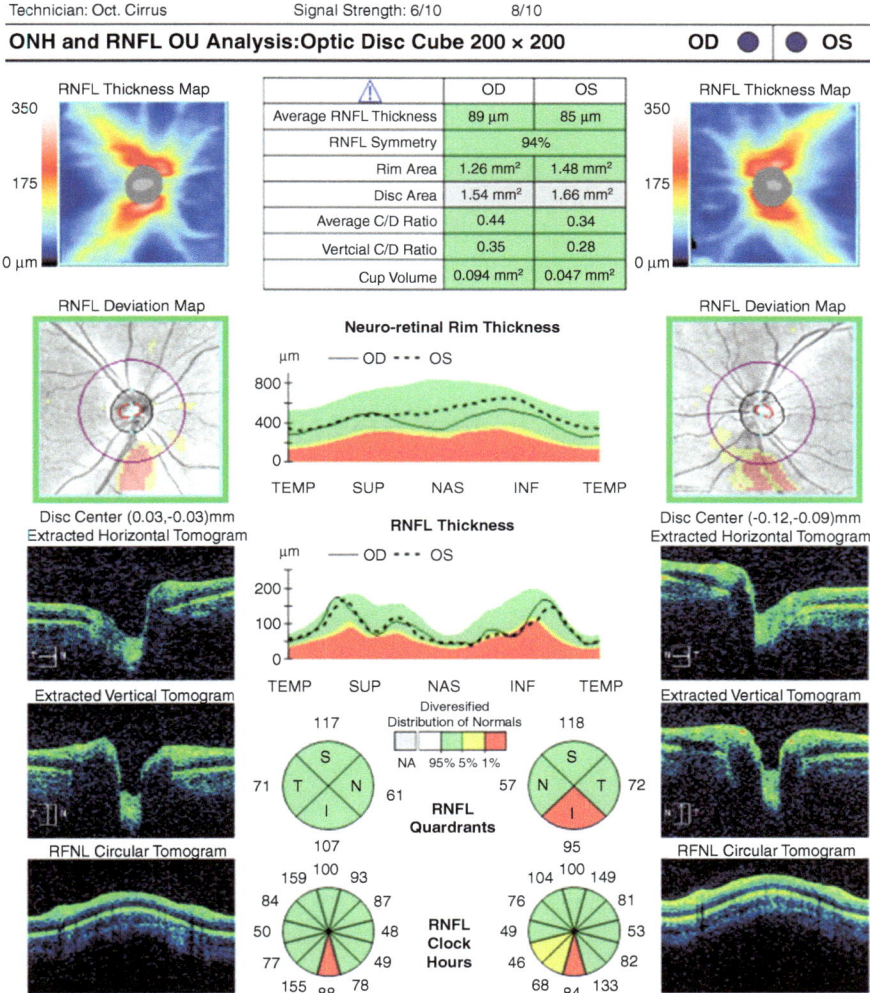

Fig. 8.28 (Cirrus HD-OCT) Unexpected OCT RNFL defects in the inferior quadrants of both eyes of a healthy, young man without any history of glaucoma. TSNIT graph shows temporal shift of the RNFL bundle both superiorly and inferiorly. The clock hour pie charts also show the 6 o'clock sectors to be "out of normal range". Evaluation of TSNIT graph reveals that both eyes have temporally shifted RNFL bundles leading to thin RNFL values at 6 o'clock sector but thicker RNFL measurements inferotemporally (at 7 o'clock sector of the right eye and 5 o'clock quadrant of the left eye). Plotting these values with a few degrees of shift away from the temporal quadrant shows that RNFL thickness values are now within the normal range (Fig. 8.29)

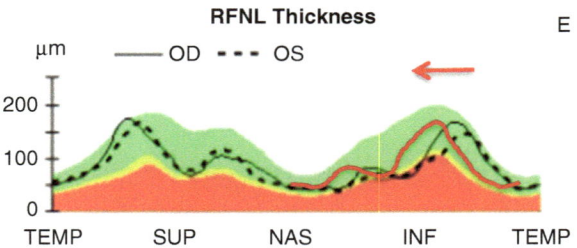

Fig. 8.29 The red profile demonstrates the RNFL thickness of the right eye moved by a few degrees nasally. This correction places the RNFL thickness values within in normal range. Both eyes have quite symmetric RNFL profiles, and the same comments are valid for the left eye as well

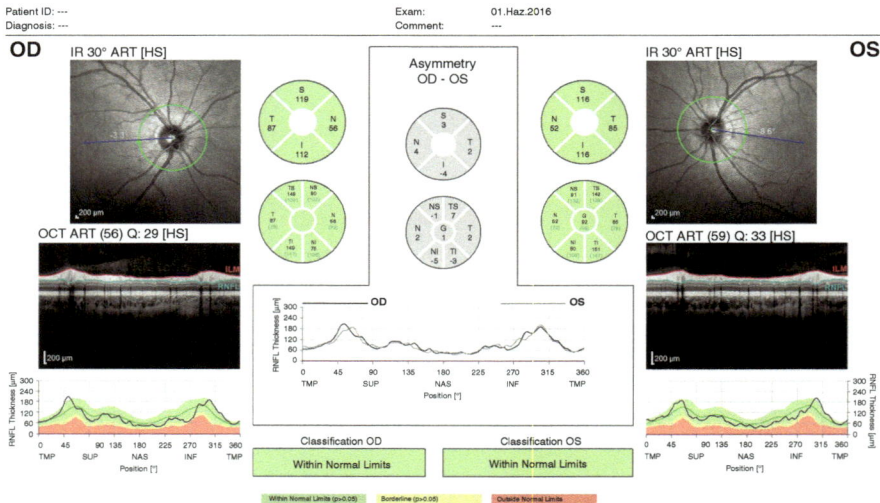

Fig. 8.30 (Spectralis OCT) The same shift is present on the TSNIT profiles on Spectralis OCT. Although the pie graphs are all flagged as green, inferotemporal quadrant values are lower than expected and TSNIT profiles show that the inferior bundle is shifted temporally. Plotting these values with a few degrees of shifting demonstrates that the RNFL thickness values are in normal range (Fig. 8.31a, b)

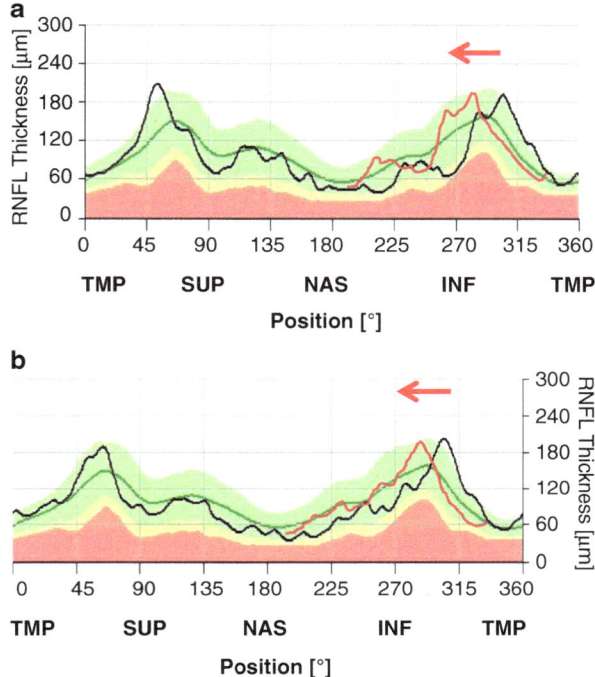

Fig. 8.31 (**a**) TSNIT profile of the right eye of the patient, (**b**) TSNIT profile of the left eye of the patient. Red lines describe how the RNFL profile would fit within the normative database green area if moved about 10°–15° nasally

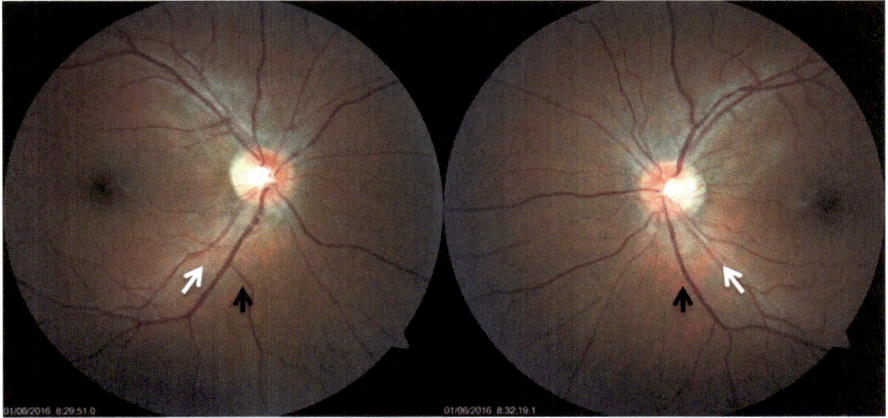

Fig. 8.32 Fundus photographs of the same patient. One can see that inferior RNFL bundles in both eyes are situated more temporally (white arrowheads) than the expected inferior location (black arrowheads)

Conclusion: This is another case with shifted RNFL configuration. On the Cirrus OCT, the TSNIT graphs show the temporal shift of the inferior RNFL bundle in both eyes. The pie charts demonstrate the RNFL to be outside of normal range at the 6 o'clock sector in both eyes. The RNFL thickness values at 7 o'clock sector for the right eye and 5 o'clock sector in the left eye are thicker than usual because of the temporal shift of the bundles.

Case 12: Split Bundle and Shifted RNFL Peaks

OCT scans of a 52-year-old female with family history of glaucoma (Figs. 8.33, 8.34, 8.35 and 8.36). Her BCVA was 20/20 with + 0.75 D OS and + 1.25 D OS. The IOP was 13 mmHg OD and 15 mmHg OS. The anterior segment exam was unremarkable OU.

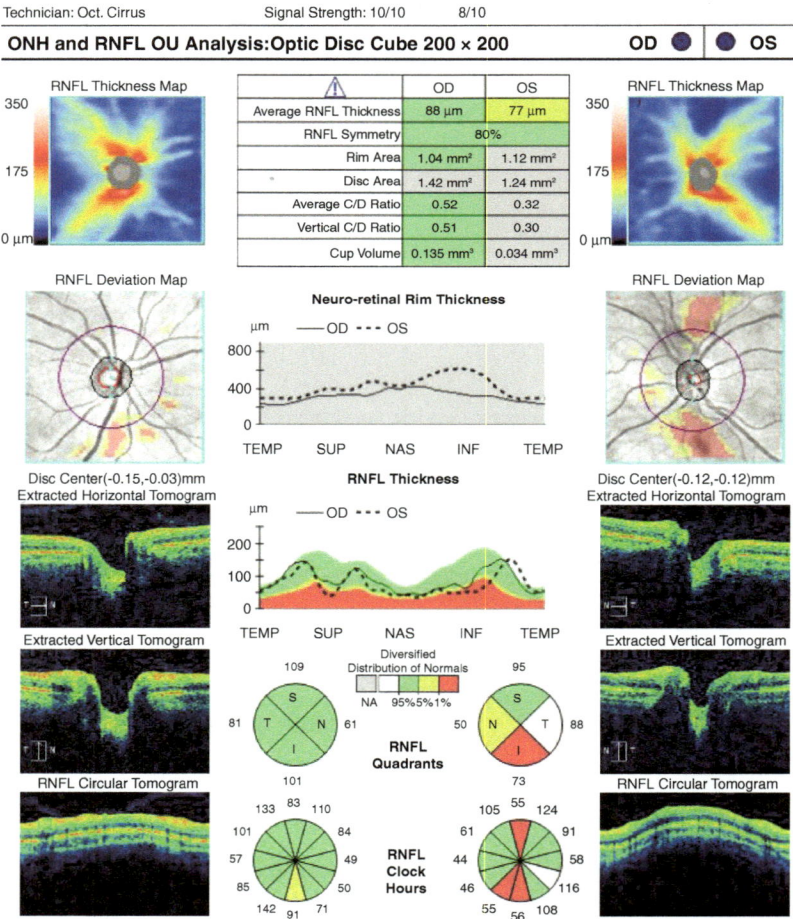

Fig. 8.33 (Cirrus HD-OCT) Good quality OCT scan showing RNFL defects in the left eye. The TSNIT profile displays shifted RNFL peaks in the inferior bundle and possible split RNFL configuration in the superior bundle

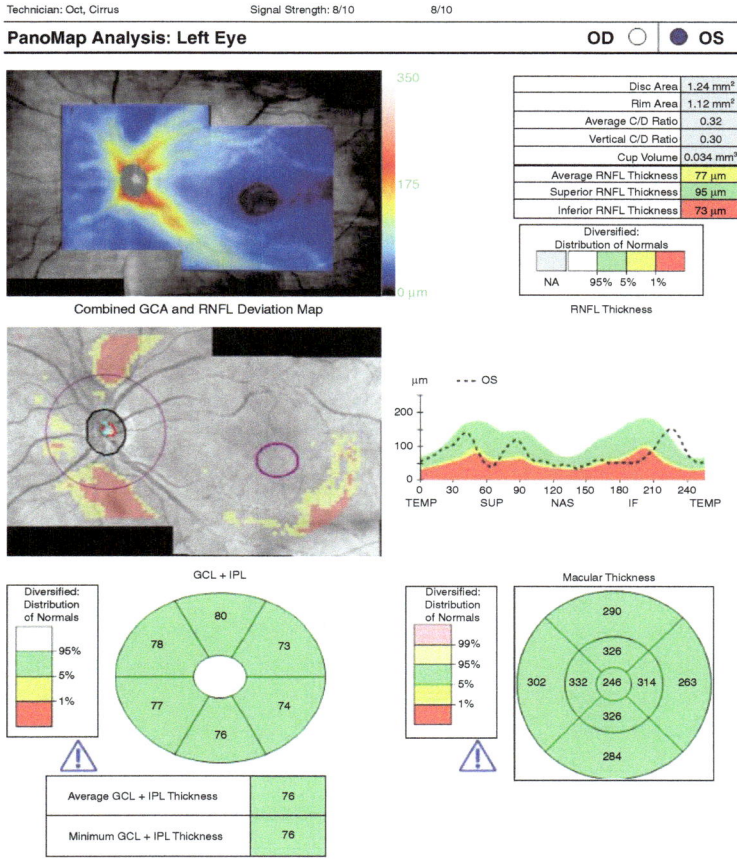

Fig. 8.34 Panomap report of the left eye shows that a possible excyclotorsion is present

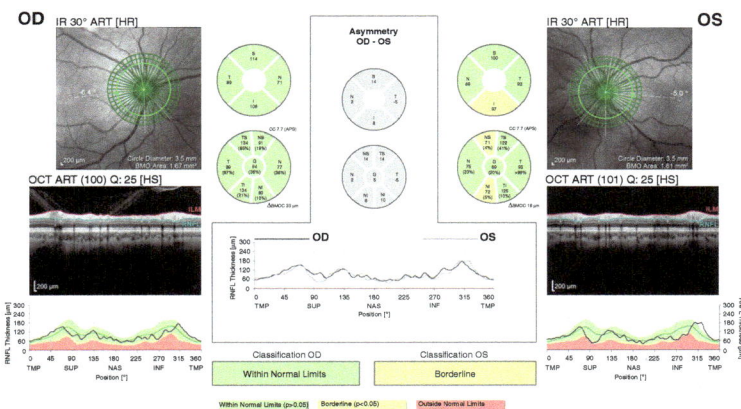

Fig. 8.35 (Spectralis, GMPE Module) Spectralis OCT with GMPE software which corrects for the FoBMO (fovea to Bruch's membrane opening) axis angle is able to correct some degree of the shift in the left eye; in addition to the torsional artifact, there is a real shift that the FoBMO correction cannot eliminate

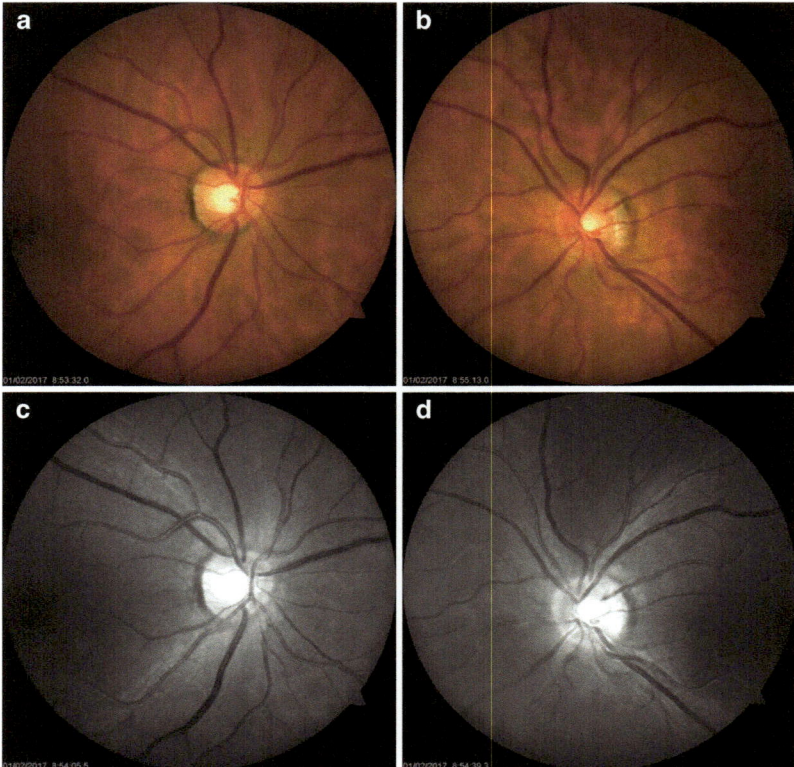

Fig. 8.36 (**a**, **b**) Color and (**c**, **d**) red-free fundus photos of the patient show that the left eye has a slightly tilted disc with peripapillary choroidal atrophy; the inferior vessels (and accompanying RNFL bundle) appear to be temporally shifted. Split RNFL bundle configuration can be observed superiorly in both eyes

Conclusion. Shifted and split RNFL bundles are two of the most common artifacts we observe on OCT images. Correction for the FoBMO axis angle by Spectralis OCT can compensate shifting of the RNFL peaks caused by the incyclotorsion or excyclotorsion of the eye. However, in most eyes, such shifts in RNFL peaks are not caused by the eye torsion. Careful examination of the TSNIT profiles can help clinicians identify these artifacts.

Development of software algorithms with smart RNFL profile matching will be able to adjust the normative database values and help address this problem [15].

8.3.2.2   Media Opacities

Floating vitreous opacities, such as Weiss rings, can cause patient-related imaging artifacts that manifest and disappear on different scans as their position changes with eye movements. They are one of the most common artifacts observed in older patients. In addition, other opacities such as cataracts, asteroid hyalosis, vitreous hemorrhages can cause various artifacts.

Case 13: Weiss Ring Over RNFL Calculation Circle

OCT scans of a 73-year-old male with bilateral cataract and ocular hypertension (Figs. 8.37 and 8.38). The BCVA was 20/40 OU, and IOP was 24 mmHg OD and 23 mmHg OS on no medications.

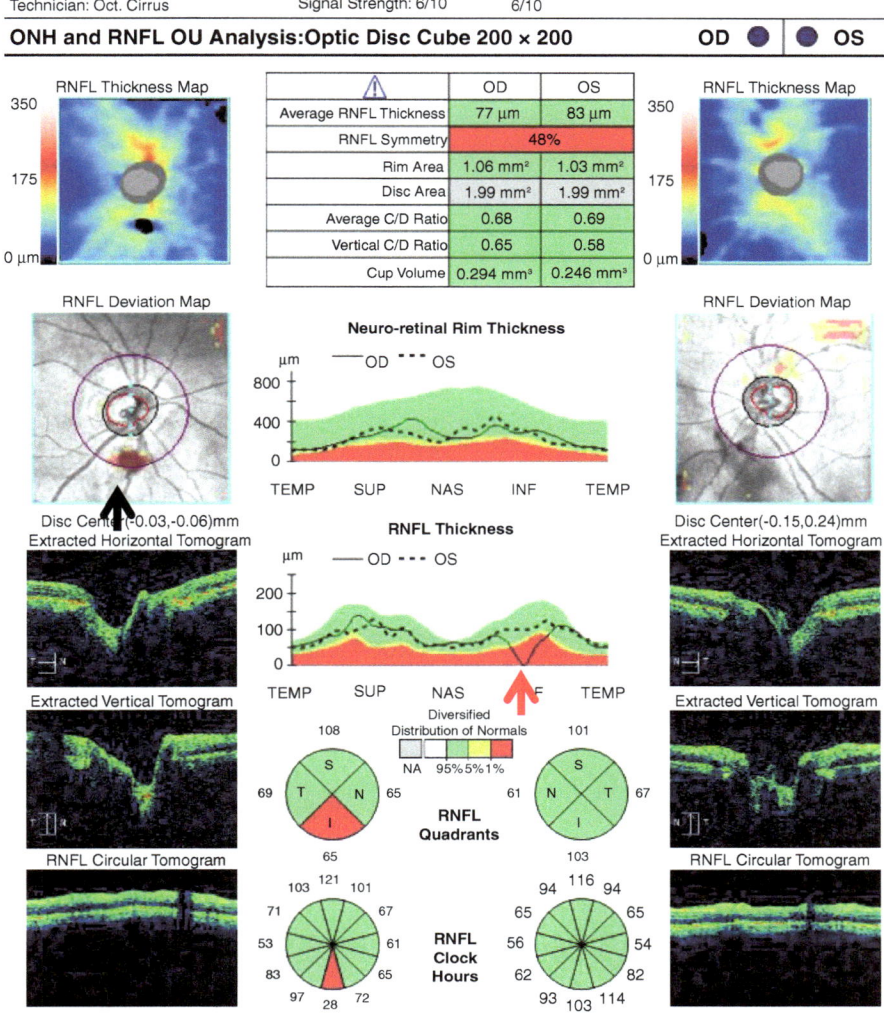

Fig. 8.37 (Cirrus HD-OCT) The SS of this scan is 6 due to presence of cataract. The position of the Weiss ring coincides with the RNFL calculation circle in the inferior quadrant in the right eye (black arrowhead). In cases where the Weiss ring blocks part of the calculation circle, it can affect the TSNIT graph and all of the pie charts. The interpreter needs to recognize this kind of artifact on the RNFL thickness map as an area of scanning failure or blockage (black arrowhead) and also on the TSNIT graph as an area of zero RNFL thickness, which is technically impossible because of the floor effect (red arrowhead)

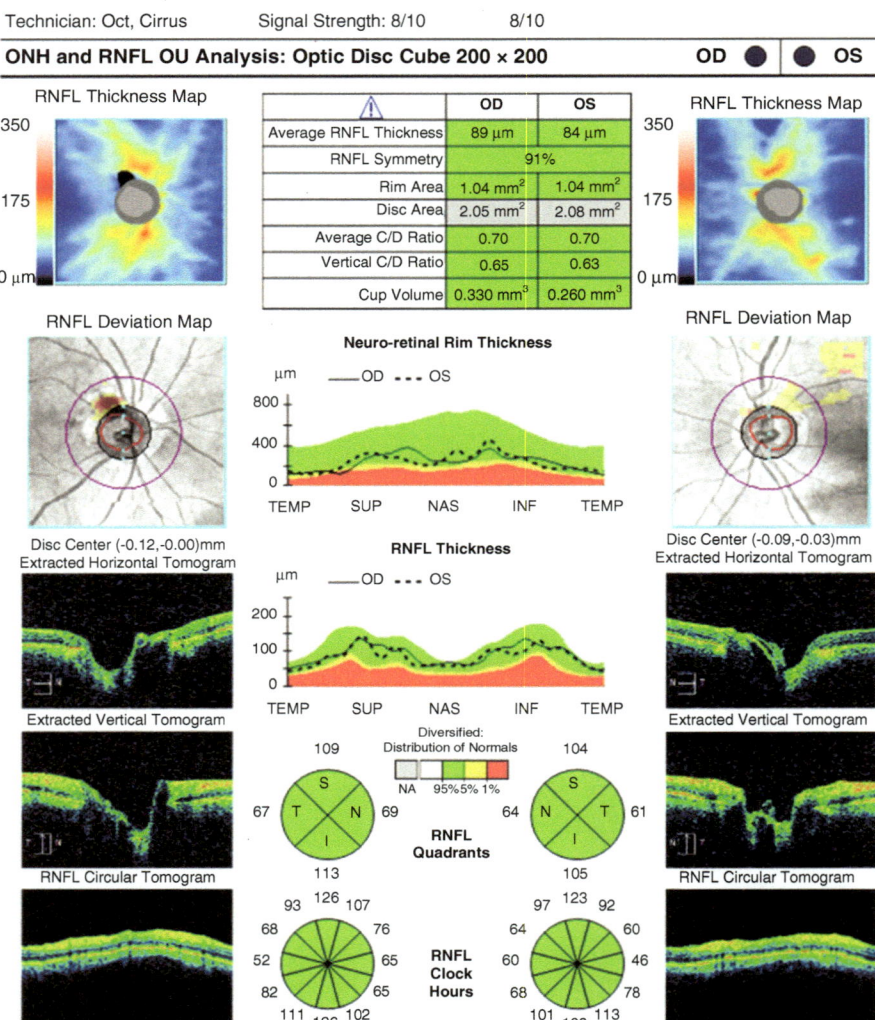

Fig. 8.38 (Cirrus HD-OCT) Same patient 2 years later: the SS in this scan is better as the patient had cataract surgery. The Weiss ring is still present in this scan, but its position during the scan does not coincide with the calculation circle and does not affect the pie charts

Conclusion. Weiss rings are common on OCT scans and can be one of the reasons for the 'red disease'. As Weiss ring moves in front of the retina, it blocks OCT signal in different areas of the ONH or retina on different scans. Careful inspection of the RNFL thickness map, the deviation map and TSNIT graph can help clinicians identify this type of artifact.

Case 14: Weiss Ring Over the Optic Nerve Head—Red Disease Artifact

The OCT scans of a 74-year-old woman with cataract and posterior vitreous detachment (Figs. 8.39 and 8.40). Her BCVA was 20/60 OU, IOP was 14 mmHg OD and 13 mmHg OS on no medications.

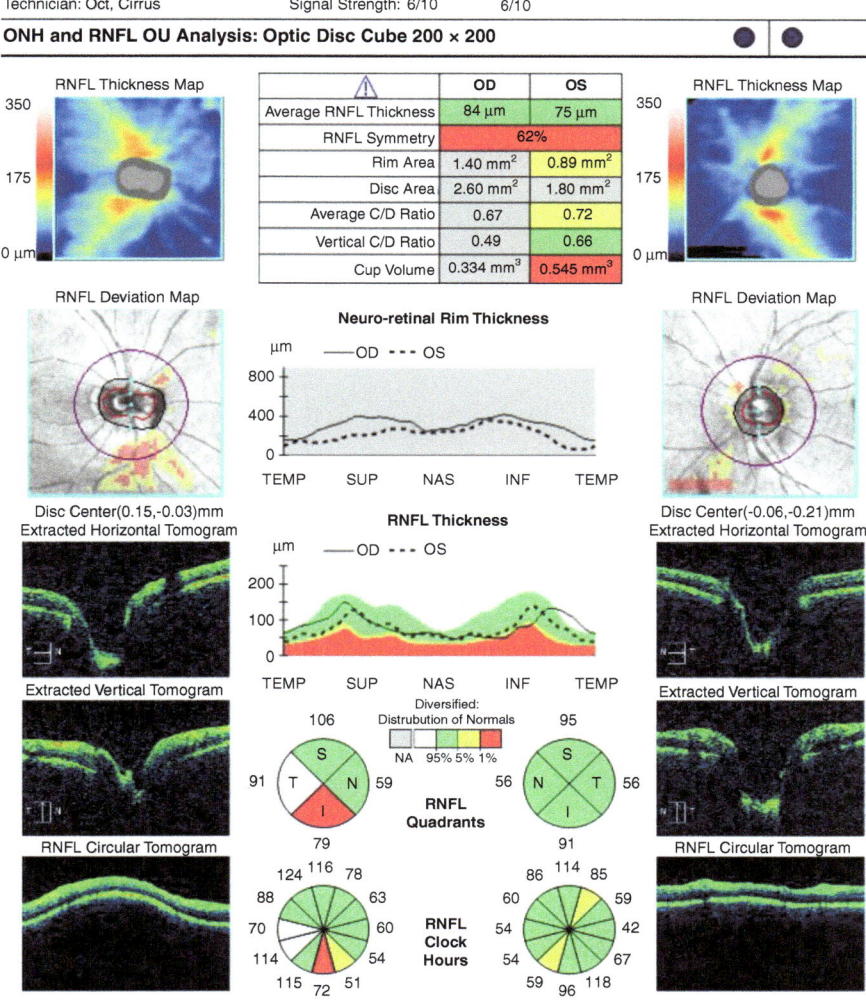

Fig. 8.39 (Cirrus HD-OCT) A Weiss ring blocking the laser light path towards the right ONH caused an artifact leading to a doubling of the disc image. Due to this artifact, the software miscalculated the disc centroid and misplaced the calculation circle, which resulted in the RNFL thickness to be flagged as outside of normal limits. Displacement of the RNFL peak also led to displaced abnormal RNFL peak. The patient needs to be rescanned after having her look around a few times

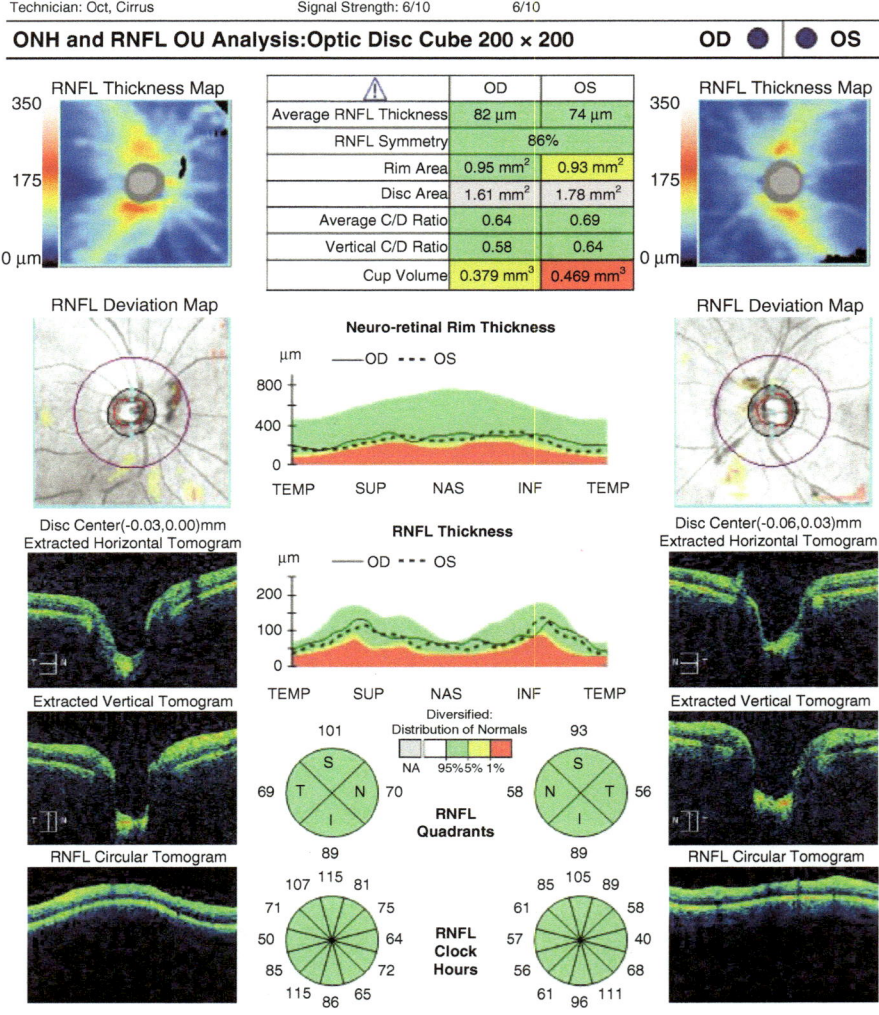

Fig. 8.40 (Cirrus HD-OCT) Rescan of the same patient with no Weiss ring over the ONH. The Weiss ring can be seen on the nasal side of the ONH. All of the ONH and RNFL parameters are within the normal range in this higher quality scan

Conclusion: Weiss rings can cause red disease artifacts even when they are not overlying the calculation circle. Checking the RNFL thickness and deviation maps are important for detecting these kinds of artifacts.

Case 15: Weiss Ring Over Optic Nerve Head—Green Disease Artifact

OCT scan of a 78-year-old female with primary open angle glaucoma who was under treatment for 10 years (Fig. 8.41). Her BCVA was 20/30 OD and 20/40 OS. Her IOP was 17 mmHg OU on the day of imaging on travoprost once daily and timolol + dorzolamide combination twice daily in both eyes.

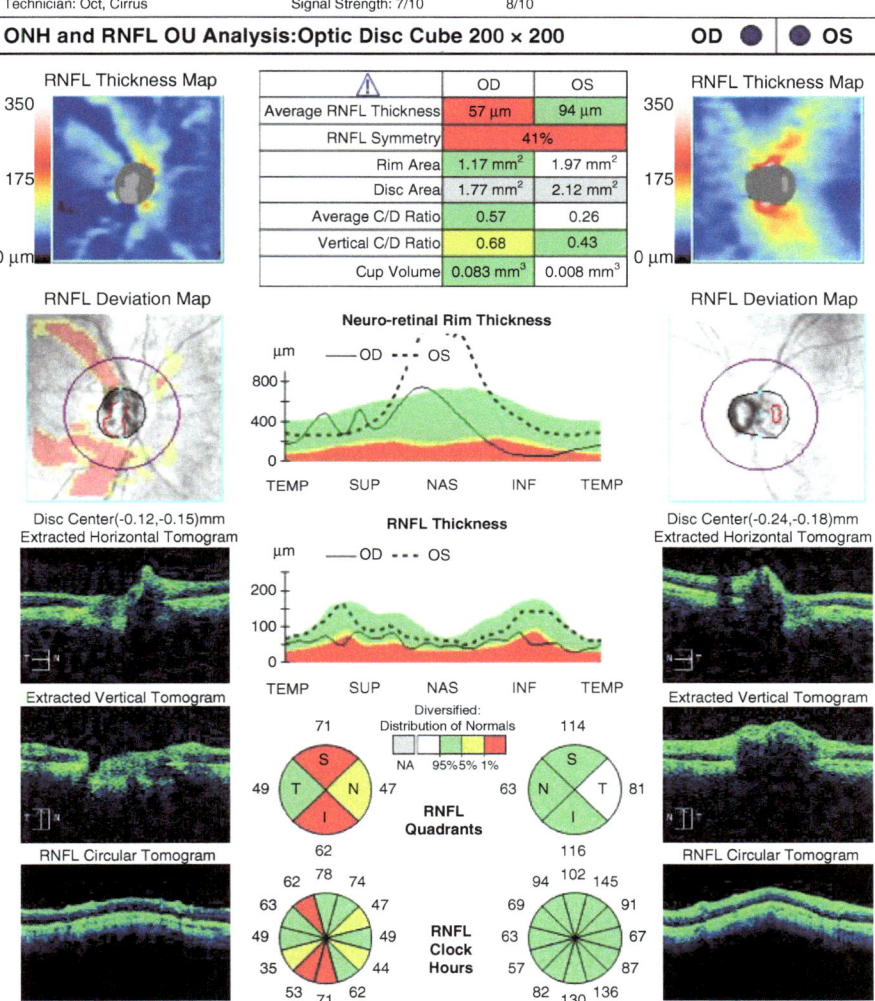

Fig. 8.41 (Cirrus HD-OCT) The OCT report of the right eye shows advanced RNFL and neuro-retinal rim damage. The Weiss ring in the left eye caused a scanning artifact, which led to incorrect placement of the calculation circle. This artifact affects both the ONH parameters and RNFL thickness measurements. It is possible that this artifact obscures RNFL defects in the left eye. The calculation circle is incorrectly placed due to the Weiss ring blocking the laser light aimed at the optic disc. As the posterior vitreous detachment was incomplete, rescanning showed similar artifacts

Conclusion: Vitreous opacities like Weiss rings generally cause red disease artifacts, but this scan is an example of a possible green disease artifact by a vitreous opacity located over the optic nerve.

Case 16: Asteroid Hyalosis

Seventy-eight-year-old, pseudophakic glaucoma suspect with asteroid hyalosis
(Fig. 8.42). BCVA was 20/30 OU. IOP was measured at 22 mmHg OD and 23 mmHg
OS.

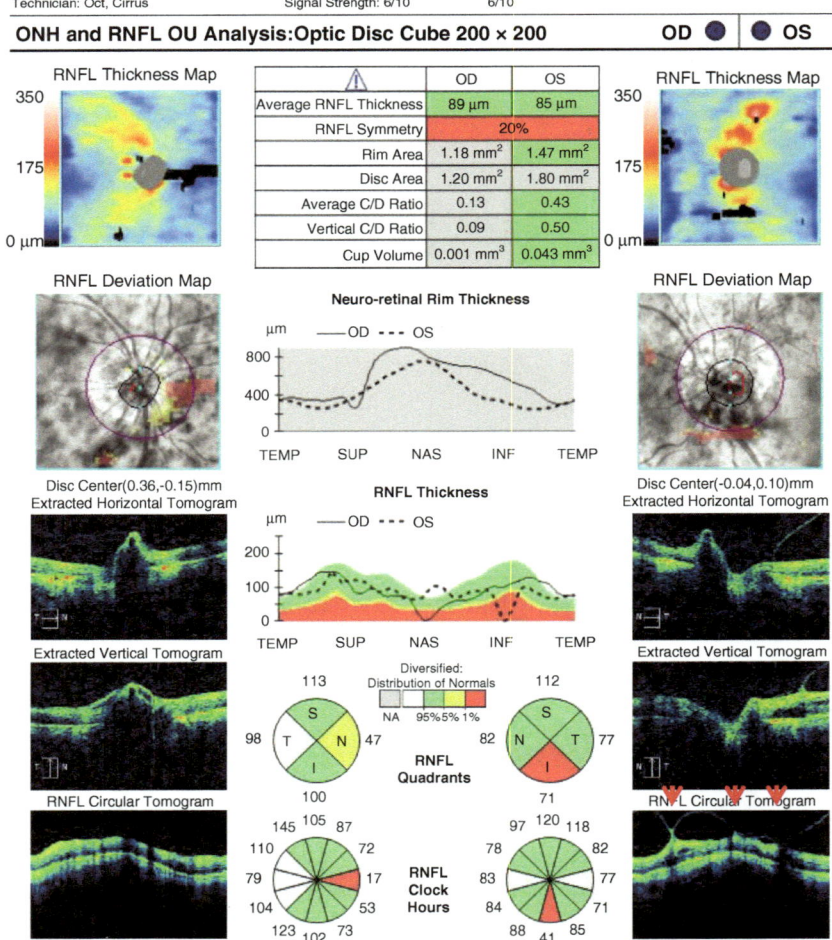

Fig. 8.42 (Cirrus HD-OCT) This is an OCT of borderline quality with a lot of artifacts. The signal
strength is 6 OU and therefore, the scan quality is not very good and a significant number of artifacts can be seen on the ONH and RNFL thickness and deviation maps. Like other vitreous opacities, asteroid hyalosis causes areas of scan defects. In addition, areas of vitreous RNFL adhesions
can be observed on the raw RNFL image leading to tractions and artificial thickening of the RNFL
along the calculation circle (red arrowheads)

Conclusion: With so many artifacts, it is impossible to use this test for either
diagnosis or follow-up of glaucoma as the moving opacities in the vitreous cause
different artifacts on repeat scans.

8.3.2.3   Vitreoretinal Interface Problems

Case 17: Peripapillary Vitreoretinal Traction

OCT scans, VFs and optic nerve photographs of a 78-year-old male with pseudoex-foliative glaucoma (Figs. 8.43, 8.44, 8.45, 8.46, 8.47 and 8.48). The patient was diagnosed with bilateral glaucoma 10 years ago. He had cataract surgery previously and his BCVA was 20/20 OU. His IOP was measured at 16 mmHg OD and 17 mmHg OS on bimatoprost and timolol/brinzolamide combination.

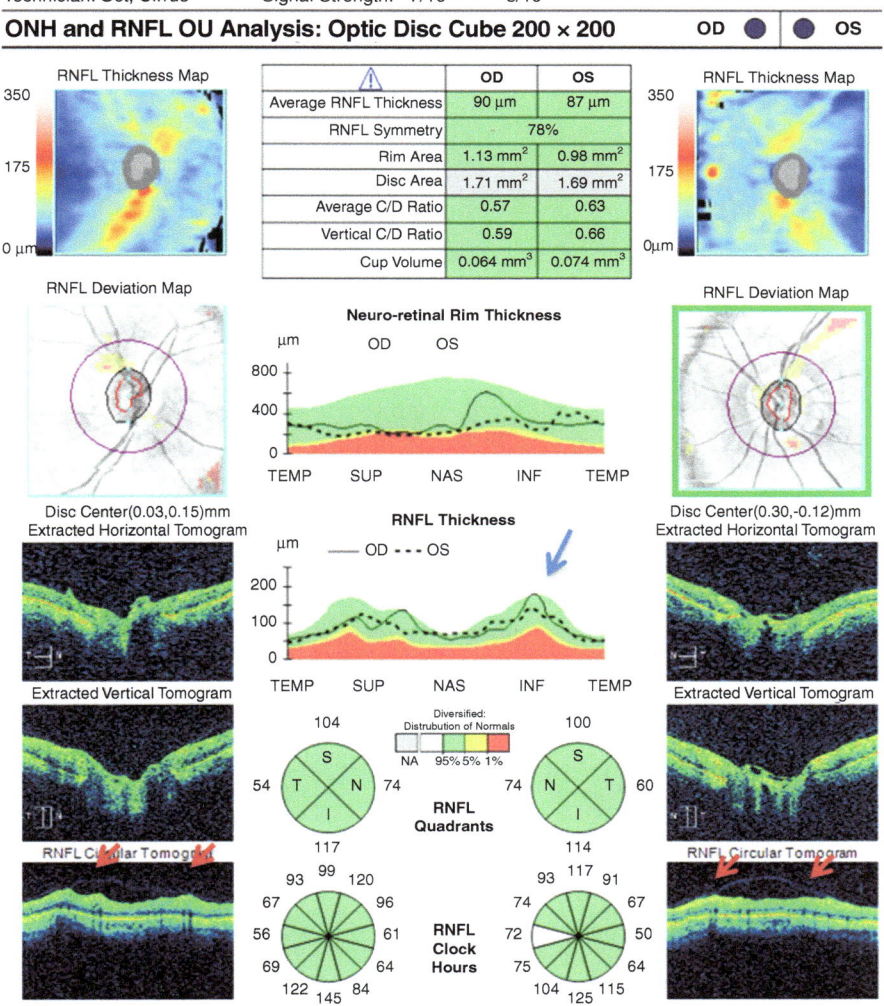

Fig. 8.43 (Cirrus HD-OCT) This OCT scan demonstrates normal RNFL and ONH parameters. The inferior quadrant RNFL thickness is high especially in the right eye (blue arrow), which is possibly caused by the vitreoretinal tractions corresponding to the calculation circles. Vitreoretinal tractions can be observed on the RNFL raw images (red arrows)

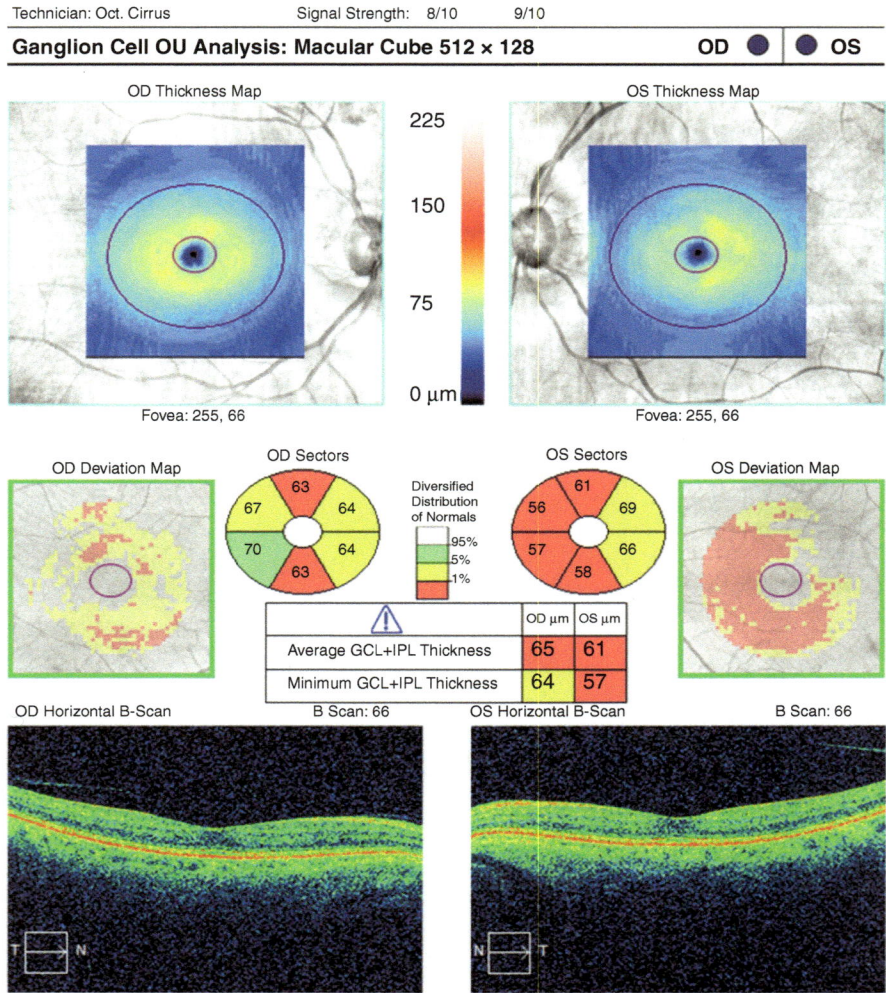

Fig. 8.44 (Cirrus HD-OCT) GCL + IPL maps of the same patient shows significant glaucomatous damage, which is not compatible with the ONH and RNFL findings on the previous OCT report

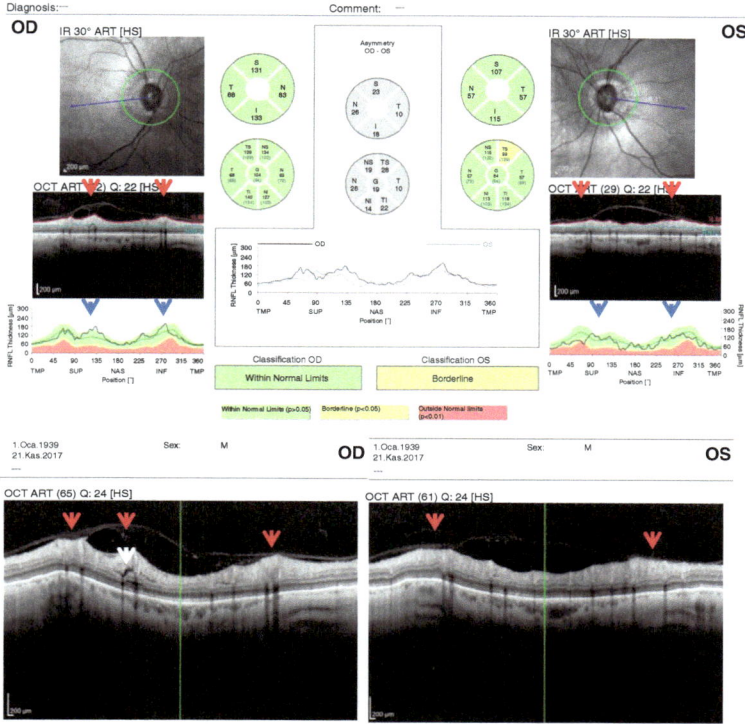

Fig. 8.45 (Spectralis OCT) RNFL thickness values again are within the normal range on Spectralis OCT. Spectralis OCT demonstrates the vitreoretinal tractions better on the raw peripapillary image (red arrowheads); the traction causes a RNFL thickness peaks in the inferior and superior quadrants (blue arrowheads). In addition, an area of peripapillary retinoschisis is present (white arrowhead) [17, 18]

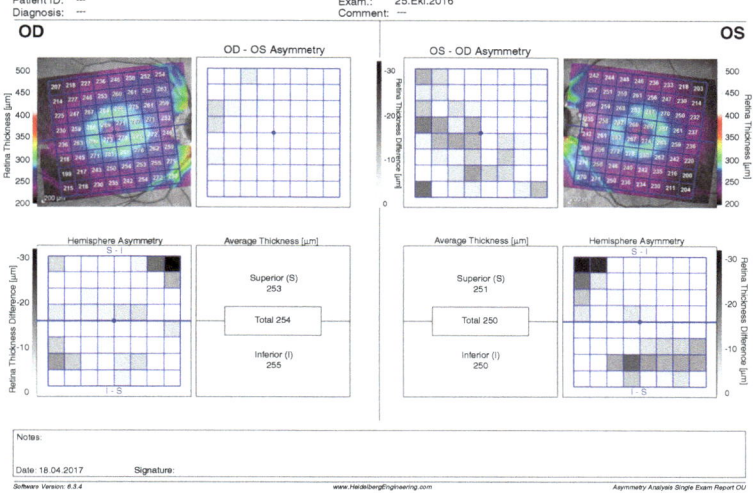

Fig. 8.46 (Spectralis OCT) Posterior pole asymmetry analysis of the Spectralis also shows areas of damage although the RNFL thickness values were normal on the previous OCT

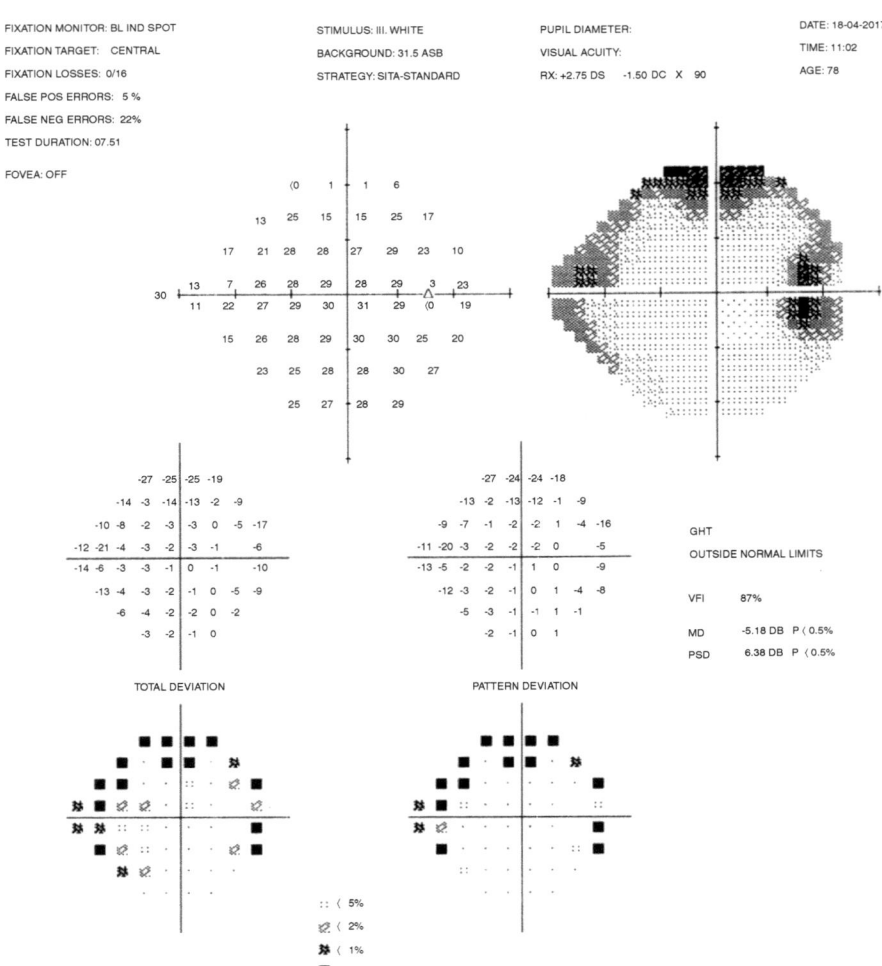

Fig. 8.47 Humphrey visual field reports of the same patient display typical corresponding glaucomatous damage in both eyes

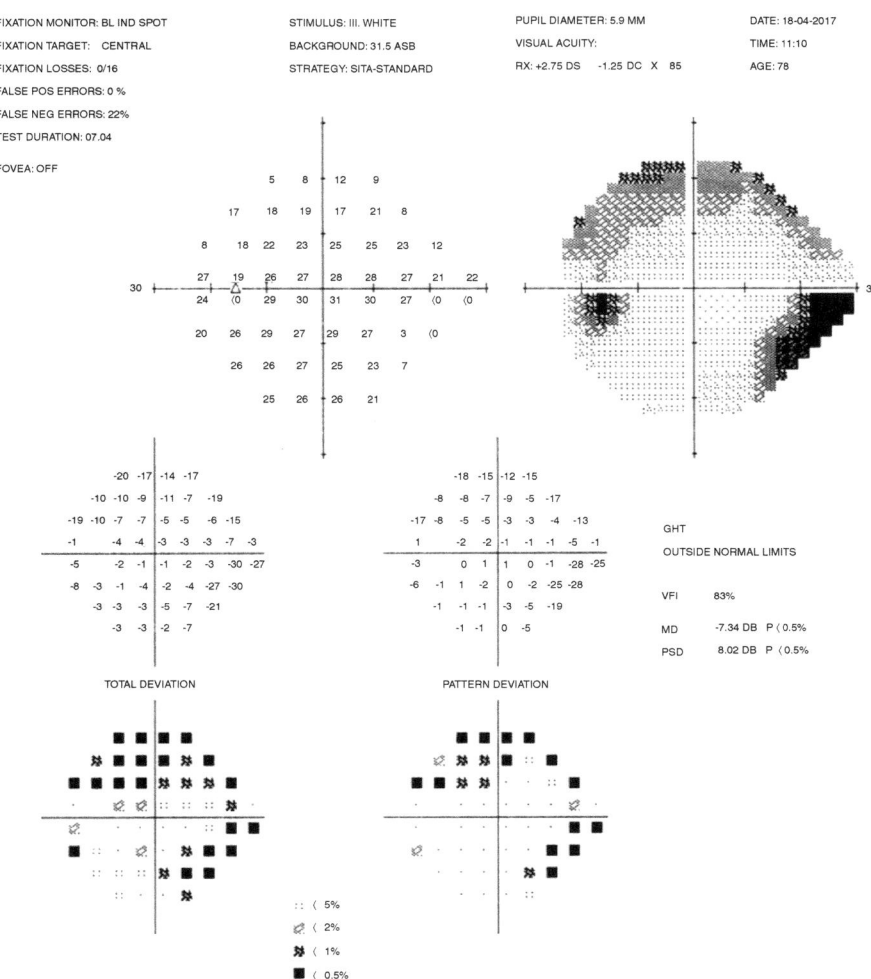

Fig. 8.47 (continued)

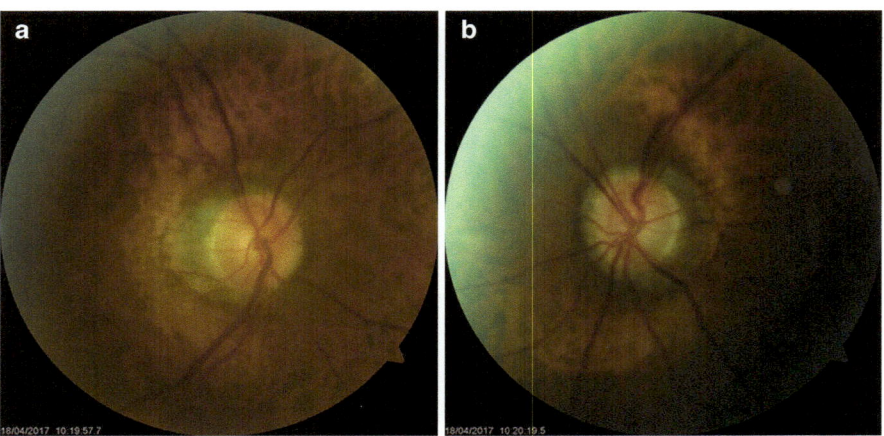

Fig. 8.48 (**a, b**) Optic nerve photographs of the same patient, neuroretinal rim thinning is present in the left eye (**b**). No indication of vitreoretinal traction around the optic nerve is identifiable in these photographs

Conclusion: Vitreoretinal traction can result in an artifactitious increase of the RNFL thickness and may lead to green disease artifact. In these eyes, OCT reports show normal peripapillary RNFL thickness values. Macular Ganglion Cell Analysis could be helpful in such eyes as it generally reflects the extent of damage. In addition, VF analysis may demonstrate glaucomatous defects. In some of these eyes, a spontaneous detachment of vitreous from the retina in the peripapillary area results in rapid reduction of RNFL thickness causing misinterpretation during follow-up. Vitreoretinal traction around the disc area is one of the most common causes of green disease artifact.

Case 18: Peripapillary Vitreoretinal Traction

Sixty-six year-old female with proliferative diabetic retinopathy and neovascular glaucoma (Figs. 8.49 and 8.50). The BCVA was counting fingers OD and 20/200 OS. The IOP was 18 mmHg in the right eye on maximally tolerated medical treatment after diode laser cyclophotocoagulation and 14 mmHg in the left eye after placement of an Ahmed Glaucoma Valve.

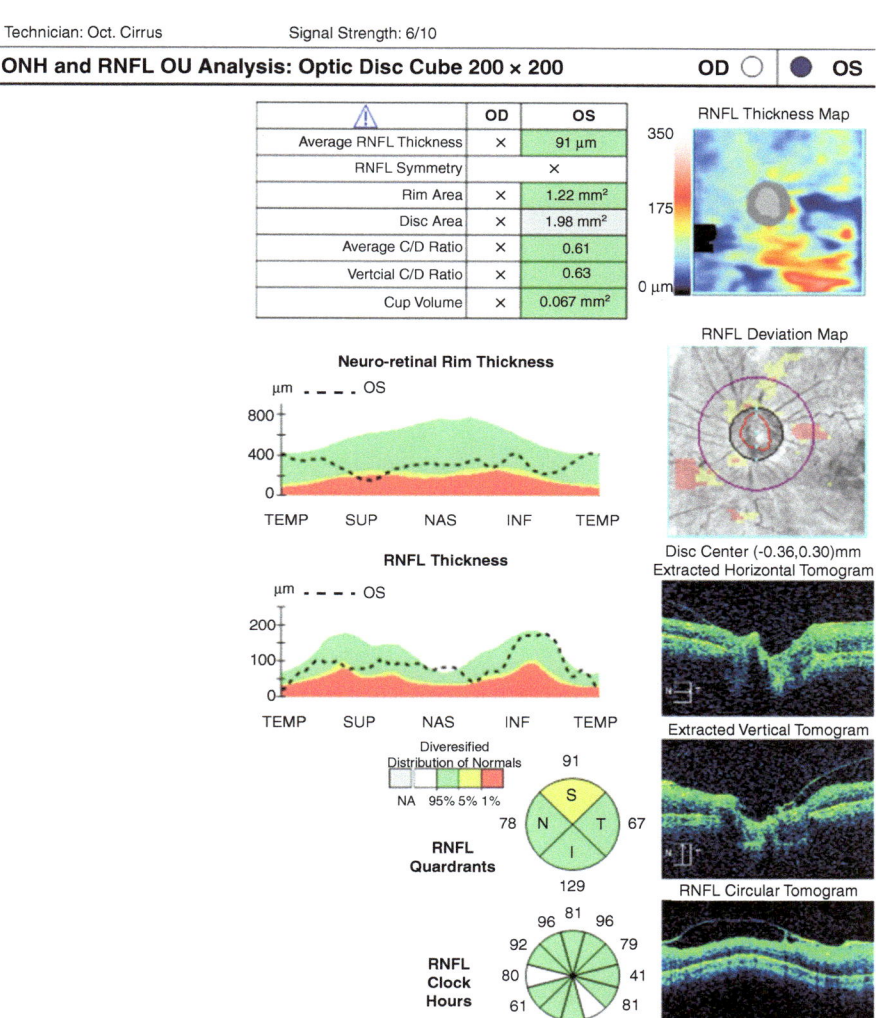

Fig. 8.49 (Cirrus HD-OCT) Only the left eye was scanned due to presence of vitreous hemorrhage in the right eye. The RNFL circular raw OCT image shows that a dense posterior vitreous face and vitreoretinal traction has led to a very thick RNFL especially inferiorly. ONH parameters are also within normal range possibly due to the adhesions between the vitreous and the optic disc

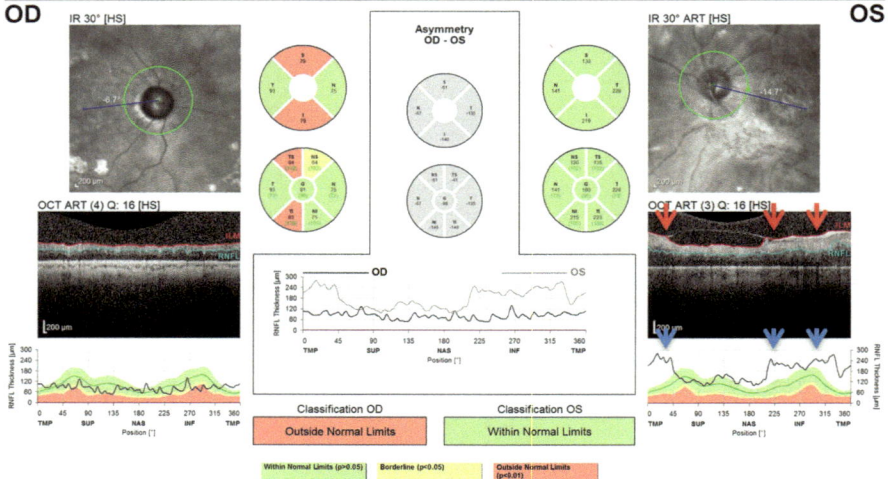

Fig. 8.50 (Spectralis OCT) An earlier Spectralis OCT of the same patient performed before development of vitreous hemorrhage in the right eye. The vitreoretinal tractions are evident on the raw
OCT image. The raw OCT image (red arrowheads) of the left eye shows areas of vitreous traction
that have led to very thick RNFL values on the TSNIT graph (blue arrowheads)

Conclusion: Vitreoretinal traction resulting from advanced diabetic retinopathy
with thickening of the posterior hyaloid face artificially thicken the RNFL, leading
to "green disease" artifact. If the vitreous completely separates form the retina,
RNFL thickness may decrease significantly and reveals the real extent of RNFL loss
in these eyes.

8.3.2.4   Optic Nerve Head Drusen

Case 19: Optic Nerve Head Drusen

The OCT scans, VFs, and fundus images of a 46-year old female glaucoma suspect (Figs. 8.51, 8.52, 8.53, 8.54 and 8.55). BCVA was 20/20 OU and the IOP was
23 mmHg OU without treatment. The anterior segment exam was unremarkable in
both eyes.

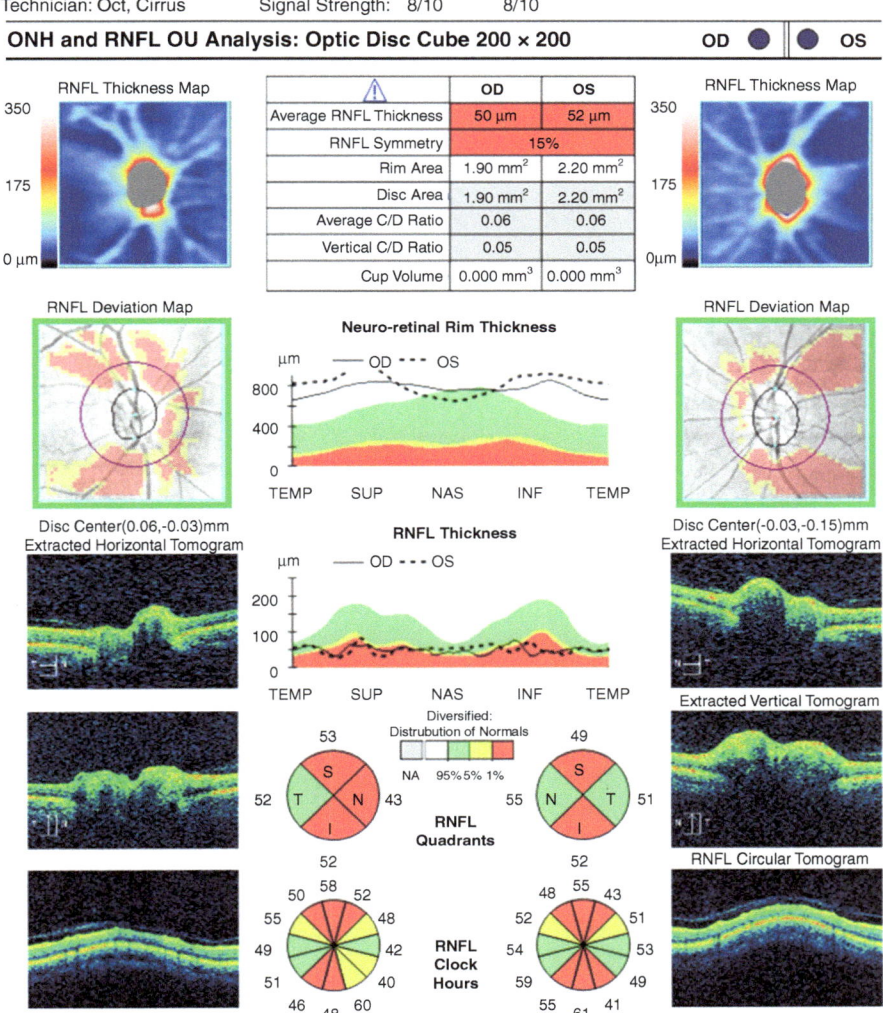

Fig. 8.51 (Cirrus HD-OCT) This is an interesting case of bilateral ONH drusen and high IOPs. The OCT scans are of high quality (SS = 8) and free of artifacts. The ONH parameters in both eyes are above the 95% prediction limits of the normative database. Although disc sizes are average, there is no cupping (cup volume = 0). RNFL analysis shows nearly end stage damage in both eyes with a very flat TSNIT graph

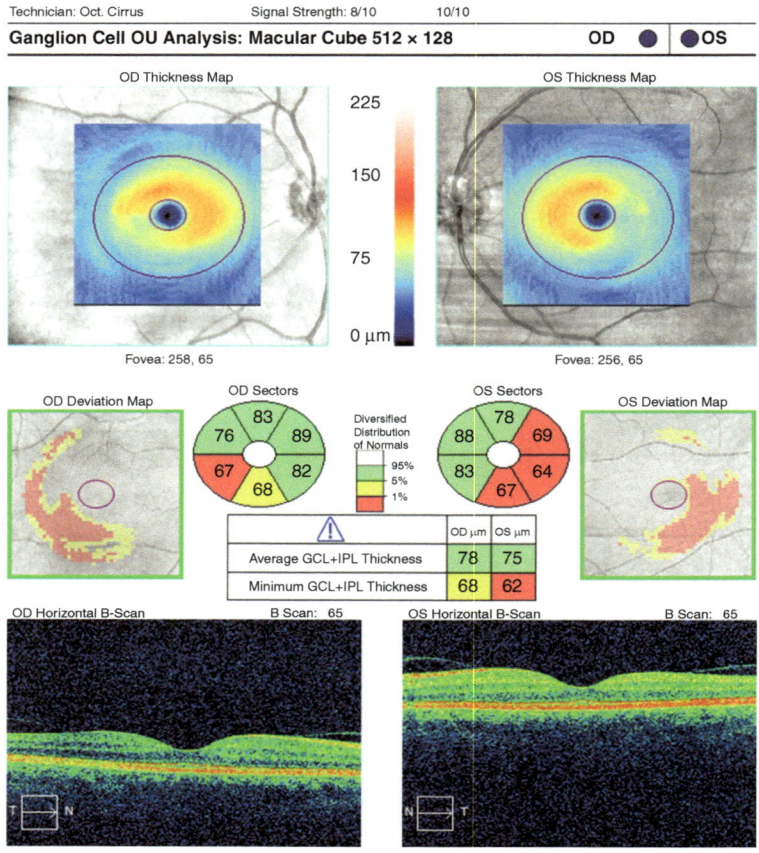

Fig. 8.52 (Cirrus HD-OCT) In contrast to the advanced RNFL damage report on previous OCT, macular Ganglion Cell Analysis reveals less severe changes in the macular area in both eyes

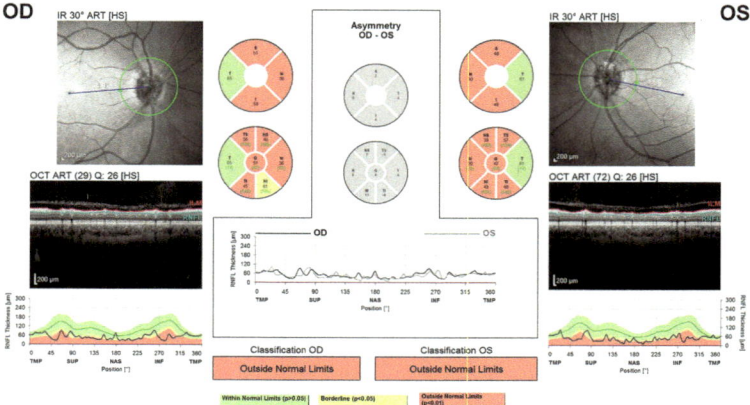

Fig. 8.53 (Spectralis OCT) Spectralis OCT demonstrates an advanced RNFL damage pattern similar to the Cirrus OCT

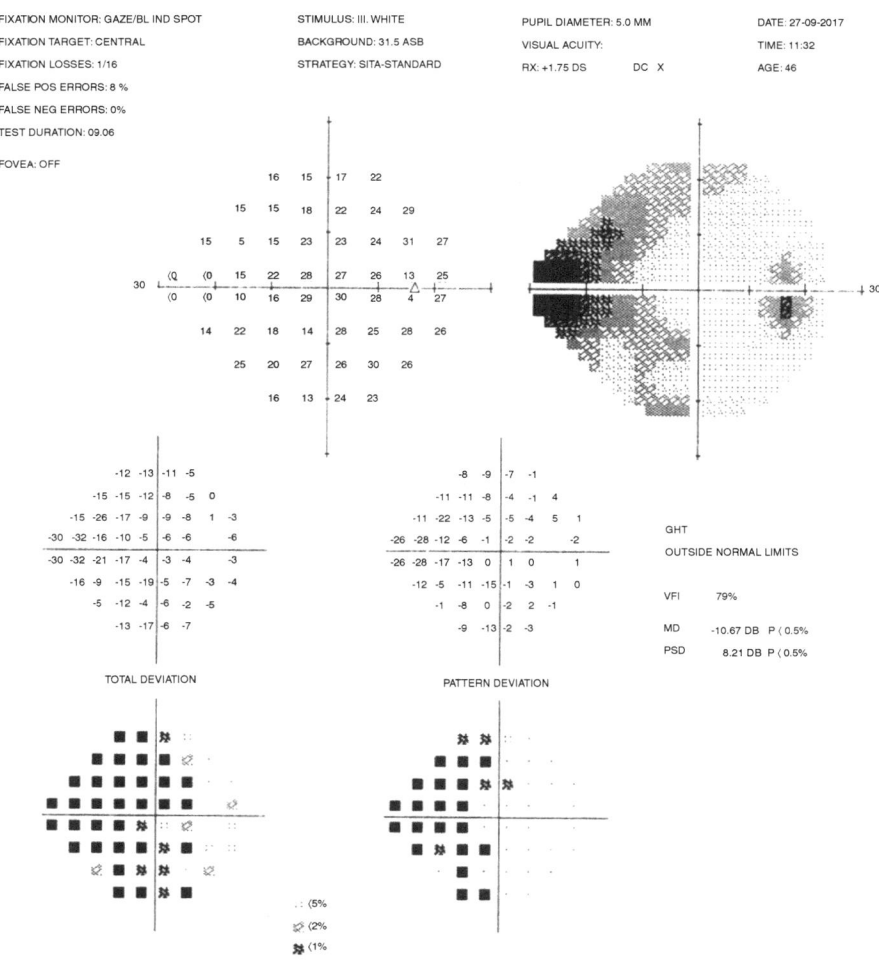

Fig. 8.54 (**a, b**) Visual field testing also reveals binasal defects in both eyes. As ONH drusen can cause various patterns of visual field loss and can be progressive, it is very difficult to discern accompanying damage due to glaucoma [19, 20]

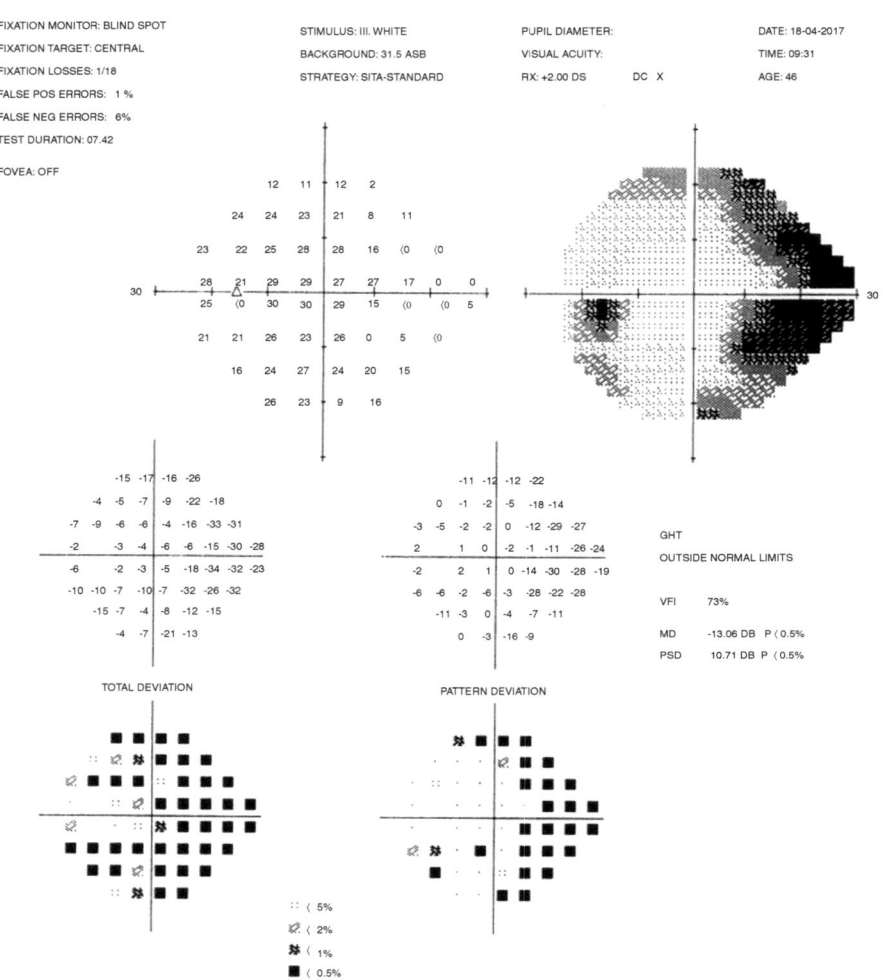

Fig. 8.54 (continued)

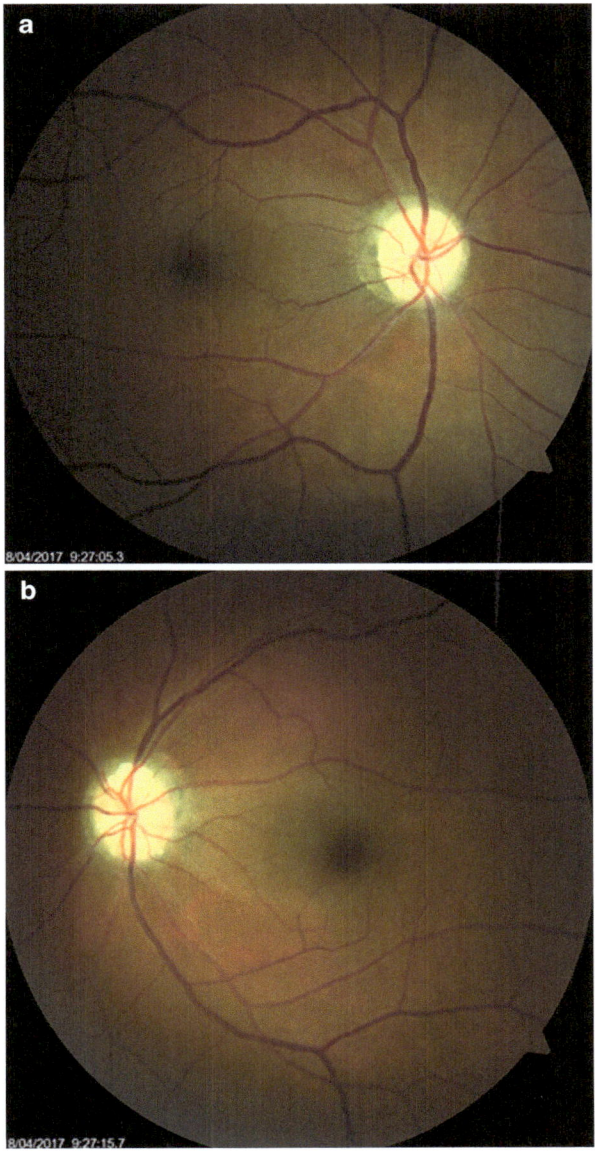

Fig. 8.55 (**a**, **b**) Color, (**c**, **d**) autofluorescence, and (**e**, **f**) red-free photographs of both eyes, showing the ONH drusen and RNFL bundle defects

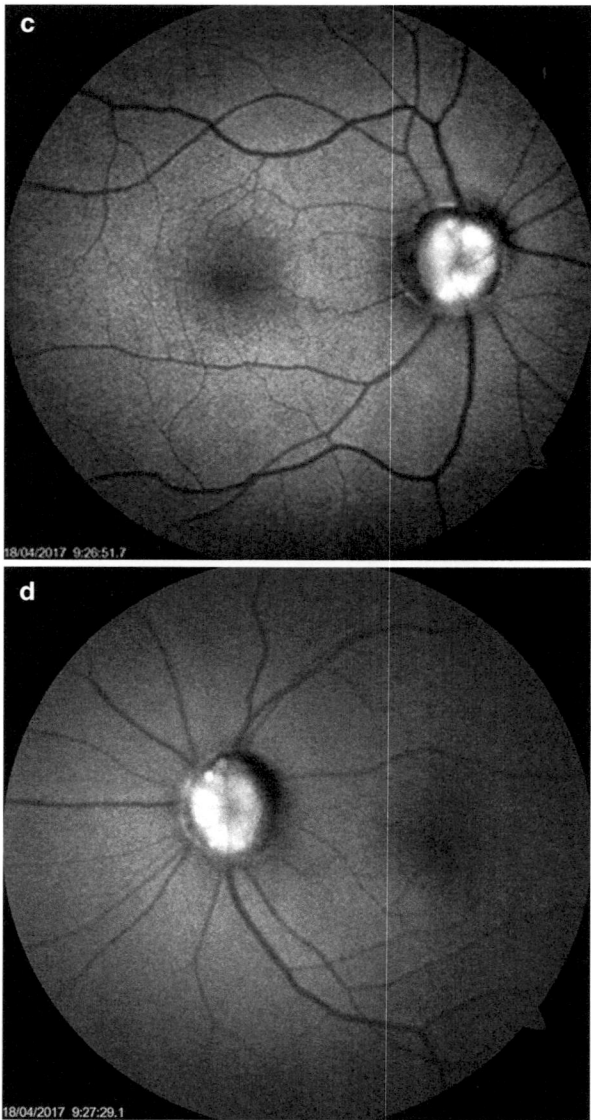

Fig. 8.55 (continued)

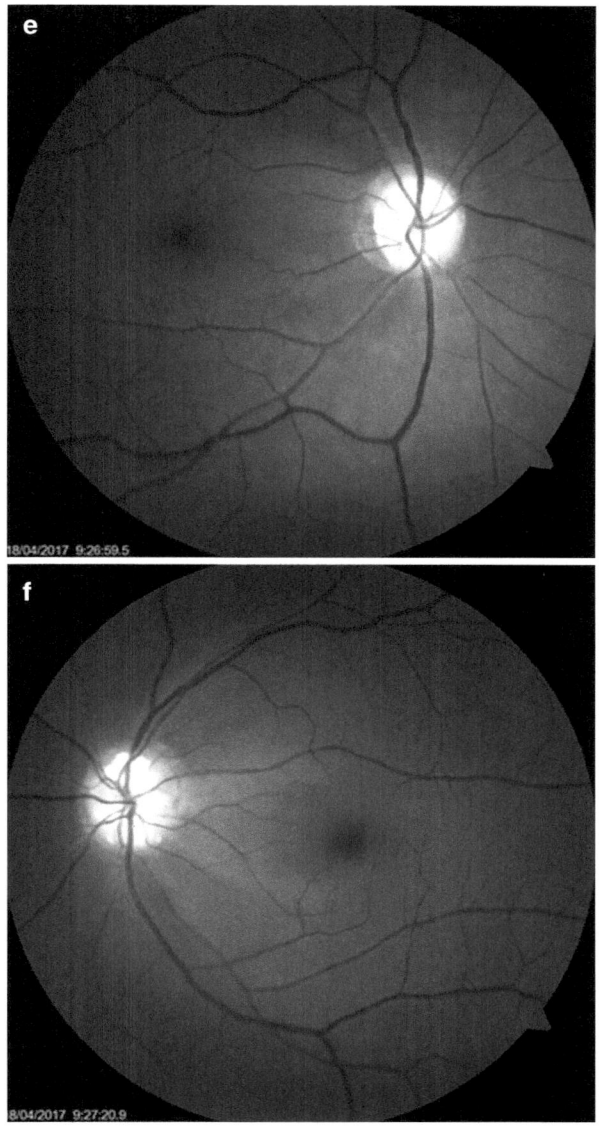

Fig. 8.55 (continued)

Conclusion: In eyes with other ONH pathologies such as ONH drusen, it can be very difficult to isolate the glaucomatous damage by structural or functional tests. Progression analysis can be helpful if the nonglaucomatous pathology is not progressive, but in the case presented above, it is well known that ONH drusen can cause progressive damage to the RNFL and visual fields similar to glaucoma [19, 20].

8.3.2.5 Other Green Disease Artifacts

In addition to above mentioned artifacts, green disease artifact can be caused by averaging in sectors that can hide a subtle notch in RNFL, or RNFL loss or notch in an eyes that started with high RNFL thickness that can lead to seemingly normal RNFL with suspected loss. Finally, RNFL can become thicker in eyes with uveitis possibly due to the RNFL edema and this can mask RNFL thinning [21].

References

1. Stein JD, Talwar N, Laverne AM, Nan B, Lichter PR. Trends in use of ancillary glaucoma tests for patients with open-angle glaucoma from 2001 to 2009. Ophthalmology. 2012;119:748–58.
2. Gabriele ML, Wollstein G, Ishikawa H, Kagemann L, Xu J, Folio LS, Schuman JS. Optical coherence tomography: history, current status, and laboratory work. Invest Ophthalmol Vis Sci. 2011;52:2425–36.
3. Dong ZM, Wollstein G, Schuman JS. Clinical utility of optical coherence tomography in glaucoma. Invest Ophthalmol Vis Sci. 2016;57:OCT556–67.
4. Asrani S, Essaid L, Alder BD, Santiago-Turla C. Artifacts in spectral-domain optical coherence tomography measurements in glaucoma. JAMA Ophthalmol. 2014;132:396–402.
5. Asrani S. Pitfalls in optical coherence tomography imaging. Glaucoma Today. 2016;(May/June):39–43.
6. Lee SY, Kwon HJ, Bae HW, Seo SJ, Lee YH, Hong S, Seong GJ, Kim CY. Frequency, type and cause of artifacts in swept-source and cirrus HD optical coherence tomography in cases of glaucoma and suspected glaucoma. Curr Eye Res. 2016;41:957–64.
7. Liu Y, Simavli H, Que CJ, Rizzo JL, Tsikata E, Maurer R, Chen TC. Patient characteristics associated with artifacts in spectralis optical coherence tomography imaging of the retinal nerve fiber layer in glaucoma. Am J Ophthalmol. 2015;159:565–76.
8. Chong GT, Lee RK. Glaucoma versus red disease: imaging and glaucoma diagnosis. Curr Opin Ophthalmol. 2012;23:79–88.
9. Sayed MS, Margolis M, Lee RK. Green disease in optical coherence tomography diagnosis of glaucoma. Curr Opin Ophthalmol. 2017;28:139–53.
10. Rao HL, Addepalli UK, Yadav RK, Senthil S, Choudhari NS, Garudadri CS. Effect of scan quality on diagnostic accuracy of spectral-domain optical coherence tomography in glaucoma. Am J Ophthalmol. 2014;157:719–27.
11. Huang J, Liu X, Wu Z, Sadda S. Image quality affects macular and retinal nerve fiber layer thickness measurements on fourier-domain optical coherence tomography. Ophthalmic Surg Lasers Imaging. 2011;42:216–21.
12. Russell DJ, Fallah S, Loer CJ, Riffenburgh RH. A comprehensive model for correcting RNFL readings of varying signal strengths in cirrus optical coherence tomography. Invest Ophthalmol Vis Sci. 2014;55:7297–302.
13. Colen TP, Lemij HG. Prevalence of split nerve fiber layer bundles in healthy eyes imaged with scanning laser polarimetry. Ophthalmology. 2001;108:151–6.
14. Kaliner E, Cohen MJ, Miron H, Kogan M, Blumenthal EZ. Retinal nerve fiber layer split bundles are true anatomic variants. Ophthalmology. 2007;114:2259–64.
15. Hong SW, Ahn MD, Kang SH, Im SK. Analysis of peripapillary retinal nerve fiber distribution in normal young adults. Invest Ophthalmol Vis Sci. 2010;51:3515–23.
16. Hood DC, Salant JA, Arthur SN, Ritch R, Liebmann JM. The location of the inferior and superior temporal blood vessels and interindividual variability of the retinal nerve fiber layer thickness. J Glaucoma. 2010;19:158–66.

17. Hwang YH, Kim YY, Kim HK, Sohn YH. Effect of peripapillary retinoschisis on retinal nerve fibre layer thickness measurement in glaucomatous eyes. Br J Ophthalmol. 2014;98:669–74.
18. Bayraktar S, Cebeci Z, Kabaalioglu M, Ciloglu S, Kir N, Izgi B. Peripapillary retinoschisis in glaucoma patients. J Ophthalmol. 2016;2016:1612720.
19. Savino PJ, Glaser JS, Rosenberg MA. A clinical analysis of pseudopapilledema. II. Visual field defects. Arch Ophthalmol. 1979;97:71–5.
20. Roh S, Noecker RJ, Schuman JS, Hedges TR, Weiter JJ, Mattox C. Effect of optic nerve head drusen on nerve fiber layer thickness. Ophthalmology. 1998;105:878–85.
21. Moore DB, Jaffe GJ, Asrani S. Retinal nerve fiber layer thickness measurements: uveitis, a major confounding factor. Ophthalmology. 2015;122:511–7.

Chapter 9
Optical Coherence Tomography in Non-Glaucomatous Optic Neuropathies

Ahmet Akman and Sirel Gür Güngör

9.1 Introduction

Non-glaucomatous optic neuropathies and a few other ocular conditions that can mimic glaucomatous optic neuropathy are called glaucoma masqueraders [1, 2]. These include ischemic optic neuropathy, optic neuritis, and degenerative diseases such as Alzheimer's and Parkinson's disease [3–5]. Retinal nerve fiber layer (RNFL) loss is a common denominator in these ailments and optical coherence tomography (OCT) findings can be confusing even to an experienced reader. The pattern of RNFL and macular ganglion cell loss and optic nerve head (ONH) topography findings on OCT scans may provide clues on differential diagnosis of these optic neuropathies. Presence or absence of ONH cupping is one of the most important findings for differential diagnosis. In eyes with RNFL and macular ganglion cell loss, absence of cupping and presence of pallor at the level of the ONH indicates a non-glaucomatous optic neuropathy. On the other hand, presence of cupping especially in eyes diagnosed as normal tension glaucoma may conceal an ischemic, hereditary or compressive pathology. In addition to OCT and clinical ONH findings, a careful clinical examination including visual acuity, color vision, pupillary light reflex and visual field (VF) testing is important for differential diagnosis.

This chapter provides a summary of the most common causes of non-glaucomatous RNFL and macular ganglion cell loss. Many other neuro-ophthalmological pathologies may also cause similar OCT findings, but most of them are rare diseases, which are beyond the scope of this book.

A. Akman (✉) · S. Gür Güngör
Department of Ophthalmology, School of Medicine, Başkent University, Ankara, Turkey

© Springer International Publishing AG, part of Springer Nature 2018   161
A. Akman et al. (eds.), *Optical Coherence Tomography in Glaucoma*,
https://doi.org/10.1007/978-3-319-94905-5_9

9.2   Common Pathologies That Can Mimic Glaucoma on OCT

9.2.1   Anterior Ischemic Optic Neuropathy

Anterior ischemic optic neuropathy (AION) is the most common acute optic neuropathy in patients over the age of 50 years. It is also the second most common cause of permanent optic nerve-related visual loss in adults after glaucoma [6]. Occasionally, patients with AION do not notice any loss of vision and, optic nerve pallor associated with an afferent pupillary defect and VF loss may be noted incidentally on clinical examination.

ONH edema is present in early stages of the disease. After a few months, ONH edema subsides leaving a pale optic disc. On OCT RNFL exam, the superior quadrant is the most commonly affected quadrant followed by the inferior, temporal and nasal quadrants. According to this loss pattern, inferior altitudinal VF defects are the most common defects observed in eyes with AION [7].

ONH cupping similar to that of glaucomatous cupping can be seen in cases of AION related to temporal arteritis [8]. On the other hand, shallow enlargement of the optic cup can be present in some of the eyes with nonarteritic AION [8]. In general, OCT patterns of RNFL thinning in AION may mimic those in glaucoma; however, the clinical history, normal IOP levels and lack of concordance between the degree of cupping and the RNFL loss/VF defects should be helpful in differential diagnosis of these two disorders.

9.2.1.1   Sample Case: Nonarteritic Anterior Ischemic Optic Neuropathy

A 76-year old female patient, with a history of nonarteritic AION, was monitored for two years. The following are the OCT and optical coherence tomography angiography (OCTA), VF reports and fundus images of the patient (Figs. 9.1, 9.2, 9.3, 9.4, 9.5 and 9.6).

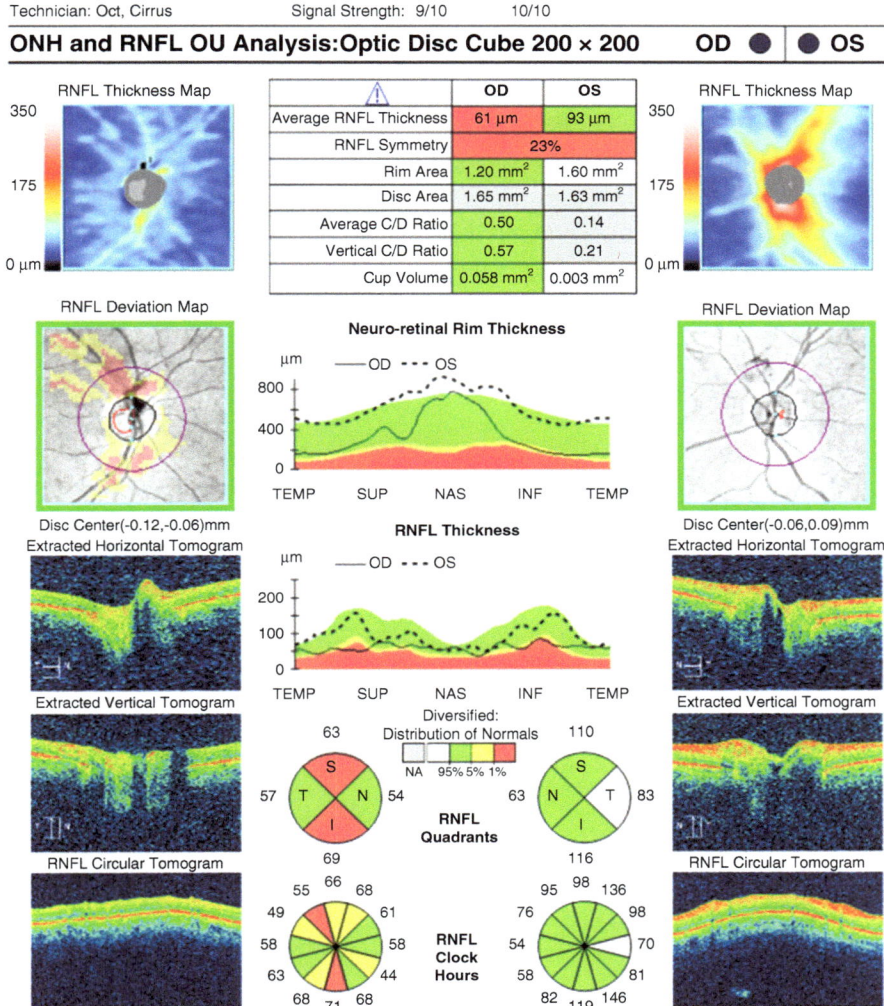

Fig. 9.1 (Cirrus HD-OCT) Peripapillary OCT scan shows significant RNFL loss in all maps and plots in the right eye. In addition, although the extracted vertical and horizontal tomograms do not show deep cupping, ONH analysis software of the Cirrus HD-OCT measured a vertical C/D ratio of 0.5. The only clue for the possibility of non-glaucomatous optic neuropathy is the small size of the optic disc and presence of a very shallow cup in the right eye. In a glaucomatous eye with this degree of RNFL loss, we would expect to see deeper excavation in the extracted tomograms. Also, the left eye has no cup at all, which is a common finding in small crowded discs

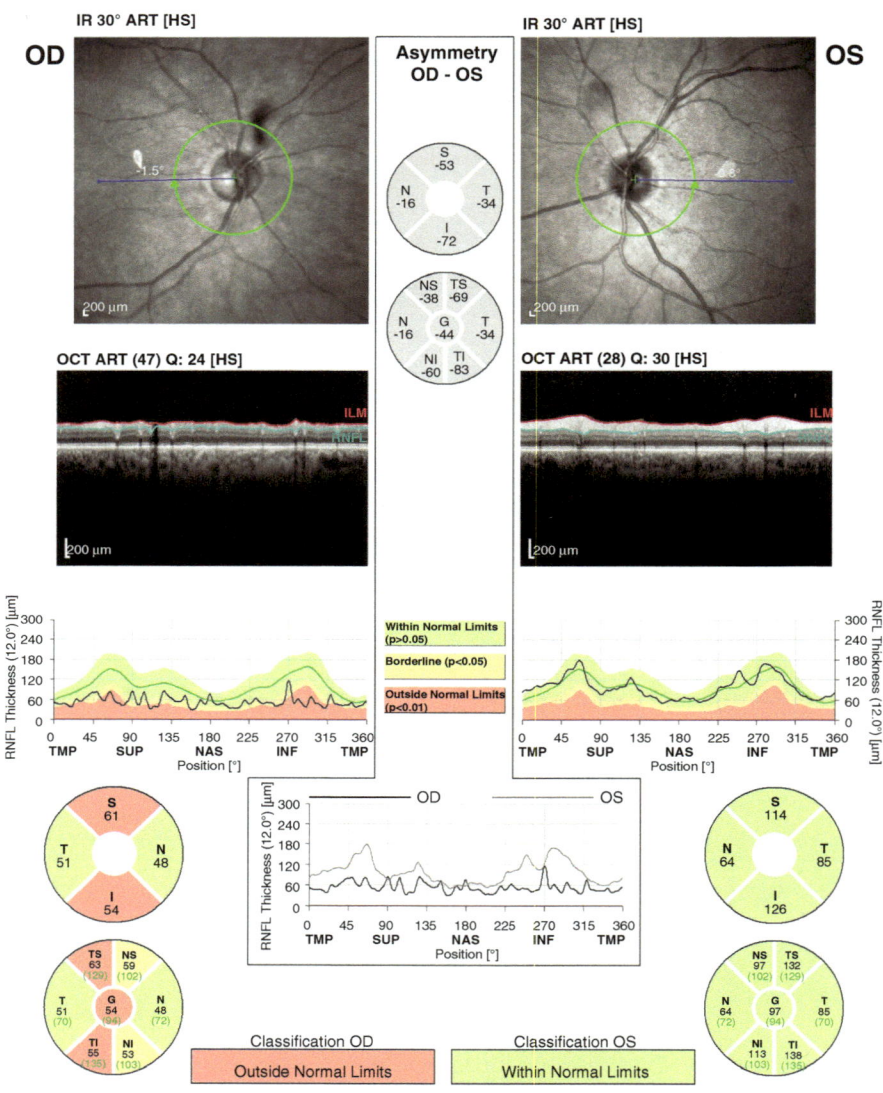

Fig. 9.2 (Spectralis OCT) Similar to Cirrus-HD OCT exam, Spectralis OCT printout shows RNFL loss in the right eye but, as there is no ONH data available in this report of Spectralis OCT, it is very difficult to make a differential diagnosis from this report. If available, ONH analysis of the Spectralis GMPE software may be helpful as it gives a detailed report about the ONH topography

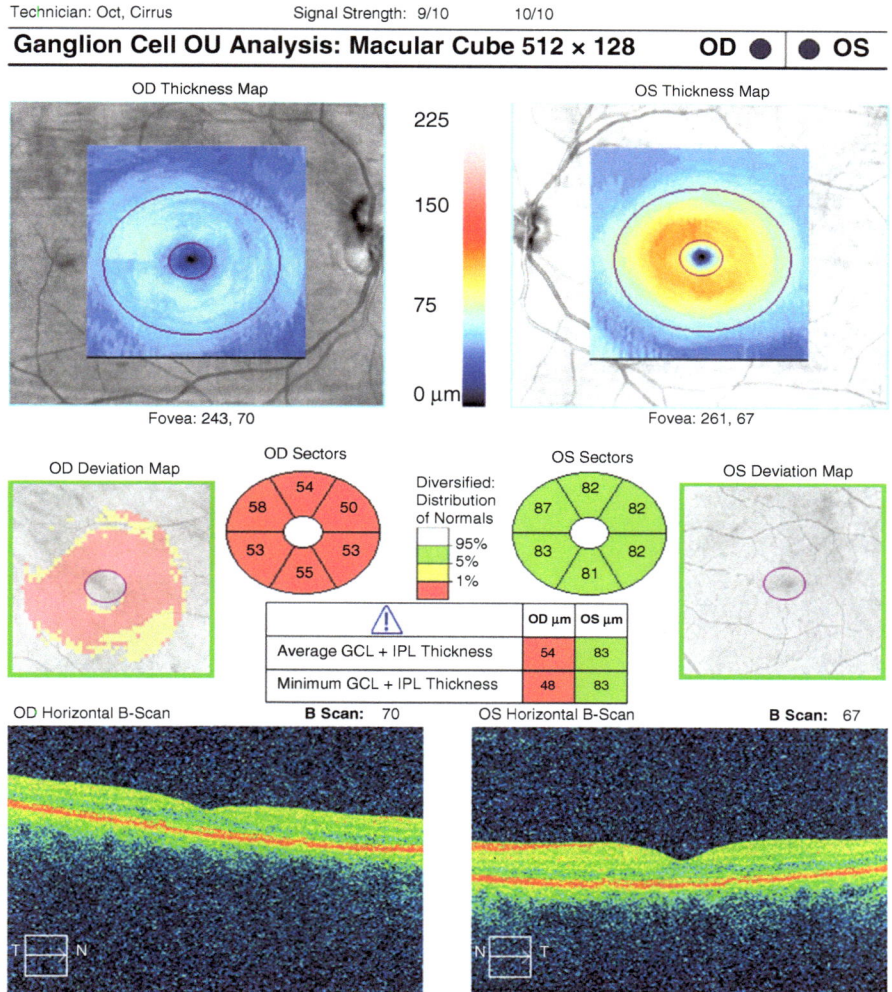

Fig. 9.3 (Cirrus HD-OCT) The macular Ganglion Cell Analysis report shows diffuse GCL + IPL loss in the right eye. There is no clue for differentiating between glaucomatous vs. non-glaucomatous GCL + IPL loss

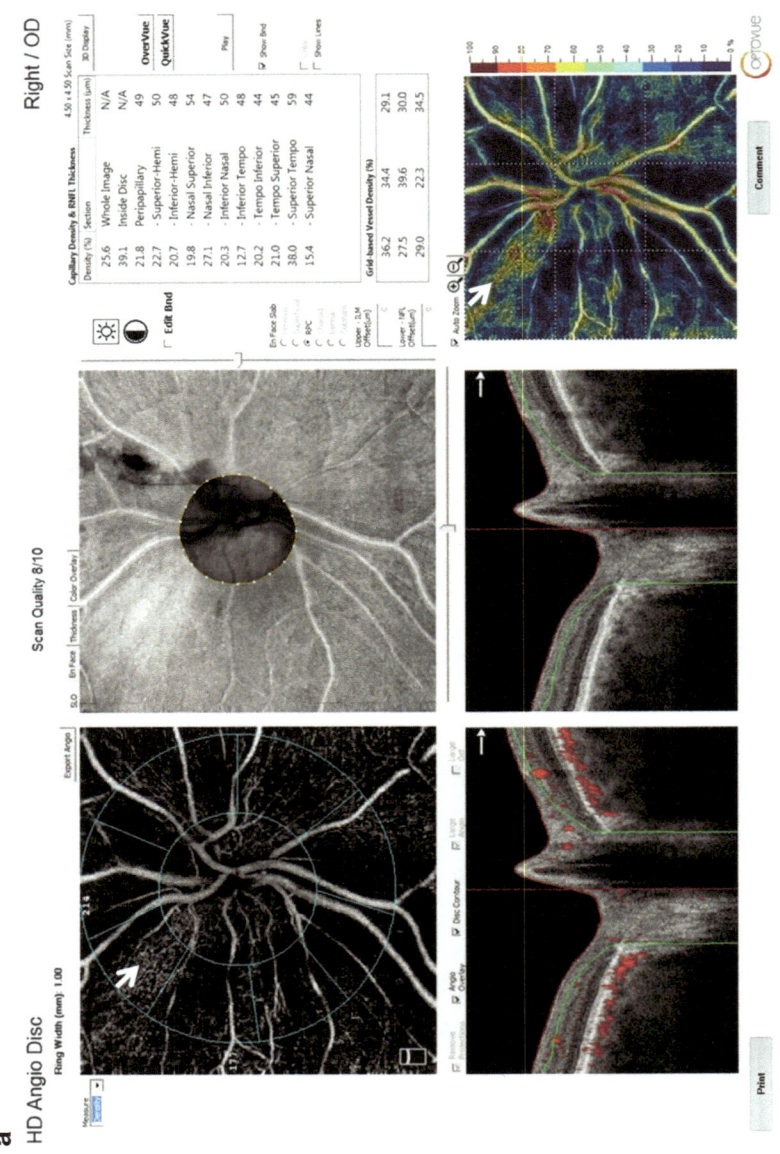

Fig. 9.4 (Optovue, AngioVue) (**a**) OCTA of the right optic nerve shows significant capillary loss in and around the ONH. Only a small sector in the superior temporal quadrant has a 38% capillary density and capillary perfusion (white arrowheads). Possibly, this is the only non-affected sector in the right ONH which is consistent with the spared VF area in the inferior hemifield of the right eye (see Fig. 9.5a) (**b**) The left eye has normal capillary perfusion in and around the ONH

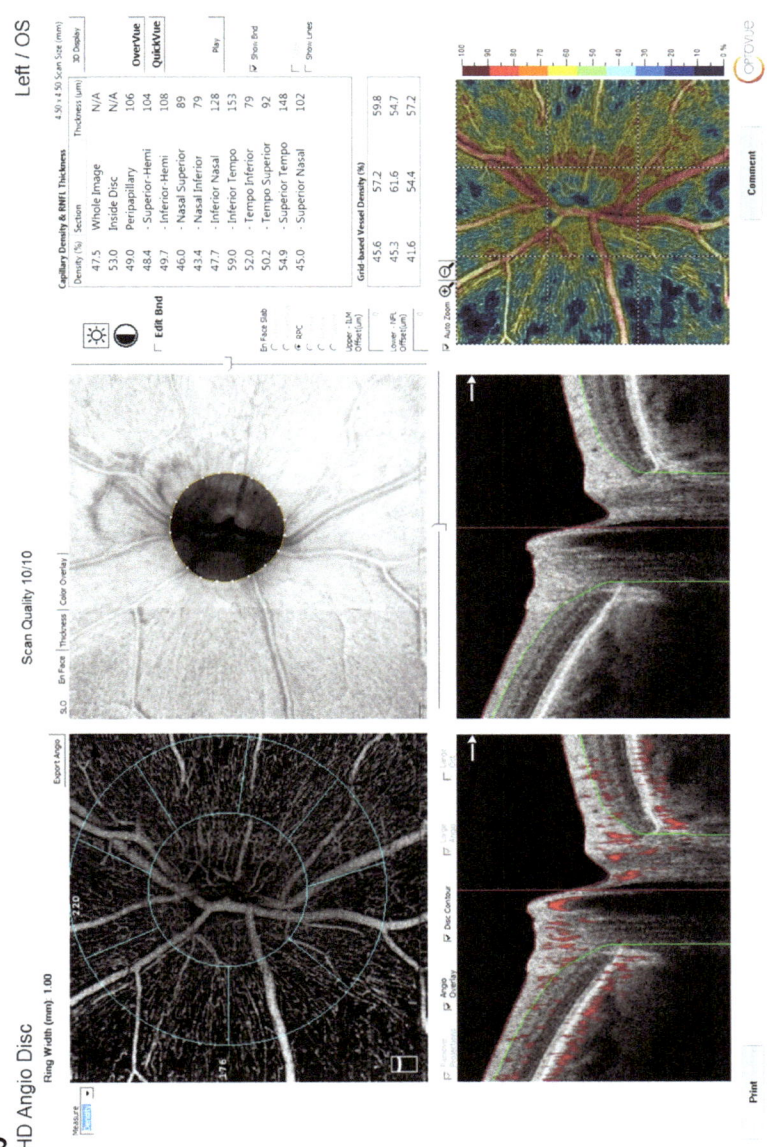

Fig. 9.4 (continued)

168   A. Akman and S. Gür Güngör

a

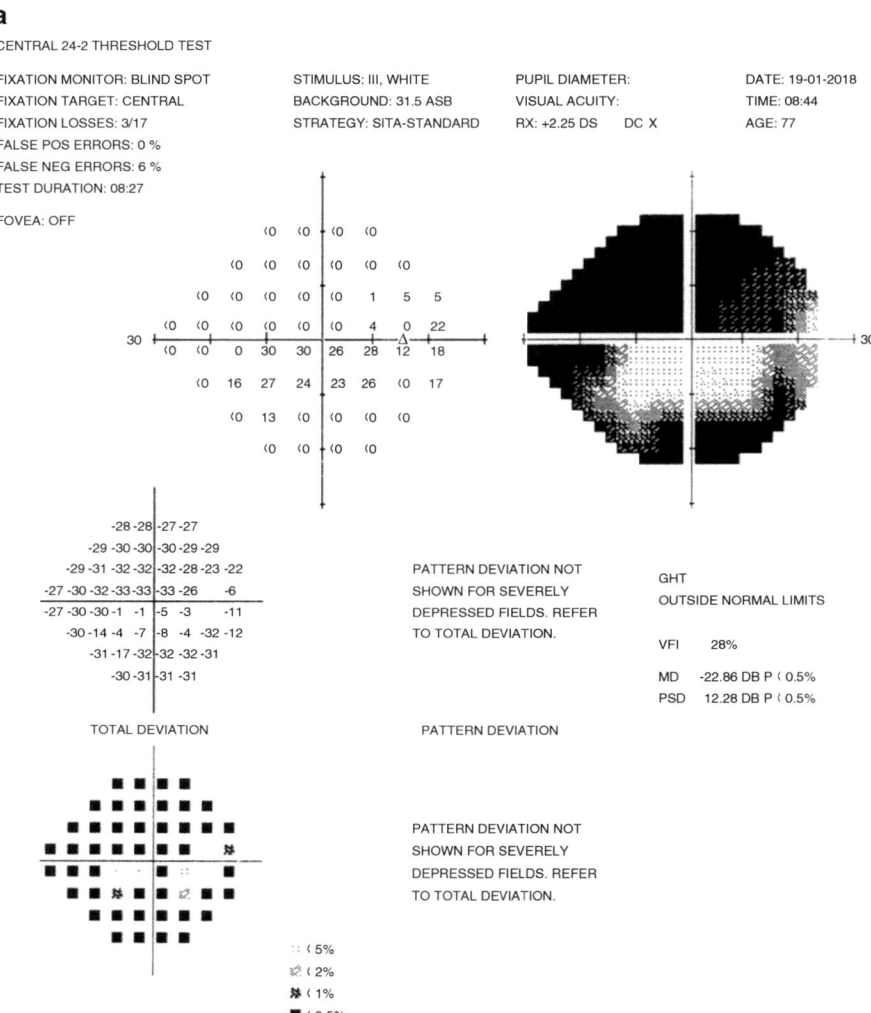

CENTRAL 24-2 THRESHOLD TEST

FIXATION MONITOR: BLIND SPOT   STIMULUS: III, WHITE   PUPIL DIAMETER: DATE: 19-01-2018
FIXATION TARGET: CENTRAL   BACKGROUND: 31.5 ASB   VISUAL ACUITY: TIME: 08:44
FIXATION LOSSES: 3/17   STRATEGY: SITA-STANDARD   RX: +2.25 DS   DC X   AGE: 77
FALSE POS ERRORS: 0 %
FALSE NEG ERRORS: 6 %
TEST DURATION: 08:27

FOVEA: OFF

PATTERN DEVIATION NOT
SHOWN FOR SEVERELY
DEPRESSED FIELDS. REFER
TO TOTAL DEVIATION.

GHT
OUTSIDE NORMAL LIMITS

VFI   28%

MD   -22.86 DB P (0.5%
PSD   12.28 DB P (0.5%

TOTAL DEVIATION   PATTERN DEVIATION

PATTERN DEVIATION NOT
SHOWN FOR SEVERELY
DEPRESSED FIELDS. REFER
TO TOTAL DEVIATION.

∷ (5%
⦰ (2%
⧣ (1%
■ (0.5%

Fig. 9.5 Humphrey VF test report of the above patient with nonarteritic ischemic anterior optic neuropathy in the right eye. (**a**) The right eye is severely affected with only a central region in the inferior hemifield spared. (**b**) The left eye has a normal VF

b

CENTRAL 24-2 THRESHOLD TEST

FIXATION MONITOR: BLIND SPOT   STIMULUS: III, WHITE   PUPIL DIAMETER: DATE: 19-01-2018
FIXATION TARGET: CENTRAL   BACKGROUND: 31.5 ASB   VISUAL ACUITY: TIME: 08:53
FIXATION LOSSES: 0/15   STRATEGY: SITA-STANDARD   RX: +2.50 DS   DC X   AGE: 77
FALSE POS ERRORS: 10 %
FALSE NEG ERRORS: 13 %
TEST DURATION: 07:13

FOVEA: OFF

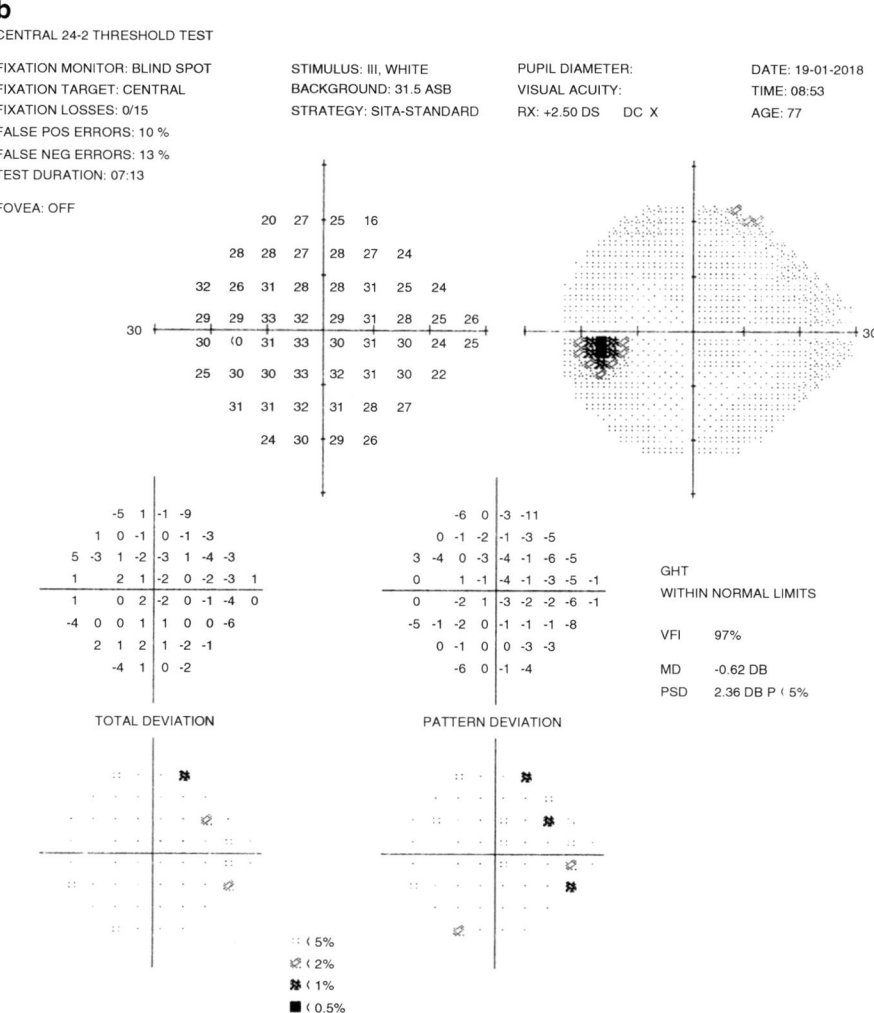

TOTAL DEVIATION   PATTERN DEVIATION

```
      -5   1 | -1  -9                        -6   0 | -3 -11
    1   0  -1 |  0  -1  -3                  0  -1  -2 | -1  -3  -5
  5  -3   1  -2 | -3   1  -4  -3          3  -4   0  -3 | -4  -1  -6  -5
  1       2   1 | -2   0  -2  -3   1      0       1  -1 | -4  -1  -3  -5  -1
  1       0   2 | -2   0  -1  -4   0      0      -2   1 | -3  -2  -2  -6  -1
 -4   0   0   1 |  1   0   0  -6         -5  -1  -2   0 | -1  -1  -1  -8
    2   1   2 |  1  -2  -1                  0  -1   0 |  0  -3  -3
      -4   1 |  0  -2                        -6   0 | -1  -4
```

GHT
WITHIN NORMAL LIMITS

VFI   97%

MD   -0.62 DB
PSD   2.36 DB P (5%

:: (5%
▨ (2%
✺ (1%
■ (0.5%

Fig. 9.5 (continued)

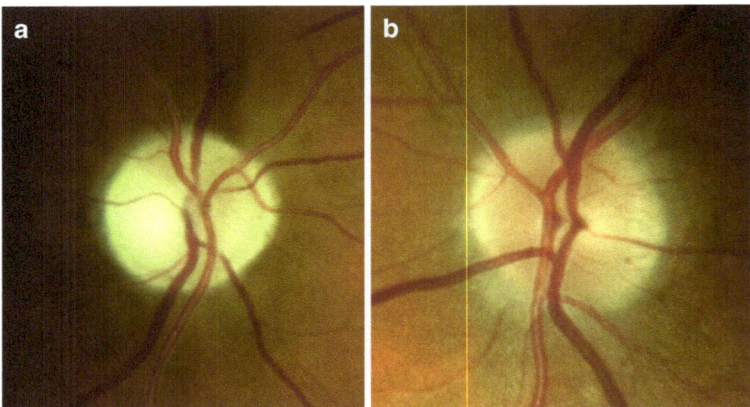

Fig. 9.6 (**a**) ONH photograph of the right eye shows pallor with shallow cupping. (**b**) ONH photograph of the left eye shows a small crowded ONH without any cupping

Conclusion: Although the peripapillary RNFL test results of Cirrus and Spectralis OCT devices show RNFL loss that can be mistaken for glaucomatous damage, the shallow ONH cupping, OCTA results, pattern of VF loss and fundus image of the right eye displaying ONH pallor not corresponding to the degree of cupping help the clinician in the diagnosis of AION.

9.2.2   Optic Neuritis and Multiple Sclerosis

Normal appearing or swollen ONH, associated with loss of vision, afferent pupillary defect and color perception deficit may be present on the initial exam in acute optic neuritis. With resolution of the acute attack, there may be pallor at the ONH associated with RNFL thinning, which may be detected with OCT.

Similar to glaucomatous optic atrophy, RNFL thinning can be observed in patients with multiple sclerosis, with or without a history of optic neuritis [9]. The temporal peripapillary quadrant is more prominently affected in patients with optic neuritis [9]. Subclinical RNFL thinning in patients with multiple sclerosis without optic neuritis has been reported [10, 11].

9.2.2.1   Sample Case: Optic Neuritis

A 43-year old woman with multiple sclerosis developed acute left visual loss clinically consistent with retrobulbar optic neuritis three years ago. Visual acuity was 20/20 in the right eye and hand motions in the left eye on presentation. The patient responded to a five-day course of 1000 mg intravenous methyl-prednisone treatment, with her visual acuity returning to 20/25 in the left eye. In her last visit, three years after the optic neuritis attack, her visual acuity was 20/20 in the right eye and 20/25 in the left eye. Following are the current OCT reports and the ONH photographs of the patient (Figs. 9.7, 9.8 and 9.9).

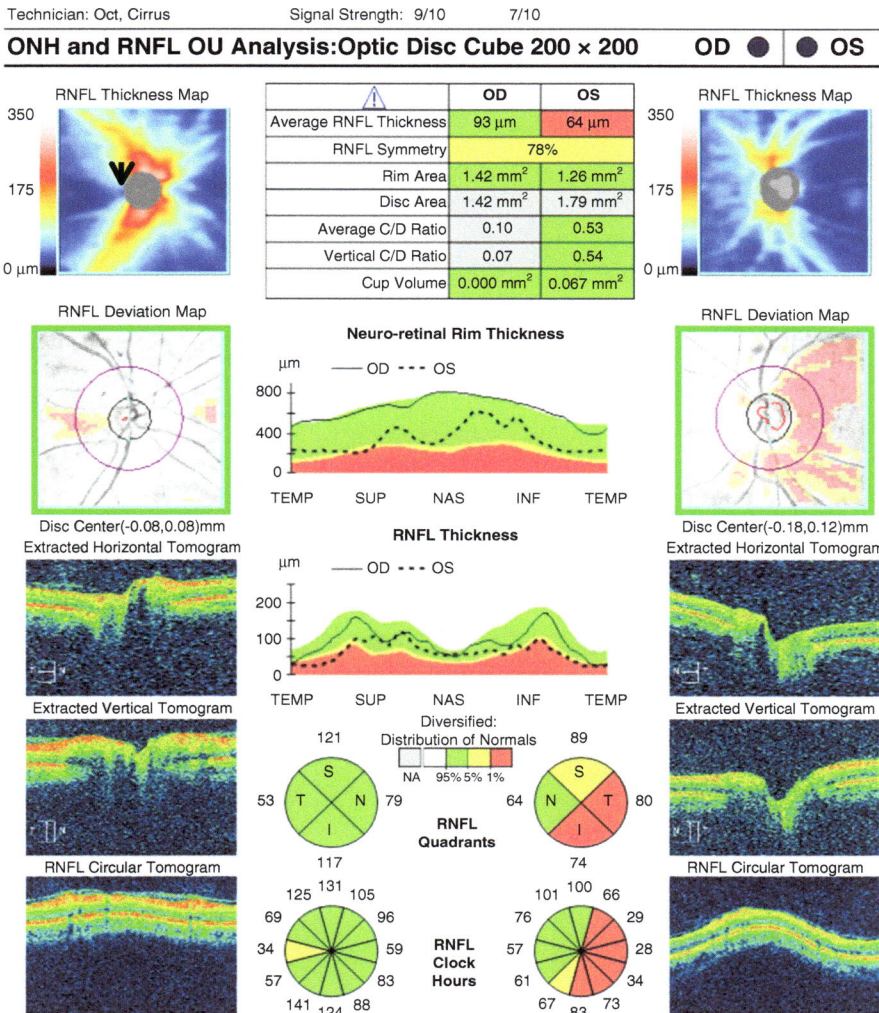

Fig. 9.7 (Cirrus HD-OCT) Peripapillary OCT scan three years after optic neuritis attack in the left eye, shows significant RNFL loss in temporal quadrant of this eye. The average cup to disc ratio is 0.53, which is not consistent with the level of RNFL loss if glaucoma were present. This is the first clue for non-glaucomatous RNFL loss. The second clue is the degree of RNFL loss in the temporal quadrant; in most glaucoma patients, inferior and superior quadrants tend to demonstrate the highest degree of damage and the temporal quadrant is spared until later stages of the disease. In this patient's RNFL deviation map of the left eye, the entire temporal quadrant demonstrates significant RNFL thinning. The RNFL thickness map of the right eye, which had no history of any ocular problems, displays a wedge-shaped area of RNFL thinning on the temporal side of the disc (black arrowhead). This area is also flagged in the RNFL deviation map. In the clock-hour pie graph, the 9 o'clock sector shows some thinning

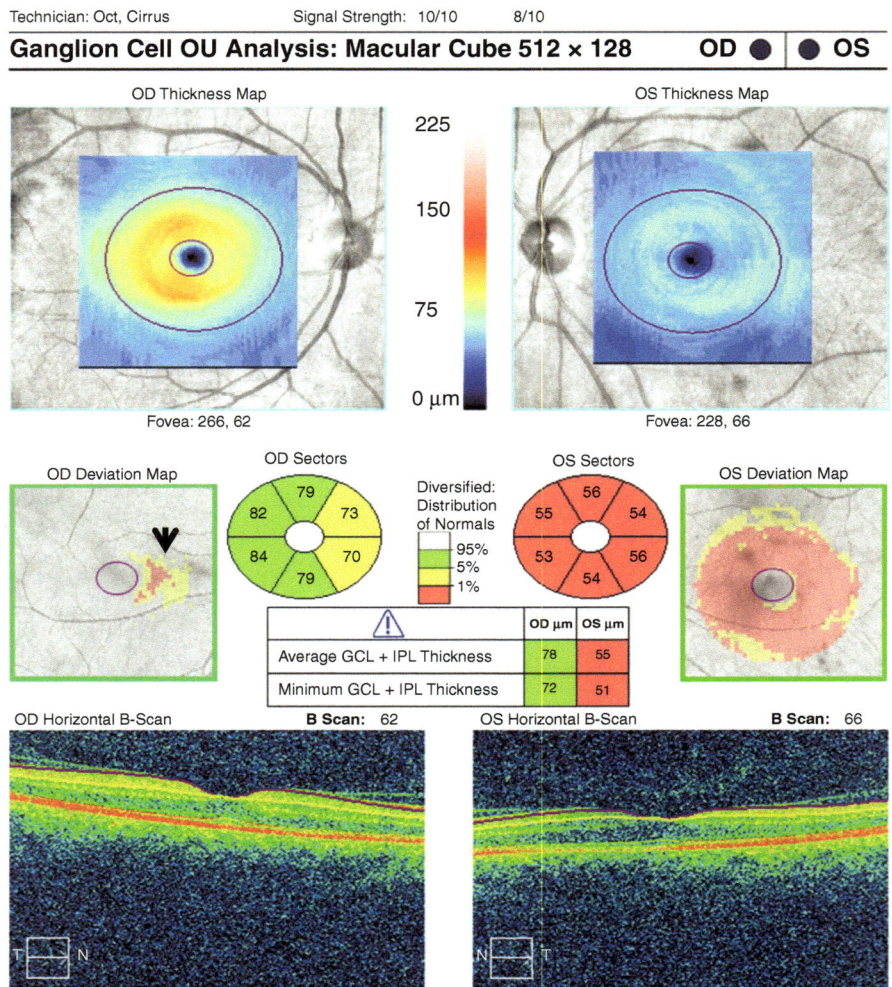

Fig. 9.8 (Cirrus HD-OCT) Macular Ganglion Cell Analysis shows significant GCL + IPL loss in the left macula, which is compatible with the peripapillary RNFL loss. GCL + IPL deviation map of the right eye also shows an area of thinning on the nasal side of the fovea, which is compatible with the wedge shaped thin RNFL area in the temporal quadrant in Fig. 9.7 (black arrowhead)

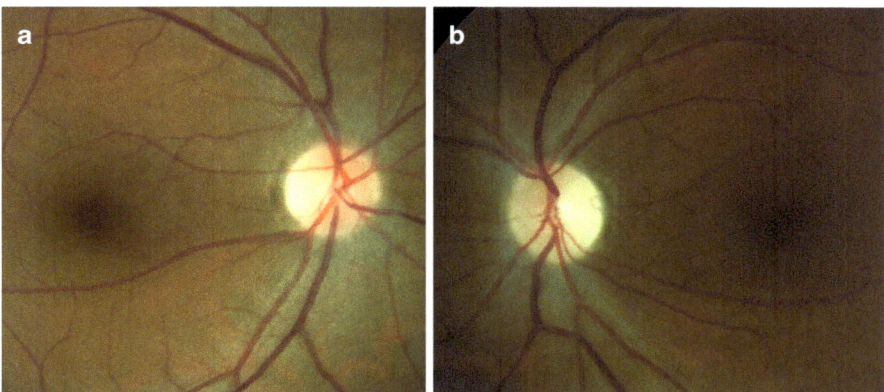

Fig. 9.9 Color disc photographs of the patient. (**a**) Note the pallor of the temporal aspect of the optic disc in the right eye. (**b**) The left disc shows temporal pallor without significant cupping

Conclusion: Similar to AION, optic neuritis causes RNFL loss without significant cupping, which is evident in the left eye of this patient. The pattern of RNFL loss, is the second clue on the peripapillary OCT scan. In contrast to glaucomatous RNFL loss, which is more concentrated in the inferior and superior quadrants, RNFL loss in optic neuritis and multiple sclerosis is more diffuse in all four quadrants with a strong propensity for the temporal quadrant [9]. ONH exam and photographs are also helpful for differential diagnosis of this patient's RNFL loss. The third interesting point in this patient is the RNFL defect extending from temporal part of the disc to the macula in the right eye. As there is no history of optic neuritis in the right eye, the first possibility is a previous, mild, subclinical optic neuritis attack in the right eye and the second possibility is subclinical RNFL thinning seen in patients with multiple sclerosis without optic neuritis.

9.2.3 Neuromyelitis Optica (Devic's Disease)

Optic neuritis and acute myelitis characterize neuromyelitis optica (NMO). The visual and neurological prognoses in NMO are poorer than in multiple sclerosis. In patients with NMO, the episodes of optic neuritis tend to recur, with severe visual impairment in at least one eye. Optic nerve pallor is common in these patients. RNFL loss in NMO is more severe than eyes with multiple sclerosis-associated optic neuritis [12, 13]. Unlike glaucomatous optic neuropathies, central vision is significantly affected in NMO.

9.2.3.1 Sample Case: Neuromyelitis Optica (Devic's Disease)

A 25-year old female was admitted to our clinic with complaints of visual impairment in her left eye in 2016. BCVA was 20/20 in the right eye and light perception in the left eye. Intravenous methyl-prednisolone was administered for seven days without any visual improvement in the left eye. She was diagnosed as NMO based on the clinical findings and serologic tests. The following are the OCT printouts at the presentation and during the follow-up (Figs. 9.10, 9.11, 9.12, 9.13, 9.14 and 9.15).

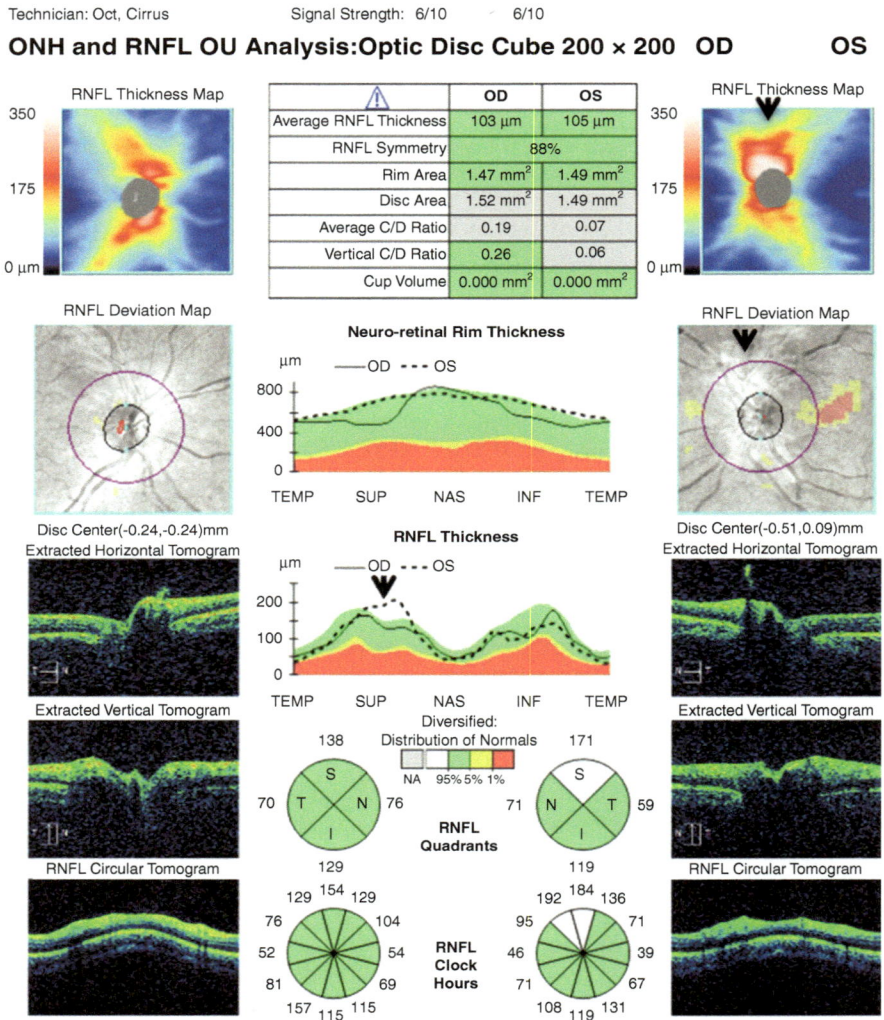

Fig. 9.10 (Cirrus HD-OCT) Peripapillary OCT report at the time of an acute left optic neuritis attack in 2016. ONH edema and RNFL thickening was present in the superior quadrant of the left ONH (black arrowheads)

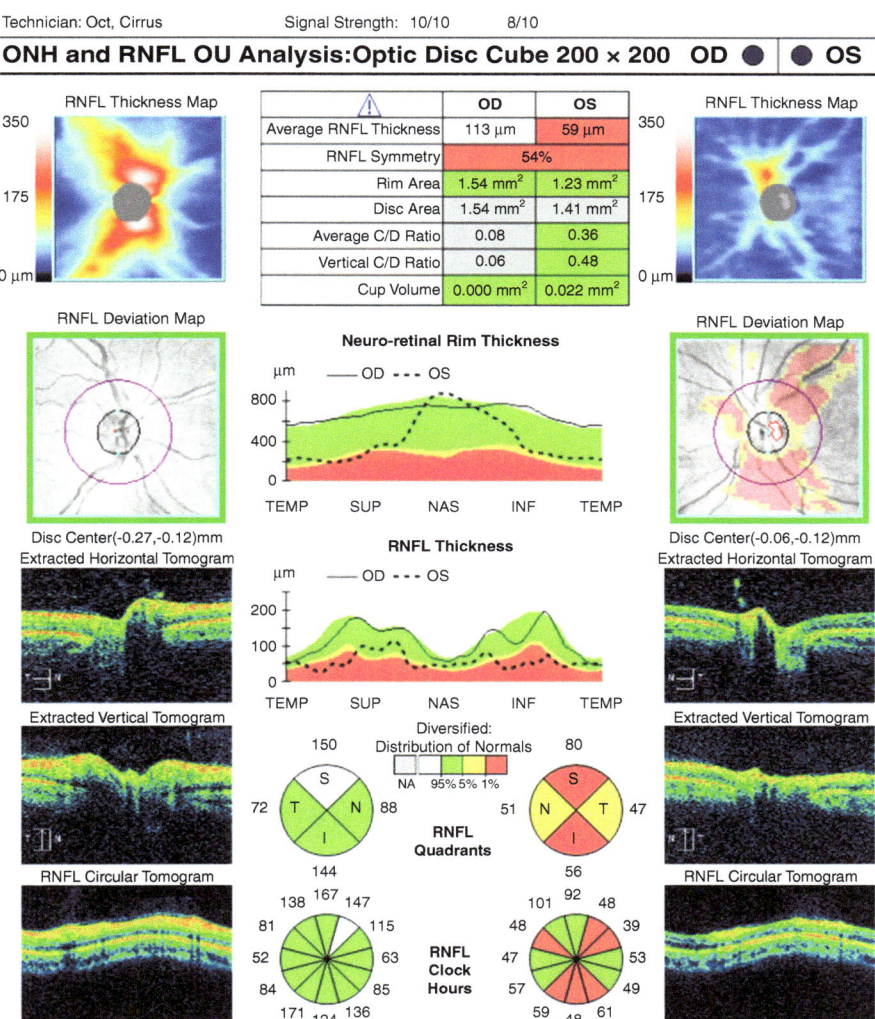

Fig. 9.11 (Cirrus HD-OCT) 1 year after the optic neuritis attack, the left eye revealed significant thinning of the RNFL, but there is no cupping in the extracted tomograms. RNFL of the right eye measured thicker in the current OCT when compared to one year earlier (Fig. 9.10). The difference with the previous OCT in the right eye is possibly related to the better quality of the current OCT, as RNFL thickness measurements increase with better signal strength which increased from 6 to 10 in this OCT

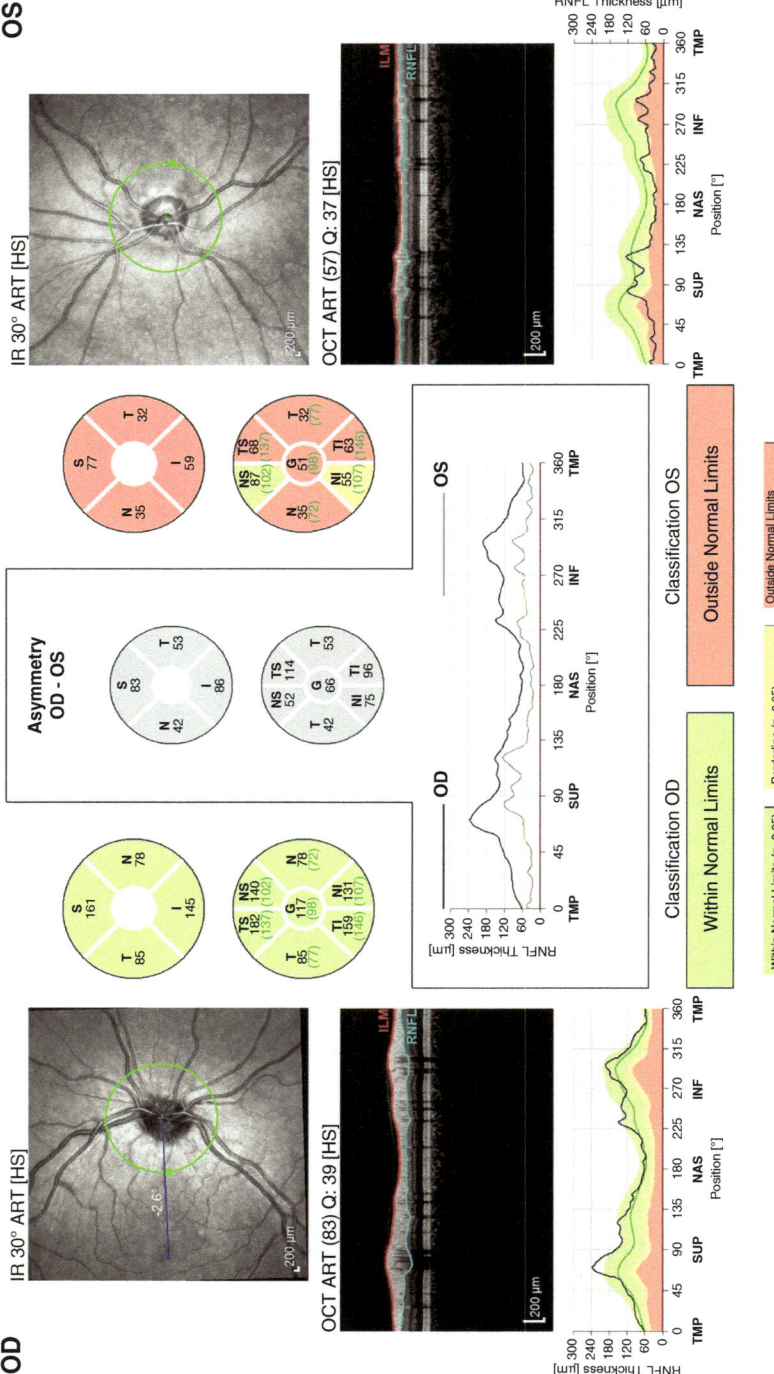

Fig. 9.12 (Spectralis OCT) Severe RNFL loss is present in the left eye. As there is no ONH data in this Spectralis printout, it is not possible to differentiate this type of RNFL loss from the glaucomatous optic neuropathy

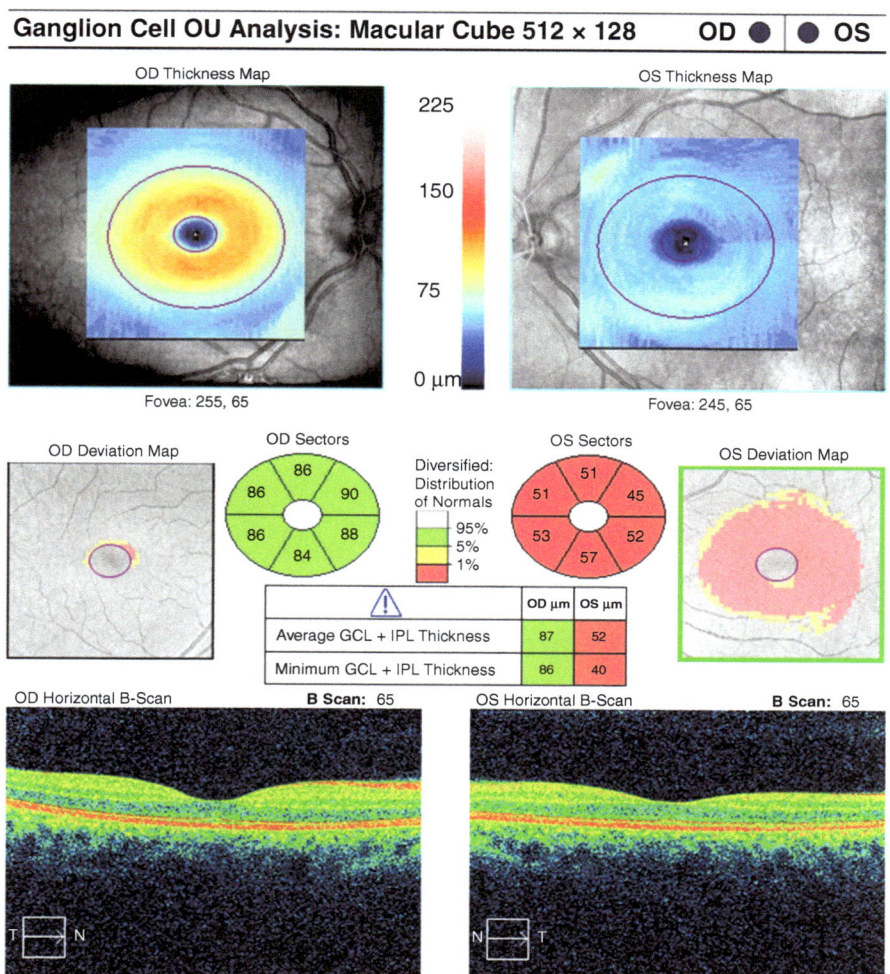

Fig. 9.13 (Cirrus HD-OCT) Macular Ganglion Cell Analysis shows significant GCL + IPL loss in the left eye, which is compatible with the peripapillary RNFL loss

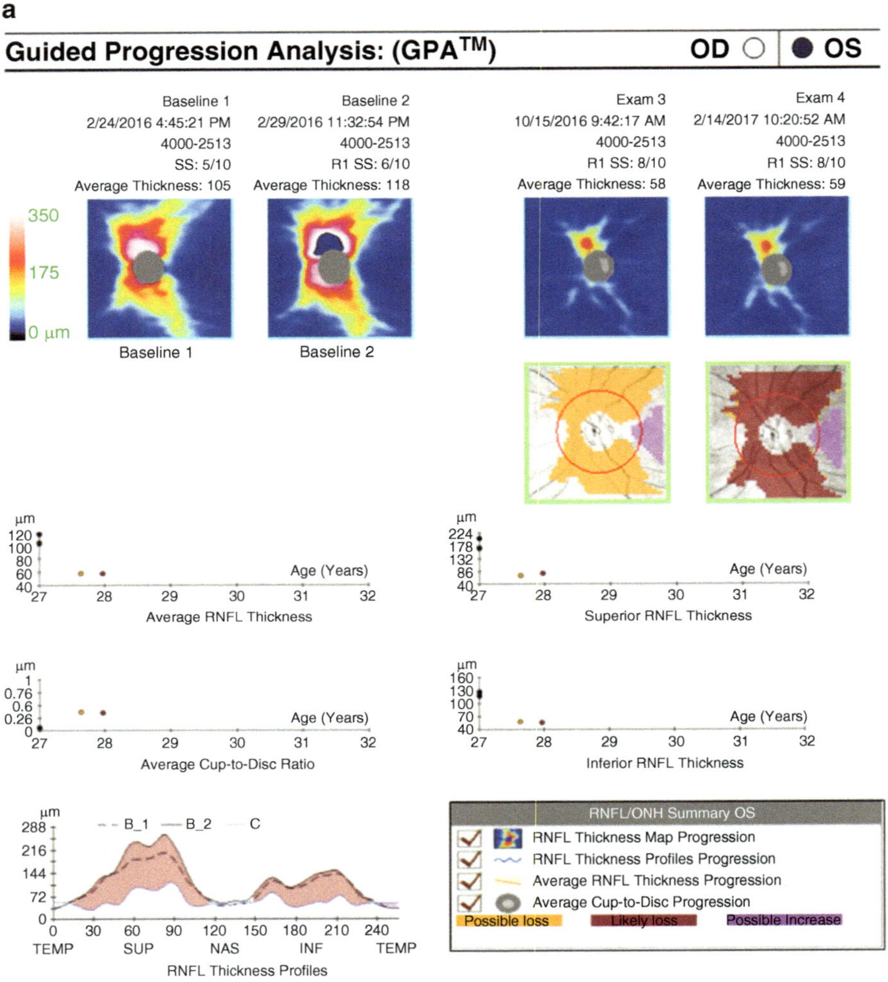

a

Guided Progression Analysis: (GPA™)   OD ○ | ● OS

Baseline 1	Baseline 2	Exam 3	Exam 4
2/24/2016 4:45:21 PM	2/29/2016 11:32:54 PM	10/15/2016 9:42:17 AM	2/14/2017 10:20:52 AM
4000-2513	4000-2513	4000-2513	4000-2513
SS: 5/10	R1 SS: 6/10	R1 SS: 8/10	R1 SS: 8/10
Average Thickness: 105	Average Thickness: 118	Average Thickness: 58	Average Thickness: 59

350
175
0 μm

Baseline 1   Baseline 2

Average RNFL Thickness

μm
120
100
80
60
40
27 28 29 30 31 32   Age (Years)

Superior RNFL Thickness

μm
224
178
132
86
40
27 28 29 30 31 32   Age (Years)

Average Cup-to-Disc Ratio

μm
1
0.76
0.6
0.26
0
27 28 29 30 31 32   Age (Years)

Inferior RNFL Thickness

μm
160
130
100
70
40
27 28 29 30 31 32   Age (Years)

RNFL Thickness Profiles

μm
288
216
144
72
0
0 30 60 90 120 150 180 210 240
TEMP   SUP   NAS   INF   TEMP

- - B_1   — B_2   — C

RNFL/ONH Summary OS

✓ RNFL Thickness Map Progression
✓ RNFL Thickness Profiles Progression
✓ Average RNFL Thickness Progression
✓ Average Cup-to-Disc Progression

Possible loss   Likely loss   Possible Increase

Fig. 9.14 (Cirrus HD-OCT GPA) (**a**) Progression analysis software of Cirrus HD-OCT shows ONH edema in two baseline scans followed by very fast RNFL damage in eight months. All four progression analysis strategies demonstrates RNFL loss in all quadrants. (**b**) *RNFL and ONH summary parameters* table shows the changes in RNFL thickness measurements

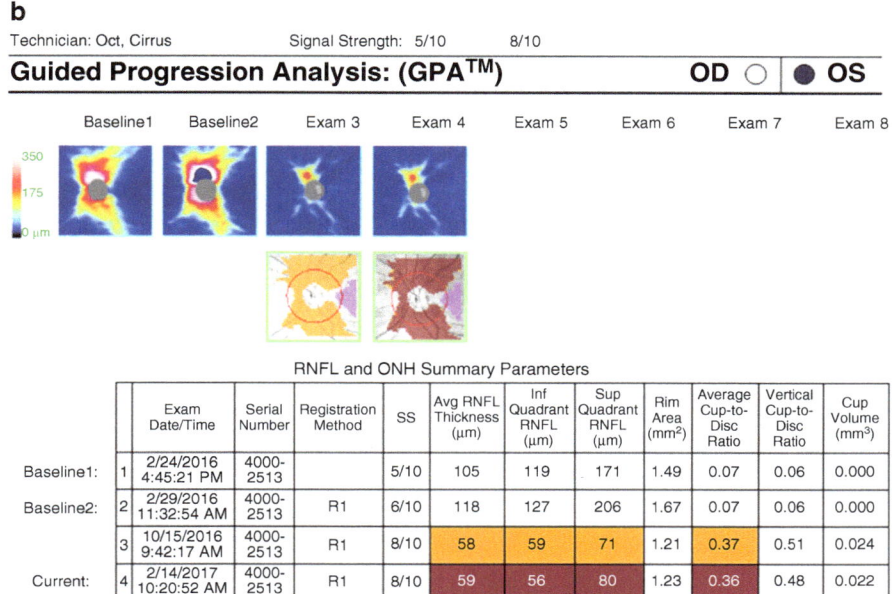

b

Technician: Oct, Cirrus   Signal Strength: 5/10   8/10

Guided Progression Analysis: (GPA™)   OD ○ | ● **OS**

RNFL and ONH Summary Parameters

		Exam Date/Time	Serial Number	Registration Method	SS	Avg RNFL Thickness (µm)	Inf Quadrant RNFL (µm)	Sup Quadrant RNFL (µm)	Rim Area (mm²)	Average Cup-to-Disc Ratio	Vertical Cup-to-Disc Ratio	Cup Volume (mm³)
Baseline1:	1	2/24/2016 4:45:21 PM	4000-2513		5/10	105	119	171	1.49	0.07	0.06	0.000
Baseline2:	2	2/29/2016 11:32:54 AM	4000-2513	R1	6/10	118	127	206	1.67	0.07	0.06	0.000
	3	10/15/2016 9:42:17 AM	4000-2513	R1	8/10	58	59	71	1.21	0.37	0.51	0.024
Current:	4	2/14/2017 10:20:52 AM	4000-2513	R1	8/10	59	56	80	1.23	0.36	0.48	0.022

Fig. 9.14 (continued)

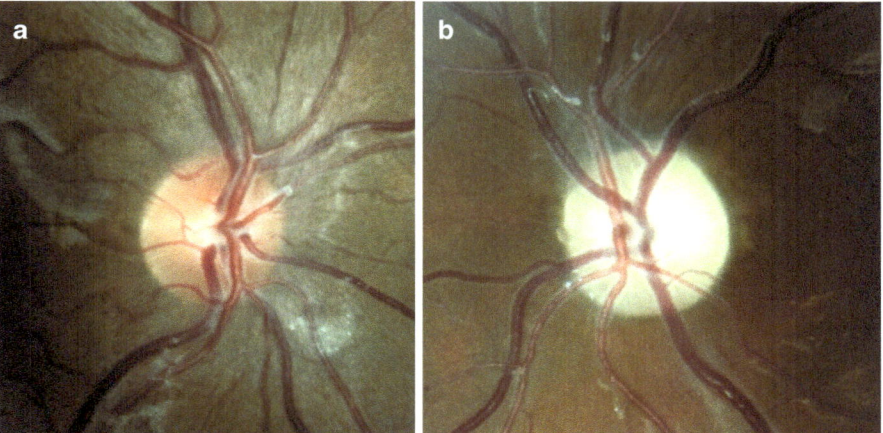

Fig. 9.15 Optic disc photographs: (**a**) The right eye has a normal ONH. (**b**) Significant pallor is present in the left ONH without any cupping

Conclusion: This patient presented as an isolated optic neuritis and later diagnosed as NMO based on clinical findings and serological tests. The clinical history of the patient and the OCT report in Fig. 9.12 facilitate the differential diagnosis from glaucoma. On the other hand, if the patient is first seen after the ONH edema has subsided, Cirrus HD-OCT reports in Figs. 9.13 and 9.15, and Spectralis OCT report at Fig. 9.14 provide few clues for differentiating this disease from glaucomatous optic neuropathy. Lack of significant cupping is the only clue in Fig. 9.13. A complete clinical exam including fundoscopy, which shows pallor without cupping and the degree of visual loss (light perception) could distinguish this case from glaucomatous optic neuropathy.

9.2.4 Compressive Optic Neuropathy

Intraorbital or intracanalicular compressive lesions usually cause slowly progressive monocular visual loss and central or diffuse VF defects. The optic disc may be normal, edematous or atrophic according to the type, stage or localization of the tumor. Non-glaucomatous cupping may also occur with tumors compressing the anterior visual pathway [14, 15]. Physical examination may disclose loss of central vision, dyschromatopsia, VF defects depending on the location of compression and an afferent pupillary defect if asymmetric compression exists. OCT-measured RNFL is thinned in compressive optic neuropathy as it is in glaucoma [16, 17].

9.2.4.1 Sample Case: Compressive Lesion

A 72-year old woman with a diagnosis of NTG was referred to our department because of progressive visual loss in the right eye (Figs. 9.16, 9.17, 9.18 and 9.19). Her visual acuity was no light perception in the right eye and 20/20 in the left eye. IOP was 16 mmHg in both eyes.

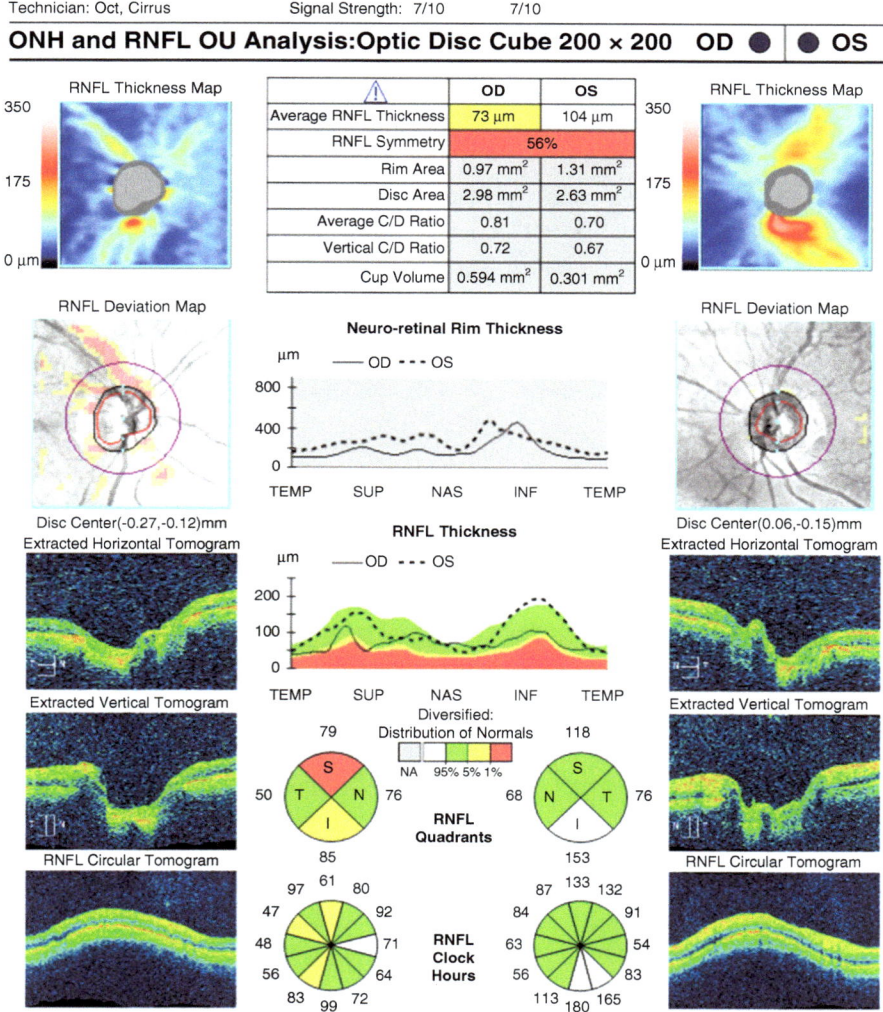

Fig. 9.16 (Cirrus HD-OCT) ONH analysis shows high average C/D ratio (0.8) and a very thin neuroretinal rim. On the other hand, RNFL loss in the RNFL deviation map looks less significant especially in the inferior quadrant. As the patient's IOP was 16 mmHg, the OCT findings of the right eye may be classified as RNFL loss secondary to NTG. Absence of RNFL loss in the left eye and high asymmetry between RNFL measurements of the two eyes (56%) must be recognized as alarming sign for a non-glaucomatous optic neuropathy in the right eye

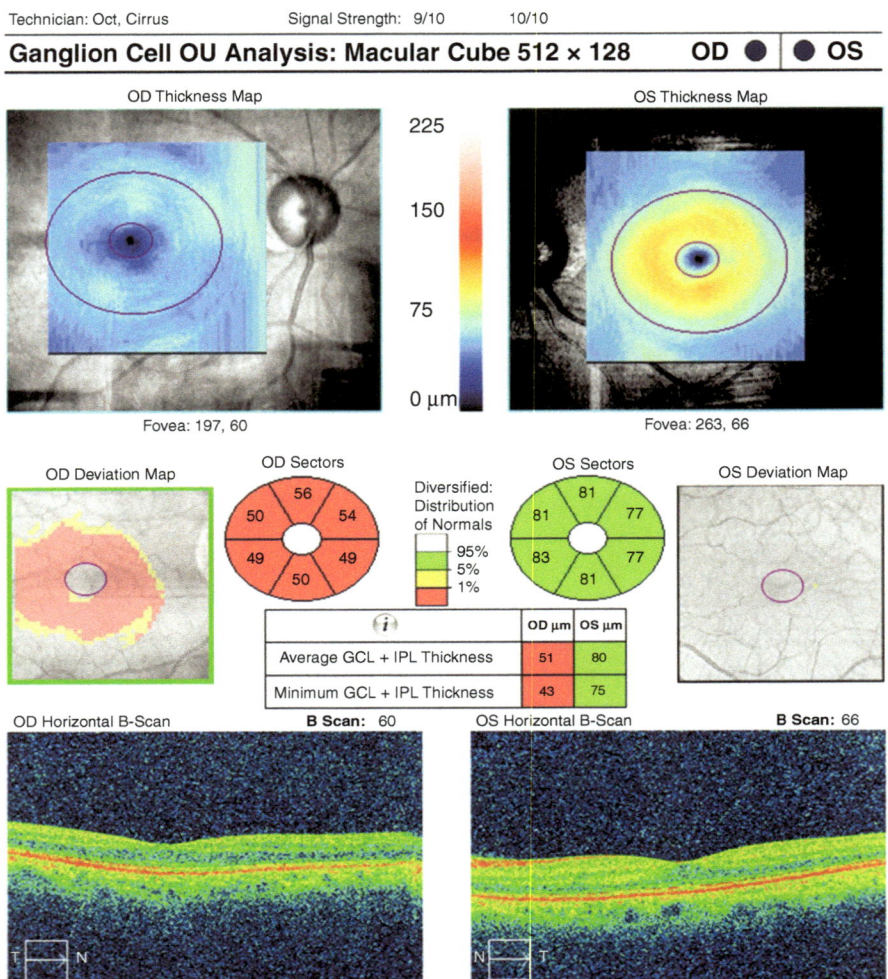

Fig. 9.17 (Cirrus HD-OCT) Macular Ganglion Cell Analysis shows a significant GCL + IPL loss in the right macula, while the left macula is completely normal. This must be another alarming finding in a patient with IOP in low teens and macular ganglion cell damage only in one eye

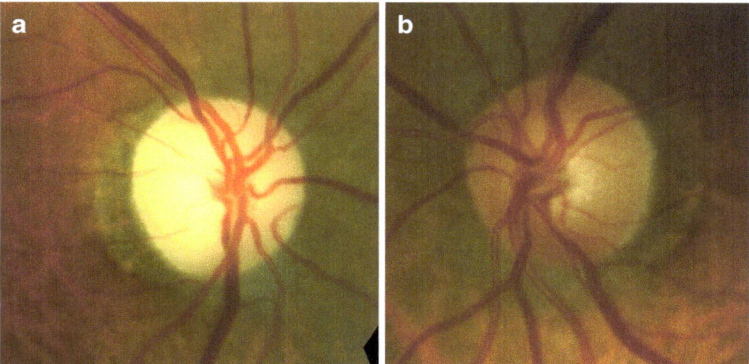

Fig. 9.18 (**a**) Fundus photograph of the right eye shows optic disc atrophy with shallow cupping and significant pallor. (**b**) The left optic disc appears normal

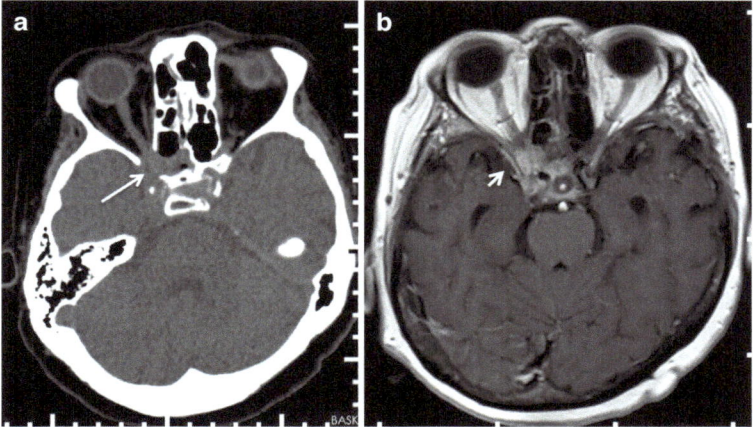

Fig. 9.19 (**a**) Transverse CT slice through skull base without contrast injection. Destruction of right ethmoid wall, sphenoid wing, anterior clinoid with soft tissue extension within the optic canal, and infiltration of the optic nerve-sheath complex posteriorly is seen (white arrow). (**b**) Post contrast fat-suppressed transverse T1 weighted magnetic resonance image. Soft tissue lesion within ethmoid posterior cell can be observed with extension into the right optic canal with optic nerve-sheath complex involvement posteriorly (white arrowhead). Accompanying bone destruction in the sphenoid wing, ethmoid wall and posterior clinoid can also be seen (Images and radiological reports are courtesy of A. Muhteşem Ağıldere, MD)

Conclusion: This case highlights the importance of CNS imaging in normal tension glaucoma patients. The patient was followed with a diagnosis of normal tension glaucoma for few years before referral and a compressive lesion was not diagnosed until recently. ONH pallor in addition to cupping and loss of vision in the right eye, absence of RNFL and macular ganglion cell loss in the left eye, and high asymmetry between RNFL measurements of the two eyes (56%) must be recognized as alarming signs for a non-glaucomatous optic neuropathy. The patient refused surgical options and there is no histopathological diagnosis available about the nature of the tumor.

9.2.4.2   Sample Case: Anterior Temporal Lobectomy

A 35-year old female with a history of epilepsy had anterior temporal lobectomy 3 years ago for control of her seizures. Her BCVA is 20/20 OU. Her IOP was measured at 23 mmHg in both eyes and she was referred to the glaucoma clinic for evaluation (Figs. 9.20, 9.21, 9.22 and 9.23).

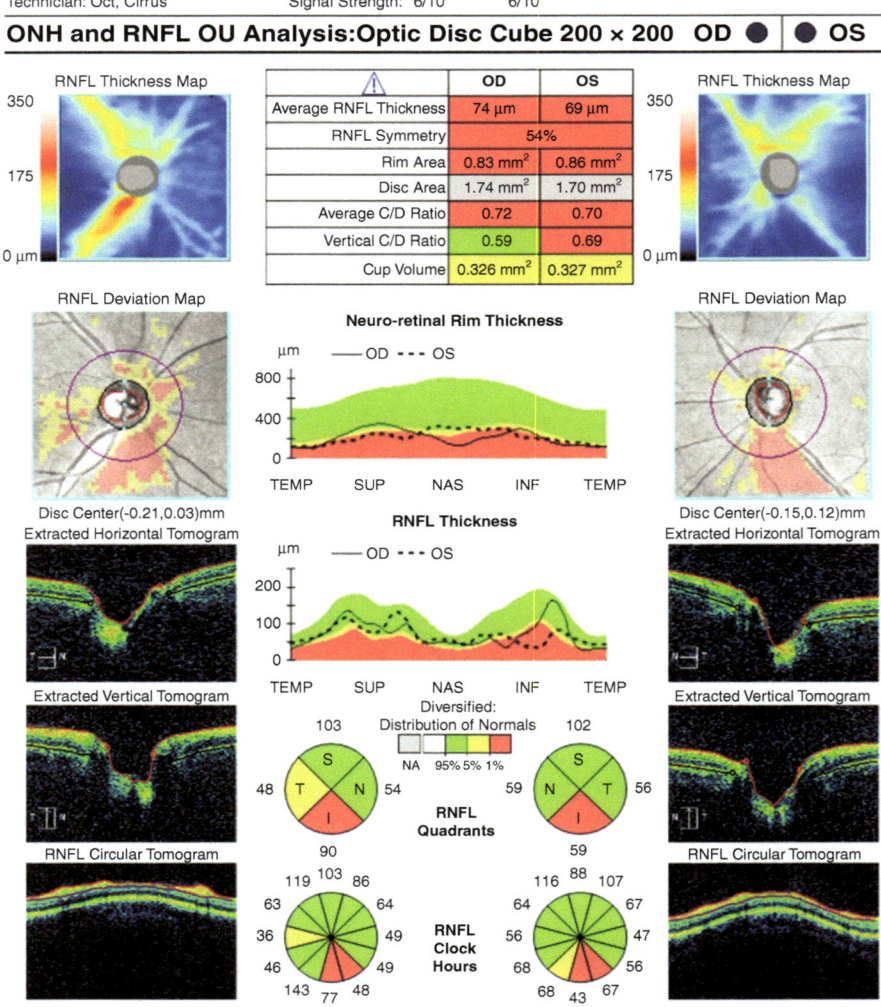

Fig. 9.20 (Cirrus HD-OCT) Peripapillary OCT shows RNFL thinning inferiorly in both eyes, which is the most common quadrant to be involved in early glaucoma RNFL loss. In addition, the average cup to disc ratio is 0.7 bilaterally. If we only looked at this OCT and did not have the medical history of the patient, we might think that this is a case of moderate glaucomatous damage

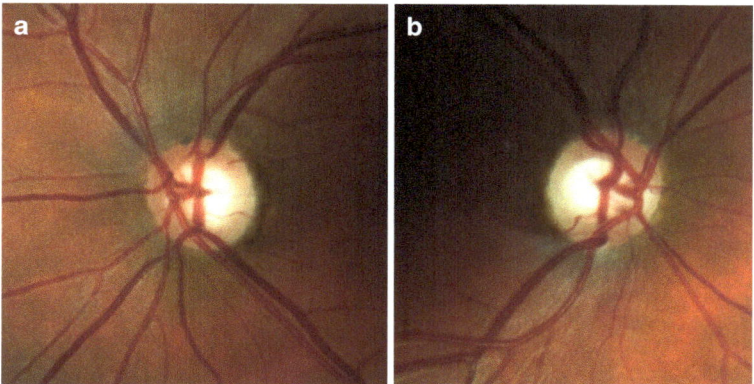

Fig. 9.21 (**a, b**) Fundus photos of both eyes show some degrees of cupping in both eyes but the neuroretinal rims appear healthy OU

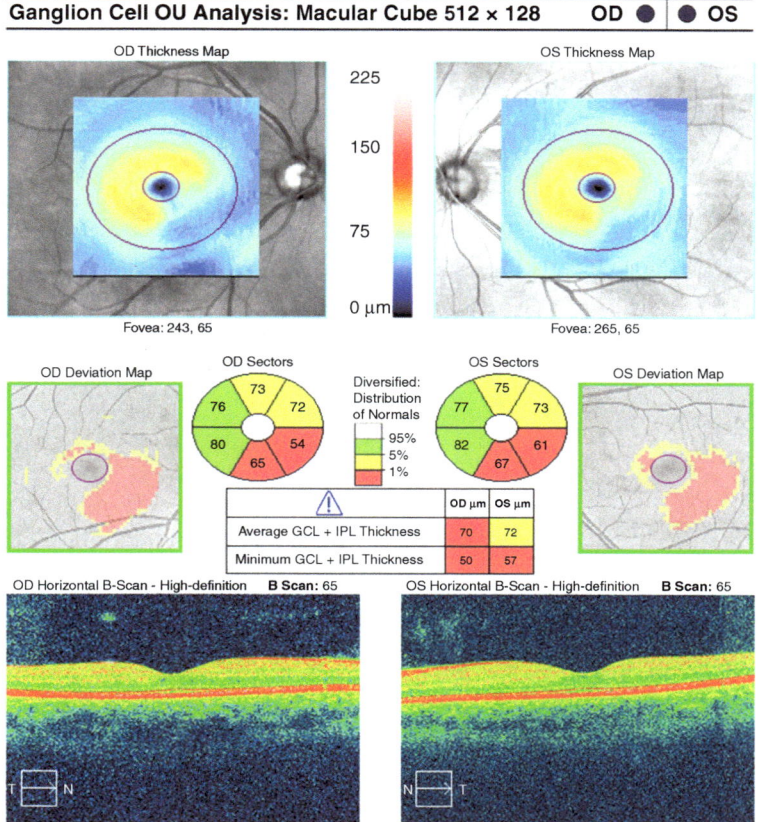

Fig. 9.22 (Cirrus HD-OCT) Macular Ganglion Cell Analysis shows congrous loss of GCL + IPL in both maculas (nasal inferior in the right eye and temporal inferior in the left eye). This is the first clue for non-glaucomatous RNFL loss, as this kind of GCL + IPL thinning is only possible in neuro-ophthalmological conditions

186   A. Akman and S. Gür Güngör

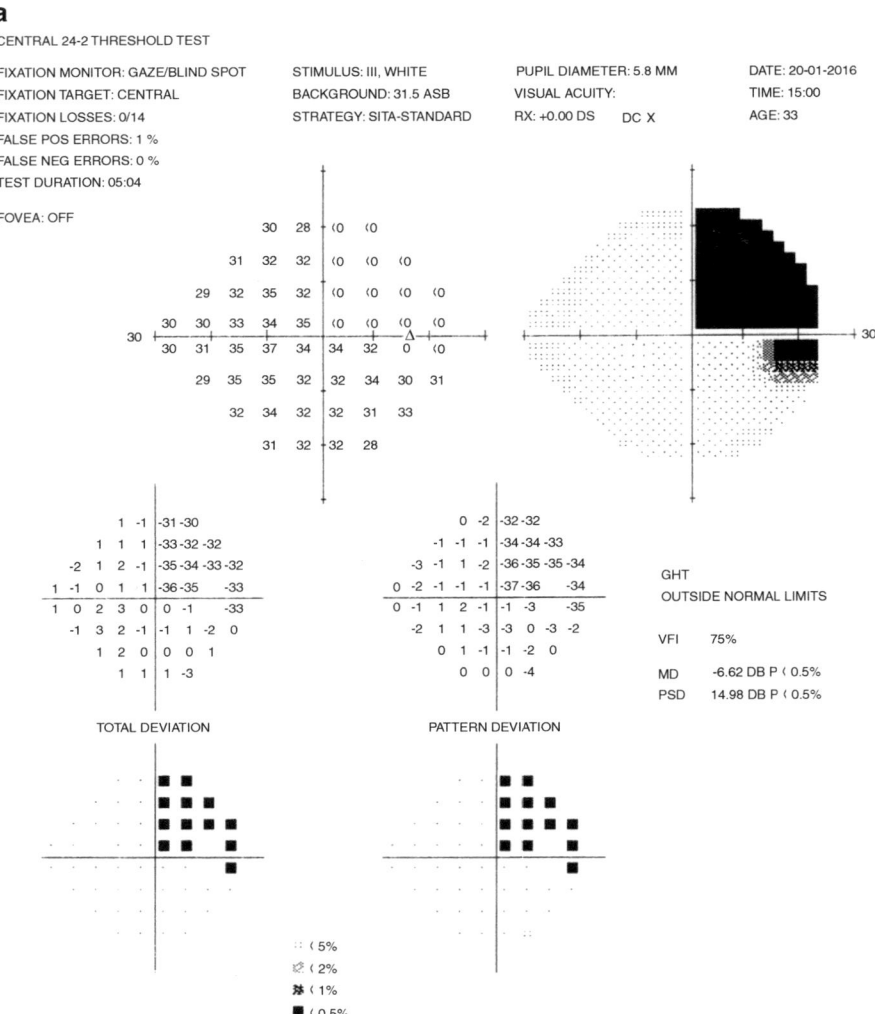

Fig. 9.23 (**a, b**) VF exam of the patient shows right homonymous superior quadrantanopia caused by the left anterior temporal lobectomy. This VF loss is in concordance with the OCT findings in Fig. 9.22

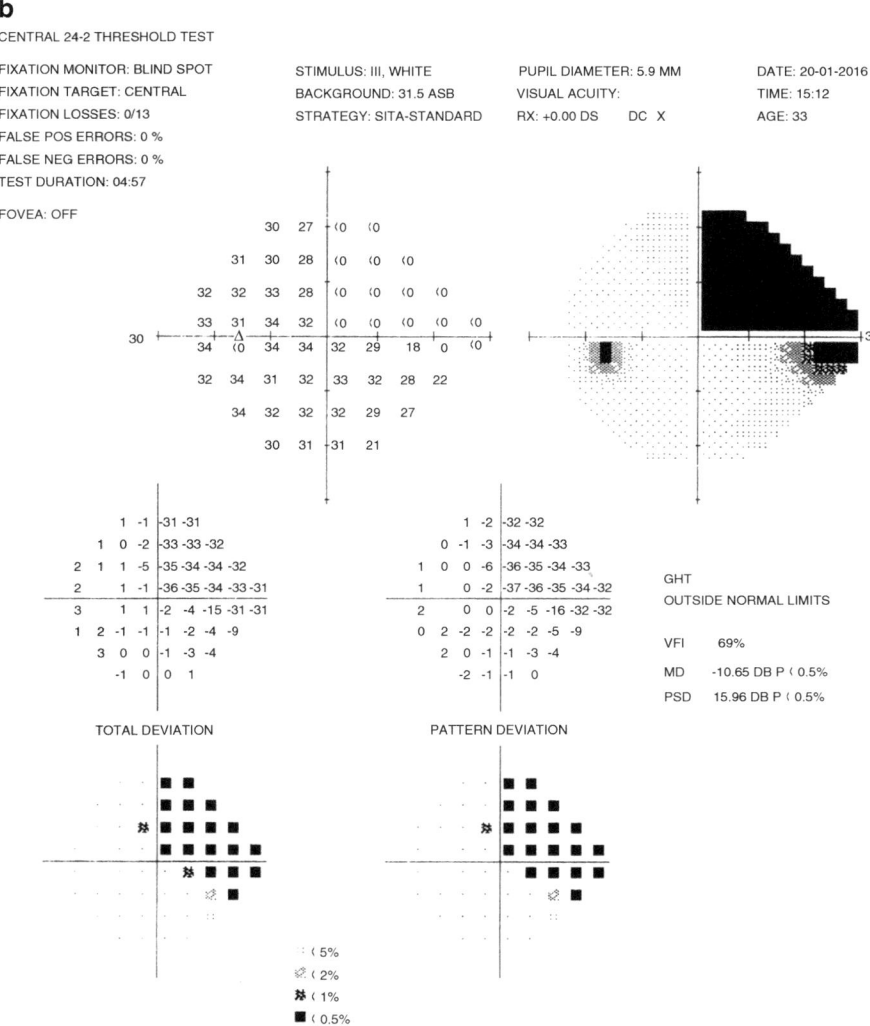

Fig. 9.23 (continued)

Conclusion: Peripapillary OCT and optic nerve findings in this ocular hypertensive patient could have been classified as glaucomatous optic neuropathy if the macular ganglion cell OCT had not been performed. The bilateral homonymous GCL + IPL damage in the macular OCT and the VF test results indicate an intracranial pathology, in this case, prior surgery. A lesion involving post-chiasmal nerve fibers whether in the optic tract, the lateral geniculate body, the optic radiation, or the visual cortex on either the left or the right side of the brain will lead to a homonymous VF loss (hemianopia or quadranopia). Following damage to the post-geniculate visual pathway, retrograde transsynaptic degeneration of the optic nerve fibers occurs, thus affecting the OCT results [18]. Another possibility for this particular case is optic tract injury during the surgery.

9.2.5   *Traumatic Optic Neuropathy*

Traumatic optic neuropathy occurs due to injury of the optic nerve from any kind of accident or trauma. The initial optic nerve examination may be normal or may show significant findings such as optic nerve avulsion. With the passage of time, ONH pallor may develop and non-glaucomatous cupping can also appear [14]. The RNFL measured by OCT reveals thinning after traumatic optic neuropathy [19, 20]. The location and magnitude of RNFL thinning likely depend on the severity of the trauma and extent of visual loss after injury. The clinical history and examination should differentiate this type of RNFL loss from glaucoma, even when the ONH shows cupping.

9.3   Conclusion

Differentiating glaucomatous and non-glaucomatous optic neuropathies can be challenging. RNFL changes on OCT in neuro-ophthalmological diseases can mimic patterns seen in glaucoma. OCT should always be used to complement the physical examination and VF testing in patients with glaucomatous and non-glaucomatous optic neuropathies.

9.4   Key Points

- OCT shows RNFL damage in non-glaucomatous optic neuropathies, but the degree of ONH cupping is generally disproportionate to the extent of RNFL damage.
- Fundus exam shows significant pallor in eyes with RNFL loss secondary to non-glaucomatous optic neuropathies.
- Patterns of RNFL loss can be different in non-glaucomatous optic neuropathies compared to glaucoma.
- Compressive CNS lesions and intracranial surgeries can cause RNFL loss and cupping similar to that observed in glaucoma.
- Visual acuity, color vision testing, VF exam, and pupillary light reflex findings are helpful in differential diagnosis.
- Macular OCT can show vertically oriented GCL + IPL thinning in CNS pathologies.
- Even in presence of seemingly typical RNFL loss and glaucomatous cupping, non-glaucomatous optic neuropathies must be ruled out especially in eyes with a diagnosis of NTG.

References

1. Dias DT, Ushida M, Battistella R, Dorairaj S, Prata TS. Neurophthalmological conditions mimicking glaucomatous optic neuropathy: analysis of the most common causes of misdiagnosis. BMC Ophthalmol. 2017;17:2–5.
2. Rosdahl JA, Asrani S. Glaucoma masqueraders: diagnosis by spectral domain optical coherence tomography. Saudi J Ophthalmol. 2012;26(4):433–40.
3. Paquet C, Boissonnot M, Roger F, Dighiero P, Gil R, Hugon JDP, Gil R, Hugon J. Abnormal retinal thickness in patients with mild cognitive impairment and Alzheimer's disease. Neurosci Lett. 2007;420:97–9.
4. Moschos MM, Tagaris G, Markopoulos I, Margetis I, Tsapakis S, Kanakis M, Koutsandrea C. Morphologic changes and functional retinal impairment in patients with Parkinson disease without visual loss. Eur J Ophthalmol. 2011;21:24–9.
5. Inzelberg R, Ramirez JA, Nisipeanu P, Ophir A. Retinal nerve fiber layer thinning in Parkinson disease. Vis Res. 2004;44:2793–7.
6. Miller RN, Arnold AC. Current concepts in the diagnosis, pathogenesis and management of nonarteritic anterior ischemic optic neuropathy. Eye. 2015;29:65–79.
7. Gerling J, Meyer JH, Kommerell G. Visual field defects in optic neuritis and anterior ischemic optic neuropathy: distinctive features. Graefes Arch Clin Exp Ophthalmol. 1998;236(3): 188–92.
8. Danesh-Meyer HV, Savino PJ, Sergott RC. The prevalence of cupping in end-stage arteritic and nonarteritic anterior ischemic optic neuropathy. Ophthalmology. 2001;108:593–8.
9. Bock M, Brandt AU, Dörr J, Kraft H, Weinges-Evers N, Gaede G, Pfueller CF, Herges K, Radbruch H, Ohlraun S, Bellmann-Strobl J, Kuchenbecker J, Zipp F, Paul F. Patterns of retinal nerve fiber layer loss in multiple sclerosis patients with or without optic neuritis and glaucoma patients. Clin Neurol Neurosurg. 2010;112:647–52.
10. Pueyo V, Ara JR, Almarcegui C, Martin J, Güerri N, García E, Pablo LE, Honrubia FM, Fernandez FJ. Sub-clinical atrophy of the retinal nerve fibre layer in multiple sclerosis. Acta Ophthalmol. 2010;88:748–52.
11. Talman LS, Bisker ER, Sackel DJ, Long DA Jr, Galetta KM, Ratchford JN, Lile DJ, Farrell SK, Loguidice MJ, Remington G, Conger A, Frohman TC, Jacobs DA, Markowitz CE, Cutter GR, Ying GS, Dai Y, Maguire MG, Galetta SL, Frohman EM, Calabresi PA, Balcer LJ. Longitudinal study of vision and retinal nerve fiber layer thickness in multiple sclerosis. Ann Neurol. 2010;67:749–60.
12. Nakamura M, Nakazawa T, Doi H, Hariya T, Omodaka K, Misu T, Takahashi T, Fujihara K, Nishida K. Early high-dose intravenous methylprednisolone is effective in preserving retinal nerve fiber layer thickness in patients with neuromyelitis optica. Graefes Arch Clin Exp Ophthalmal. 2010;248:1777–85.
13. Ratchford JN, Quigg ME, Conger A, Frohman T, Frohman E, Balcer LJ, Calabresi PA, Kerr DA. Optical coherence tomography helps differentiate neuromyelitis optica and MS optic neuropathies. Neurology. 2009;73:302–8.
14. Trobe JD, Glaser JS, Cassady J, Herschler J, Anderson DR. Non-glaucomatous excavation of the optic disc. Arch Ophthalmol. 1980;98:1046–50.
15. Greenfield DS. Glaucomatous versus non-glaucomatous optic disc cupping: clinical differentiation. Semin Ophthalmol. 1999;14:95–108.
16. Costa-Cunha LV, Cunha LP, Malta RF, Monteiro ML. Comparison of Fourier-domain and time-domain optical coherence tomography in the detection of band atrophy of the optic nerve. Am J Ophthalmol. 2009;147:56–63.
17. Monteiro ML, Cunha LP, Costa-Cunha LV, Maia OO Jr, Oyamada MK. Relationship between optical coherence tomography, pattern electroretinogram and automated perimetry

in eyes with temporal hemianopia from chiasmal compression. Invest Ophthalmol Vis Sci. 2009;50:3535–41.
18. Goto K, Miki A, Yamashita T, Araki S, Takizawa G, Nakagawa M, Ieki Y, Kiryu J. Sectoral analysis of the retinal nerve fiber layer thinning and its association with visual field loss in homonymous hemianopia caused by post-geniculate lesions using spectral-domain optical coherence tomography. Graefes Arch Clin Exp Ophthalmol. 2016;254:745–56.
19. Cunha LP, Costa-Cunha LV, Malta RF, Monteiro ML. Comparison between retinal nerve fiber layer and macular thickness measured with OCT detecting progressive axonal loss following traumatic optic neuropathy. Arq Bras Oftalmol. 2009;72:622–5.
20. Medeiros FA, Moura FC, Vessani RM, Susanna R Jr. Axonal loss after traumatic optic neuropathy documented by optical coherence tomography. Am J Ophthalmol. 2003;135:406–8.

Chapter 10
Utility of OCT for Detection or Monitoring of Glaucoma in Myopic Eyes

Atilla Bayer and Kouros Nouri-Mahdavi

10.1 Introduction

Myopia is one of the most common ocular conditions worldwide and its association with glaucoma is well recognized [1–4]. Myopia has been increasing at a rapid rate in the younger population, and a dramatic rise in the prevalence of myopia is expected as this population ages [2]. It is accompanied by various degenerative changes in the posterior segment structures of the eye including the sclera, optic nerve head (ONH), choroid, Bruch's membrane, retinal pigment epithelium (RPE), and neurosensory retina. Thorough understanding of anatomic changes in the ONH and retinal nerve fiber layer (RNFL) is important especially considering the fact that myopic eyes are 2–3 times more likely to develop glaucoma compared to non-myopic eyes [3, 5]. In a recent study by Shim and associates, OAG developed earlier in participants with high myopia than in others [1]. There was a high prevalence of OAG in participants with high myopia, even in those 19–29 years of age.

Optical coherence tomography (OCT) has enabled recognition of morphological changes in glaucoma, which was not previously possible on clinical examination [6]. OCT studies of altered biometry and topography of the ONH, retina and choroid has allowed evaluation of their relationship with demographic factors, visual function, and fundoscopic findings in myopia [7]. As the normative databases of current OCT devices largely comprise data collected from normal eyes with no or low degrees of myopia, the deviation maps or classification charts provided by such devices are likely to be inaccurate in highly myopic eyes. Volume scans acquired with most commercial OCT instruments have a depth of focus of about 2 mm. The posterior eye

A. Bayer (✉)
Department of Glaucoma, Dünyagöz Eye Hospital, Ankara, Turkey

K. Nouri-Mahdavi
Stein Eye Institute, University of California Los Angeles, Los Angeles, CA, USA
e-mail: nouri-mahdavi@jsei.ucla.edu

© Springer International Publishing AG, part of Springer Nature 2018
A. Akman et al. (eds.), *Optical Coherence Tomography in Glaucoma*,
https://doi.org/10.1007/978-3-319-94905-5_10

wall of a highly myopic eye has sometimes curvatures that exceed this limit. Other characteristics of myopic eyes mentioned above also create difficulties on OCT imaging. This chapter provides updated information on the current uses, limits, and keypoints of OCT imaging in myopic eyes with suspected or definitive glaucoma.

10.2 Ocular Features of Myopia and Implications in Glaucoma

10.2.1 Challenges in Detecting and Managing Glaucoma

Glaucoma is assessed clinically mostly by evaluating changes in the ONH or in the visual field (VF). Myopia may affect these measurements. Uneven expansion of the posterior globe wall leading to tilting of the disc and subsequent oval shape of the disc, shallow enlarged cupping, peripapillary atrophy (PPA), and poor media are some of the characteristics of myopic eyes that make disc evaluation challenging (Fig. 10.1) [5, 6]. Degenerative changes in the peripapillary region in degenerative myopia could lead to VF defects that can mimic those observed in glaucoma.

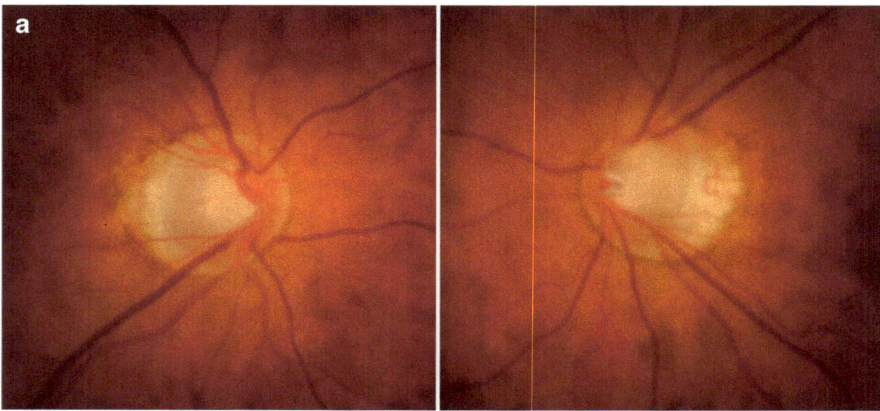

Fig. 10.1 (a) Optic disc photographs of a female patient with moderate to high myopia (−5.00 D, SE) and suspected of glaucoma. Suspicious looking tilted large optic discs can be observed with peripapillary atrophy (PPA) and enlarged cups bilaterally. (b) Visual field tests are classified as "within normal limits" bilaterally. (c) Spectralis OCT baseline retinal nerve fiber layer (RNFL) tests in year 2011 were classified as "borderline" and "outside normal limits" in the right and left eyes, respectively. However, the findings are due to displaced RNFL peaks and the RNFL Change Report is stable in both eyes over 5 years of follow-up. (d) In the Posterior Pole Asymmetry Analysis tests, there is suspected thinning in the baseline hemisphere asymmetry charts but both eyes are stable during the 5 years of follow up as indicated back the lack or regions of thinning retinal thickness that would be flagged in red on the right bottom subtraction image

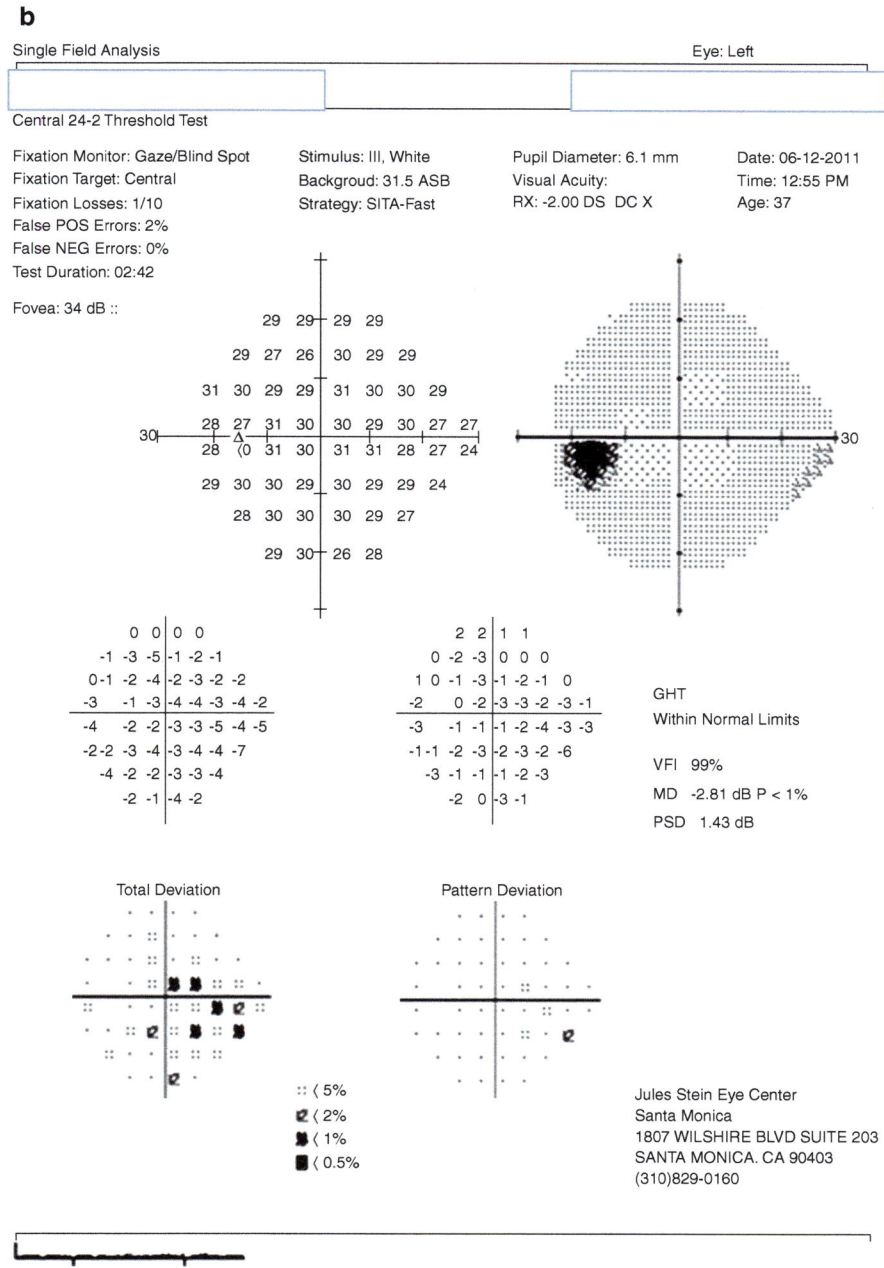

Fig. 10.1 (continued)

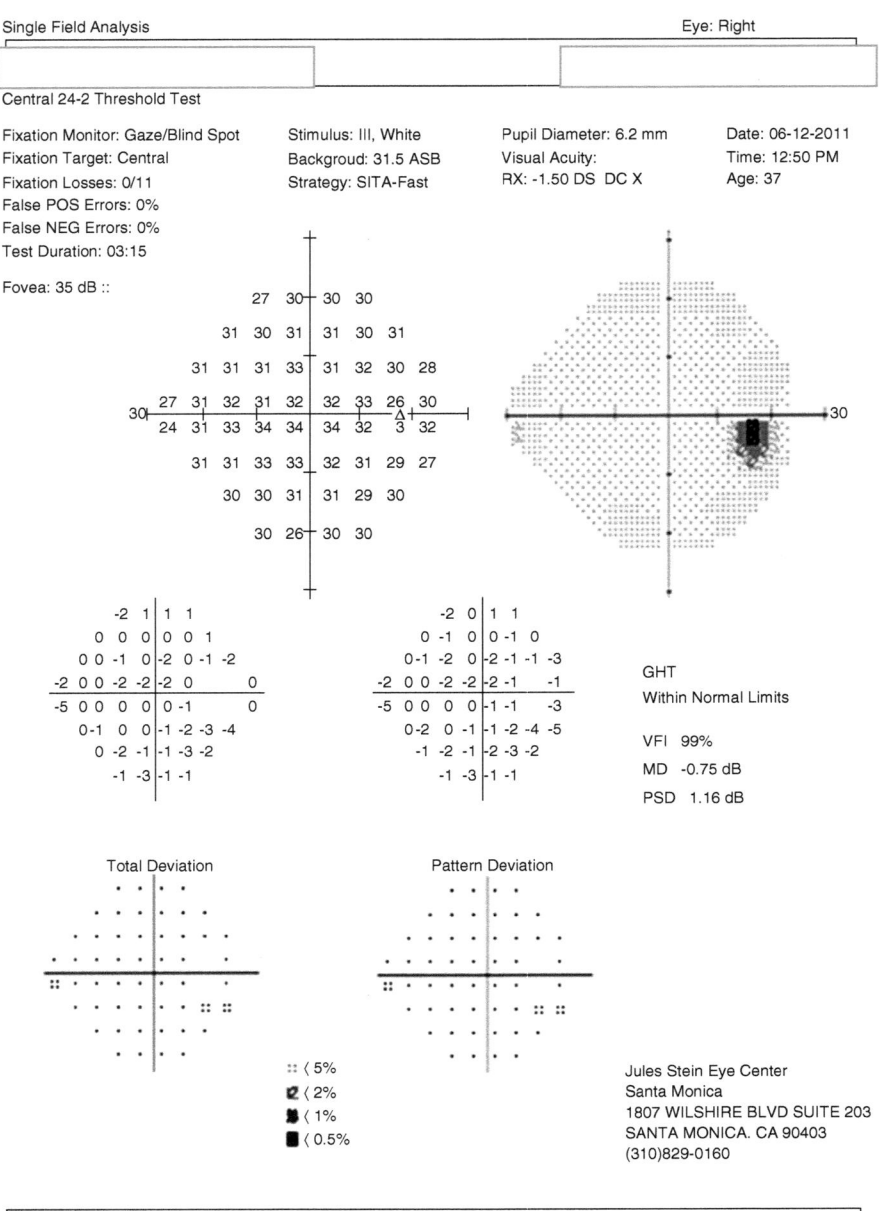

Fig. 10.1 (continued)

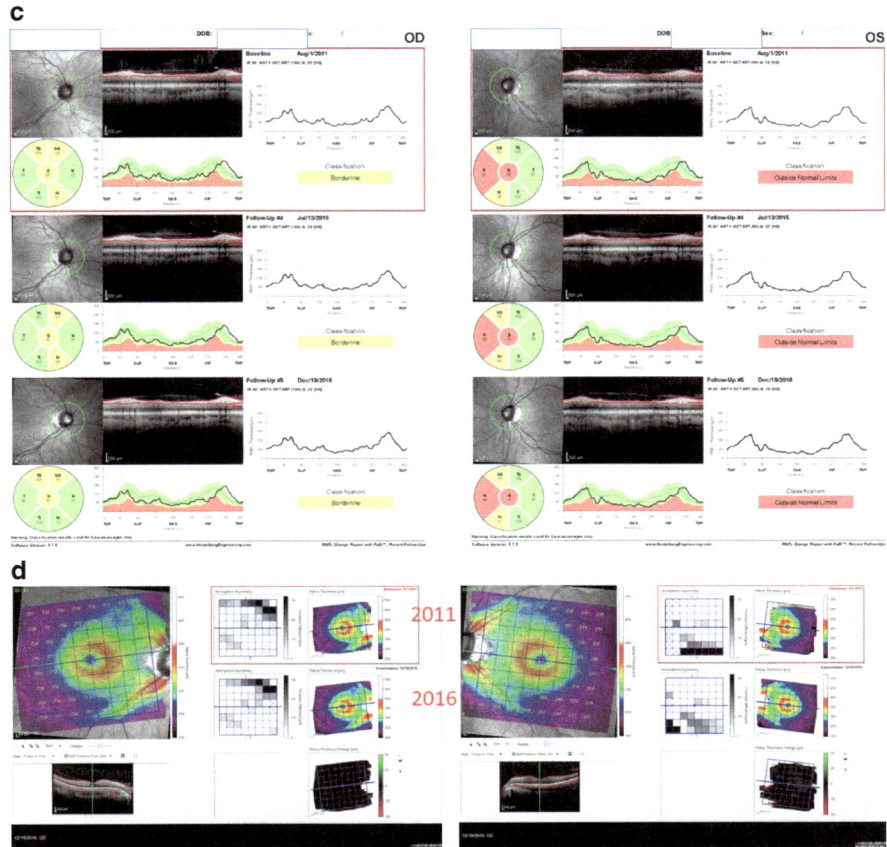

Fig. 10.1 (continued)

Thinning of the eyewall layers in myopia changes the scleral rigidity. Lower corneal hysteresis has been reported as another characteristic of myopic eyes affecting IOP measurements [8–10]. These characteristics of myopic eyes can make an accurate glaucoma diagnosis challenging, since there is no proven biomarker for the disease. Preventive treatment can be bothersome and expensive and have potential side effects. Given that a correct diagnosis before VF damage emerges is difficult at best, some myopes are probably overtreated while others with glaucoma are being undertreated or go completely untreated.

10.2.2 Optic Nerve Head Changes

Detecting glaucoma in eyes with low to moderate myopia is not more challenging than emmetropic eyes, since the appearance of the ONH is more or less similar [11]. In high axial myopia, including the highly myopic form of primary open angle glaucoma, the eyewall stretches and the axial length increases. During this process, the ONH is pulled towards the temporal direction, which eventually results in an optic disc with a temporally tilted appearance with elevation of the nasal disc margin and temporal flattening [11–13]. Jonas and associates recently reviewed the histological changes of high axial myopia [14]. In their study, scleral thinning started at or behind the equator with maximal thinning in the posterior pole. They also reported presence of an elongated scleral flange (defined as the canal between the optic nerve border and the point where dura mater merges with the sclera) and stretching and thinning of the lamina cribrosa with decreased distance between the retrobulbar cerebrospinal fluid space with the IOP compartment. Morgan and associates found that the pressure difference between the intraocular and retrobulbar spaces was distributed over a shorter length, resulting in steeper pressure gradient across the lamina cribrosa [15]. Development of large pores in lamina cribrosa has been reported as characteristic of eyes with primary open angle glaucoma [16].

Although a tilted disc appearance refers to the ONH being rotated around the vertical axis from a two-dimensional fundoscopic view, tilting of the disc can occur along horizontal or oblique axes (Fig. 10.2). The degree of the ONH tilt is estimated by the disc 'ovality' index, which is measured as the ratio of the longest to shortest

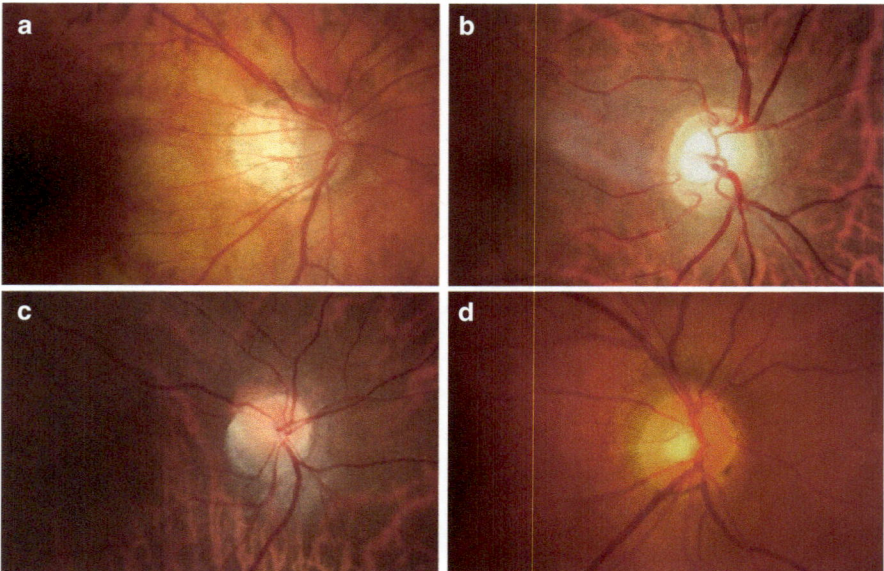

Fig. 10.2 Examples of tilted discs; (**a**) temporal tilt, (**b**) nasal tilt, also called disc dysversion, (**c**) inferotemporal tilt, (**d**) superotemporal tilt

diameters of the disc. On the other hand, the index of tilt is defined as the ratio of the shortest diameter to the longest diameter [17]. The course of ONH vessels also changes in tilted discs. The second geometric variable in the optic discs is the rotation about the sagittal axis of the ONH. This is defined as ONH torsion. However, disc torsion is now considered as tilting of the disc occurring along an oblique axis.

In a morphometric study conducted by Jonas and associates, optic discs of highly myopic eyes (>-8.0 diopters) were found to be significantly larger and shaped more oval than those of non-highly myopic eyes [12]. In another clinical observational study, ONH area was significantly larger in a subset of highly myopic eyes (>-8.0 diopters) [18]. The optic disc cup can also be remarkably shallow in myopic eyes.

10.2.3   Peripapillary Atrophy

Peripapillary atrophy, has classically been divided into a peripheral α-zone, and a central β-zone based on clinical findings. The latter has been known to be associated with glaucomatous optic neuropathy and myopia. The α-zone is characterized by irregular hypopigmentation and hyperpigmentation of the RPE and slight thinning of the choroidal tissues. The hallmark of β-zone is a complete loss of the RPE, marked atrophy of the photoreceptor layer and the choriocapillaris, clear visibility of large choroidal vessels and sclera. It is marked by a sharp boundary along the adjacent α-zone and abuts the peripapillary scleral ring [19, 20] (Fig. 10.3). Recent histological and clinical investigations revealed that the peripapillary region in highly myopic eyes showed additional features. In some myopic eyes, between the β-zone and the clinical disc margin, there is an area lacking the Bruch's membrane called the γ-zone [21]. The γ-zone has traditionally been recognized as the myopic temporal crescent or conus [22, 23]. It is defined as a whitish area temporal to the

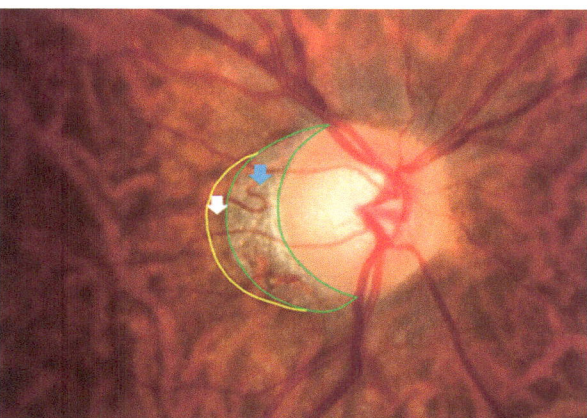

Fig. 10.3 The two zones of peripapillary atrophy defined clinically as the central β-zone (blue arrowhead) and a peripheral α-zone (white arrowhead)

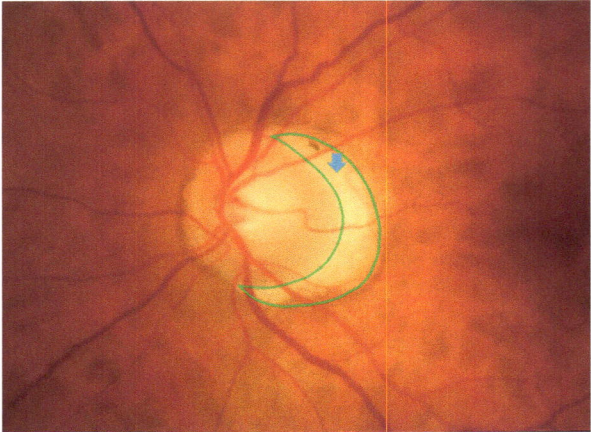

Fig. 10.4 Peripapillary γ-zone in a myopic eye (blue arrowhead)

disc margin without underlying choriocapillaris vessels and without any signs of RPE (Fig. 10.4). This zone of PPA must be differentiated from the β-zone which serves as a marker of glaucomatous disease and progression [21, 24].

10.2.4 The Macular Area and Posterior Pole Changes

Changes in the posterior wall and macular area of the eye may affect clinical evaluation of the retina especially in highly myopic cases. These changes can be summarized as posterior precortical vitreous pockets, precursor changes of posterior vitreous detachment, retinoschisis, peripapillary intrachoroidal cavitation, dome-shaped macula, and changes in the inner curvature of the sclera [25]. Fortunately, most of these changes can be diagnosed with OCT imaging. Details of these changes are outside the scope of this chapter. A few examples of changes that might affect detection of glaucoma are shown in Fig. 10.5.

10.3 OCT Findings in Myopia

10.3.1 The Optic Nerve Head

The anatomic changes in the ONH and surrounding structures of eyes in high myopia have been identified in vivo with OCT imaging. The angle of ONH tilting can be measured with OCT [26]. Other features of glaucomatous optic neuropathy that can be observed on OCT imaging include, enlargement of laminar pores (Fig. 10.6), dehiscence of the lamina cribrosa (seen as an acquired pit of the ONH in extreme cases), expansion of the dural attachment posteriorly with enlargement of the subarachnoid

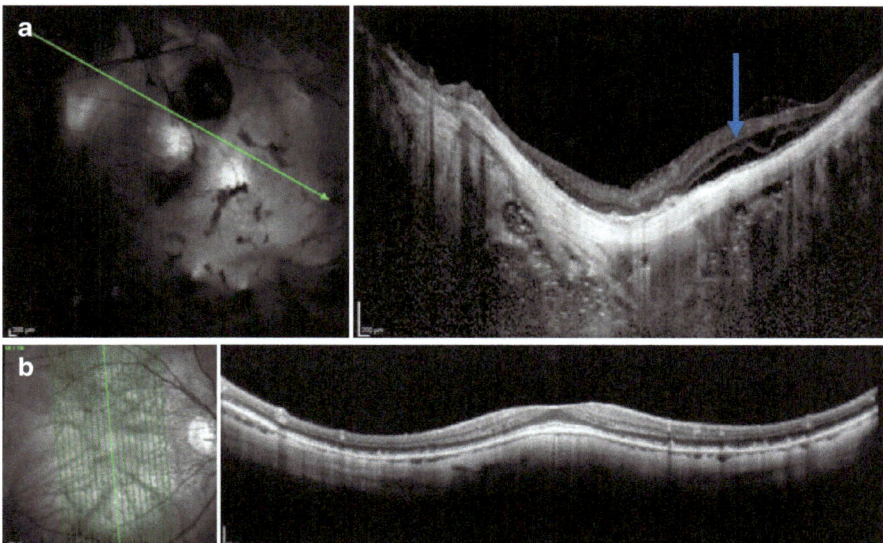

Fig. 10.5 (**a**) Posterior pole optical coherence tomography scan of a highly myopic eye with an axial length of 30.84 mm. Note that sclera is bowed posteriorly (top right, posterior staphyloma). The hyporeflective space (blue arrow) represents an area of retinoschisis, another finding observed in highly myopic eyes, which may interfere with glaucoma evaluation. (**b**) In some highly myopic eyes, convexity of the posterior staphyloma causes inward bulge of the macula, which is known as dome-shaped macula

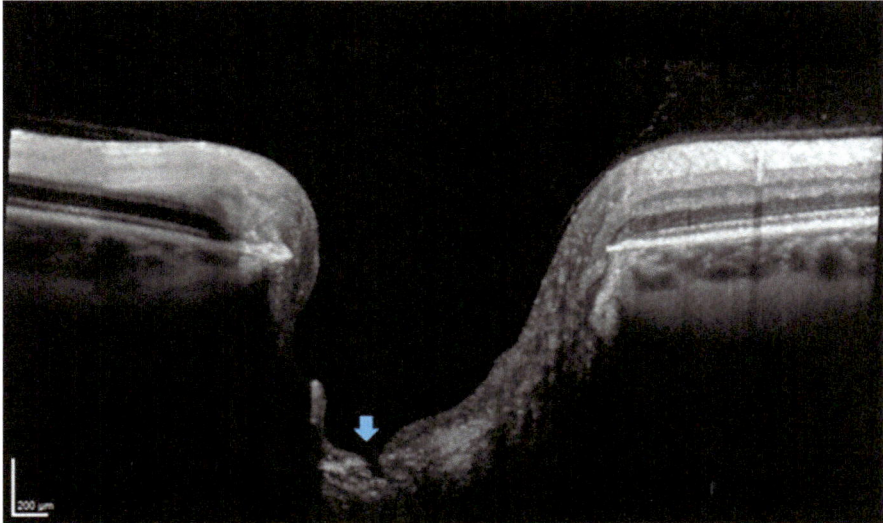

Fig. 10.6 Optical coherence tomography imaging of an enlarged laminar pore in a myopic eye (blue arrowhead)

space immediately behind the sclera and expansion of the circle of Zinn-Haller, with potentially compromised circulation of the prelaminar portion of the ONH [27].

Minimum rim width analysis with Glaucoma Module Premium Edition (GMPE) software of Spectralis OCT (Heidelberg Engineering Inc., Heidelberg, Germany) device may be helpful in myopic eyes when PPA or tilted ONH pose challenges to RNFL measurement.

10.3.2   The Retinal Nerve Fiber Layer

There are various sources of error with RNFL measurement in myopic eyes. These can be summarized as temporal displacement of RGC axons and blood vessels and torsional changes in the RNFL topography, problems with correct centering of the measurement circle on a myopic disc, variable focusing effect caused by tilting of the ONH, magnification issues related to myopic refraction, and segmentation errors. Peripapillary retinoschisis is also observed more frequently in myopic eyes.

Leung and associates measured the angle between the temporal superior and temporal inferior RNFL bundles on Cirrus HD-OCT images, and reported a reduction of this angle with increasing axial length [7]. As the axial length increases, the retina is dragged temporally and the RGC axons are compressed against the bundles originating from the opposite hemisphere temporal to the disc. This effect results in the thickening of the RNFL in the temporal quadrant and its thinning in the other quadrants especially nasally [28]. Temporal displacement of the vessels and RNFL peaks is typically observed in this scenario (Figs. 10.7 and 10.8).

Most of the current OCT devices automatically identify the optic disc or BMO centroid and center the calculation or scan circle on this centroid. Presence of a myopic tilted optic disc can make it challenging to determine the BMO centroid, therefore, confounding peripapillary RNFL analysis with OCT. For example, nasal displacement of the calculation circle causes thickening of the RNFL in the temporal region and decreases RNFL thickness in the other regions. In eyes with myopic tilted discs, the clinician should check the RNFL profile as well as the raw data and look for artifacts or other imaging issues, such as data being cut off due to marked height difference along the peripapillary the retina on the circular tomogram (Fig. 10.9). Raw images of the circular tomogram may also provide hints on the magnitude and axis of ONH tilt.

Location of the main temporal superior and inferior blood vessels is correlated with the RNFL thickness profile. In patients with ONH torsion, direction of torsion influences the location of blood vessels and peripapillary RNFL thickness, whereas the macular sectoral ganglion cell/inner plexiform layers (GCIPL) thickness is not affected [29]. Thickening of the temporal RNFL with temporal shifting of the superior peak in eyes with temporal (counterclockwise) ONH torsion can lead to interpretation errors because OCT devices provide sectorial analysis of the peripapillary RNFL based on their normative database. In this situation, ganglion cell or posterior pole analysis algorithms would be more helpful.

The average RNFL thickness may be affected by magnification of the ocular optical system, especially when myopia exceeds −4.0 diopters (D) [28, 30]. Current OCT

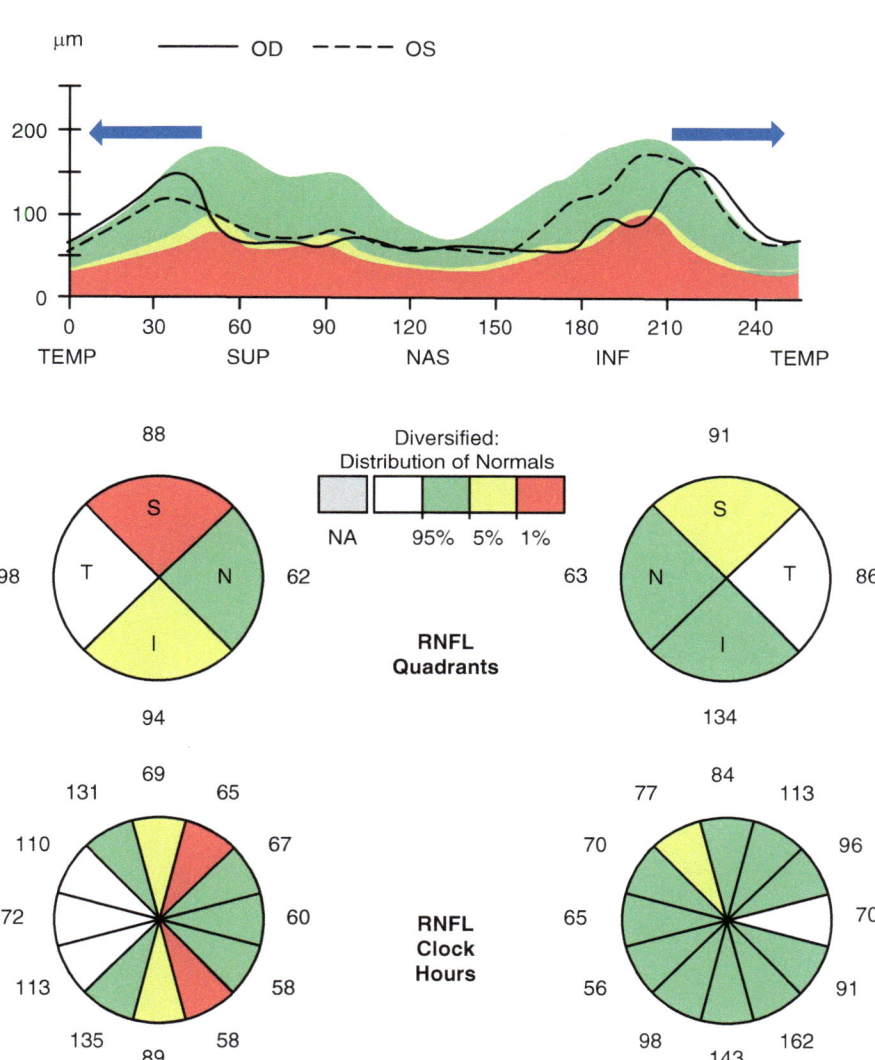

Fig. 10.7 Retinal nerve fiber layer (RNFL) analysis by Cirrus HD-OCT shows abnormally reduced thickness in superior and inferior sectors of the right eye and superior quadrant of the left eye of a myopic young patient suspected of glaucoma. The RNFL peaks on the thickness plots are temporally displaced in both eyes (blue arrows) leading to thickening of the RNFL (>95th percentile) in the temporal quadrants and apparent thinning superiorly in both eyes and inferiorly in the right eye

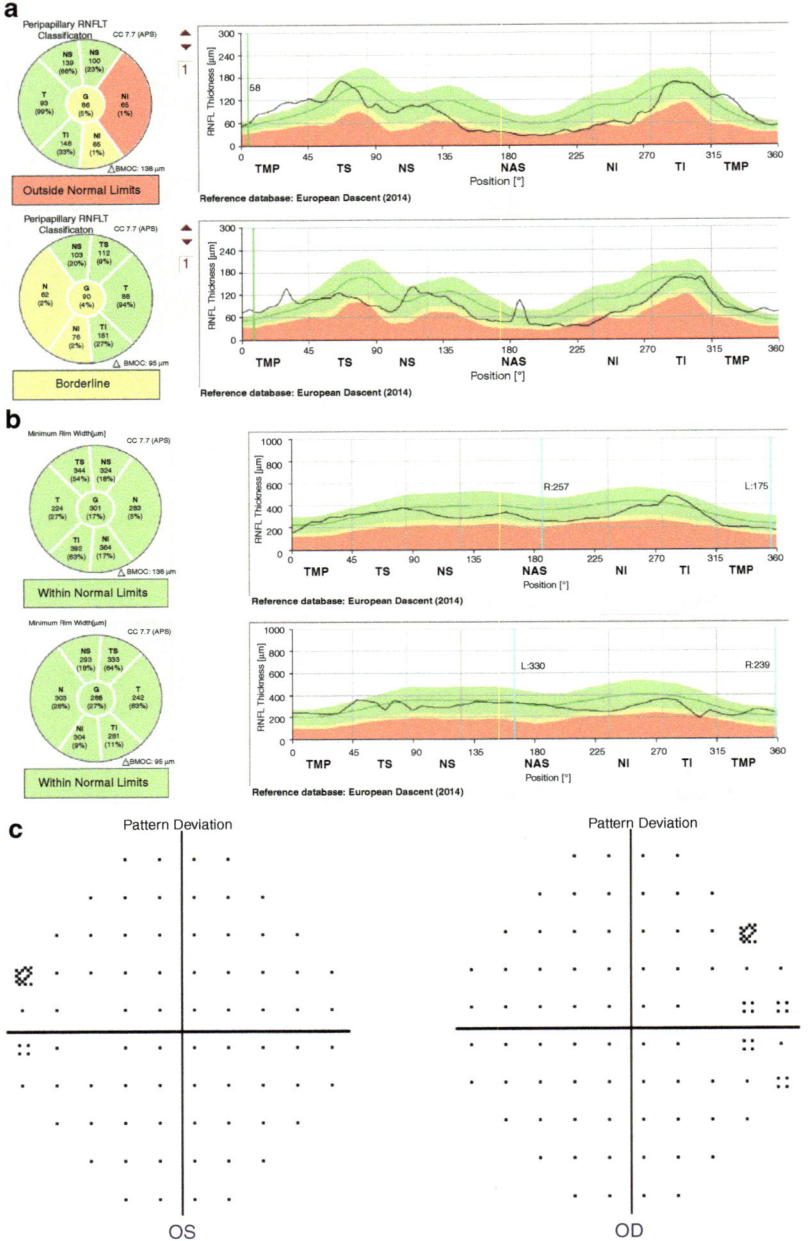

Fig. 10.8 This glaucoma suspect patient had myopia of −9 diopters (D) and −8.50 D in the right and left eyes, respectively. (**a**) Retinal nerve fiber layer (RNFL) thickness plots and classification charts showed thinning in the nasal sectors of both eyes with classification of 'outside normal limits' in the right eye, and borderline in the left eye based on sectoral analyses. (**b**) Minimum rim width analysis revealed measurements within normal limits in all sectors for both eyes. (**c**) Central 24-2 visual field tests were classified as within normal limits in both eyes

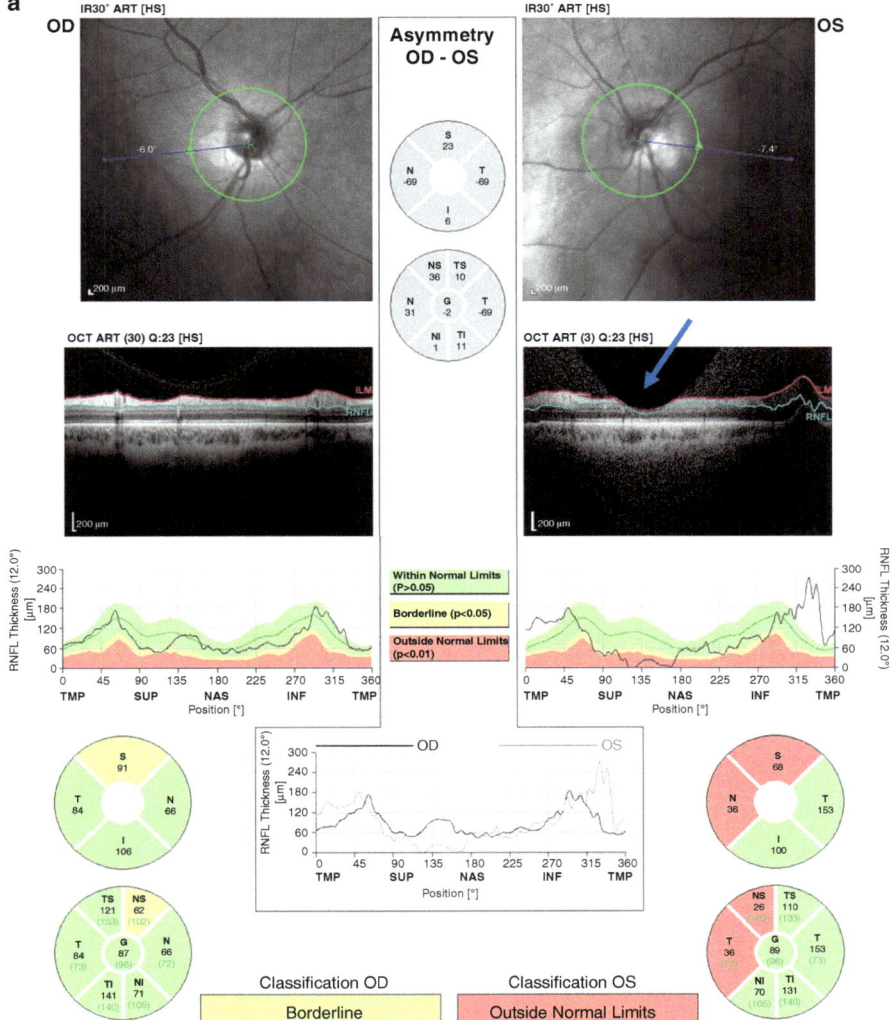

Fig. 10.9 (**a**) Spectralis optical coherence tomography (OCT) retinal nerve fiber layer (RNFL) printout of a patient with high myopia of −10.00 diopters spherical equivalent in both eyes, where classification was borderline in the right eye and outside normal limits in the left eye. When the RNFL profile of the left eye is carefully reviewed, one can see a crescent shaped defect in the retinal layers in the nasal superior area (see blue arrow). There is also artefactual thickening in the inferior temporal area; the likely cause is that because of the extreme curvature, the RNFL thickness is not measured perpendicularly. Classification is outside normal limits in the superior and nasal quadrants. (**b**) When the raw data is checked, one can see that the patient has inferotemporally tilted optic nerve head and the apex of the RNFL profile is out of the scanning zone, i.e., the difference between the retinal surface peak and trough almost exceeds the 2-mm depth of focus of the OCT device. (**c**) The test was repeated taking care that all the RNFL profile was fit within the scanning zone; the OCT classification is now within normal limits in the superior and nasal quadrants, although borderline thinning is present in the nasal superior sector, which is symmetrical in both eyes. (**d**) Raw image after the second test where RNFL profile is fit within the scanning zone

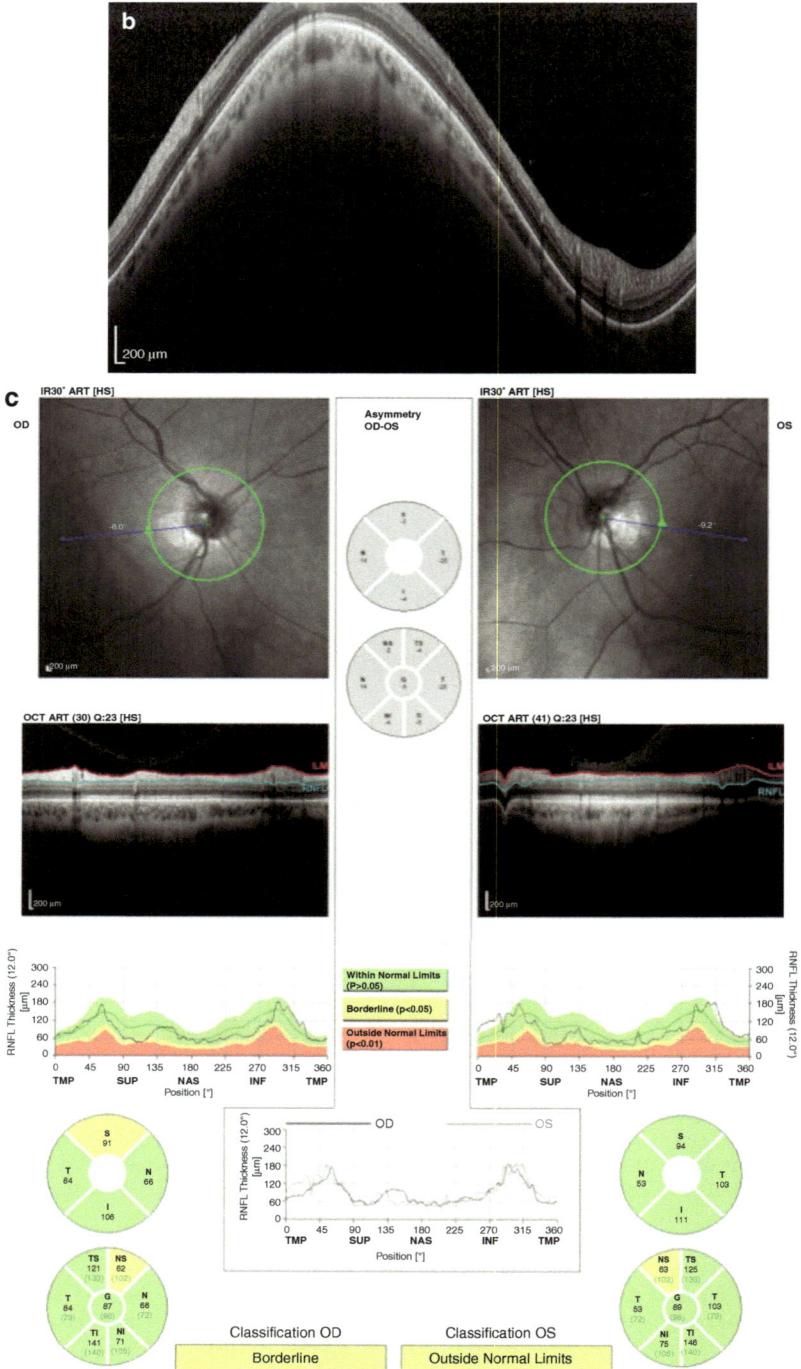

Fig. 10.9 (continued)

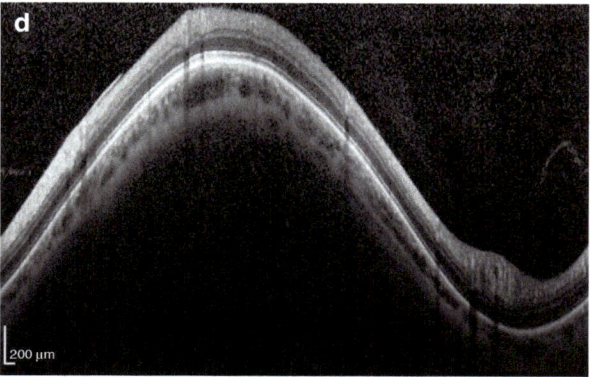

Fig. 10.9 (continued)

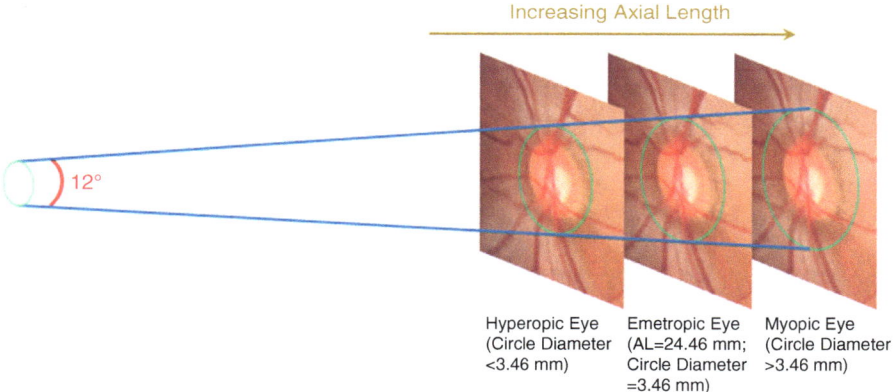

Fig. 10.10 Effect of axial length (AL) on the scan circle diameter. Scan circle is 3.46 mm in diameter in an emmetropic eye with average AL. Scan circle diameter directly affects the RNFL thickness measurements resulting in thinner measurements in a longer eye and thicker ones in a shorter eye

devices have been set to measure RNFL thickness at a fixed angular distance (approximately 12°) centered on the optic disc. However, the magnification effect of the eye is known to impact the actual size and hence, location, of the scan circle on the peripapillary retina [31]. The SD-OCT measurements are not thoroughly corrected for the magnification of the ocular optical system. Some devices such as Spectralis OCT require the corneal curvatures to be entered into the system before scanning. The additional focusing mechanism of the OCT devices also partially compensates for the axial length of the eye. A longer eye will result in a larger measurement circle diameter, thereby measuring the RNFL at a farther distance from the optic disc or BMO centroid. The reverse would apply to small eyes [32] (Fig. 10.10). Measurement circle's standard diameter of 3.46 mm in an emmetropic eye (considered as an eye with an axial length of 24.46 mm in Cirrus HD-OCT) decreases to 2.78 mm in a 20 mm long eye and increases to 4.00 mm in a 28 mm long eye [33].

In some myopic eyes, the automatic segmentation algorithms cannot accurately measure the RNFL thickness most commonly due to a larger area of PPA. In these cases, the lack of contrast between the RNFL and the remaining eyewall layers (typically only sclera) causes erroneous measurements. This is another issue that creates difficulty in the evaluation of glaucoma patients with high myopia [28]. Larger scan circles (4.1 and 4.7 mm in diameter) are available on the GMPE software of Spectralis, which may circumvent this issue.

To avoid misdiagnosis and to improve the sensitivity and specificity of glaucoma detection by OCT, a separate normative RNFL profile for myopic eyes is needed. The implementation of a myopic normative database in OCT instruments would potentially allow more precise interpretation of OCT printouts when used in myopic eyes. Recently, Seol and associates reported that the diagnostic ability of OCT significantly improved for detection of glaucoma in myopic eyes after incorporation of a customized myopic normative database into Cirrus HD-OCT (Fig. 10.11) [34].

In eyes with peripapillary retinoschisis, a transient increase in the RNFL thickness measurements is commonly observed (Fig. 10.12); after the resolution of retinoschisis, the RNFL thickness decreases remarkably. We propose that clinicians should examine the thickness maps as well as the raw OCT images in order to rule out retinoschisis so as not to overestimate the RNFL thickness or misinterpret the resolution of retinoschisis as a rapid structural progression. An area with supernormal RNFL thickness is oftentimes a clue to the presence of schisis areas. The schisis cavity can occasionally be observed as a darker, more or less localized, area on the *en face* IR images. More studies on this topic are needed to clarify whether a collapse of the schisis cavity represents a significant event in the course of RNFL deterioration.

10.3.3   Peripapillary Atrophy

In the infrared (IR) images, ONH can be surrounded by an area of hyper-reflectance, more commonly visible in the temporal area. This area corresponds to the PPA observed on fundus exam and is a possible source of OCT artifacts in myopic eyes as mentioned above. Proper identification of PPA zones is important for a correct diagnosis of glaucoma.

The conventional β-zone has, to date, been defined as visible sclera along with visible large choroidal vessels on fundus exam. It therefore included the (new) β-zone and the (new) γ-zone (see Sect 10.2.3). Since the new β-zone has been associated with glaucoma, whereas the γ-zone has been found to correlate with myopia rather than glaucoma, one may infer that clinical differentiation between these two zones may increase the diagnostic utility of β-zone for glaucoma [24].

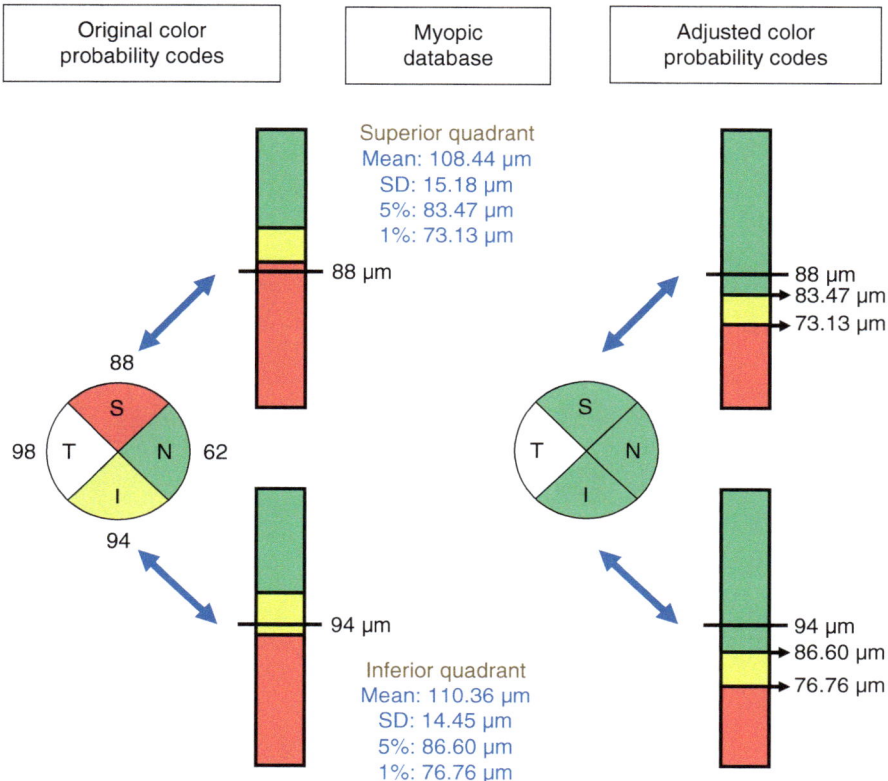

Fig. 10.11 The right eye of a 36-year-old glaucoma suspect woman with moderate myopia monitored in our clinic. Original color probability codes of retinal nerve fiber layer (RNFL) thickness display red color (p < 1%) in the superior quadrant and yellow color (1% < p < 5%) in the inferior quadrant. After applying the criteria derived from the myopic database, the superior (88 μm) and inferior RNFL thickness (94 μm) are shown in green (within normal limits). For the superior quadrant, the 5% cutoff point is 83.47 μm and the 1% value is 73.13 μm. For the inferior quadrant, the 5% cutoff point is 86.60 μm and the 1% value is 76.76 μm. Adjusted color probability codes of RNFL thickness show improved color probability codes in the superior and inferior quadrants. The bar graphs indicate the percentile values of the superior and inferior quadrants for the original and adjusted color probability codes [34]

An overview of the various peripapillary zones is provided in Figs. 10.13, 10.14, 10.15 and 10.16.

In eyes with wide PPA area, the standard 3.46 mm RNFL measurement circle may include the PPA area resulting in segmentation errors. Other OCT algorithms including a larger size scan with the GMPE software of Spectralis OCT, or macular imaging may be used as complementary or alternative options (Fig. 10.17).

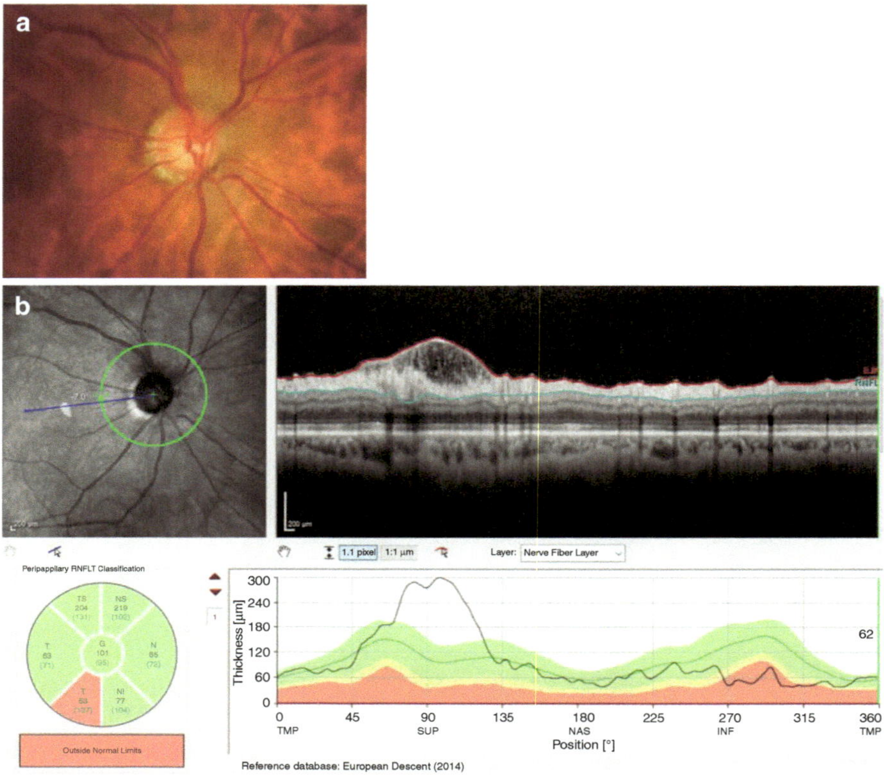

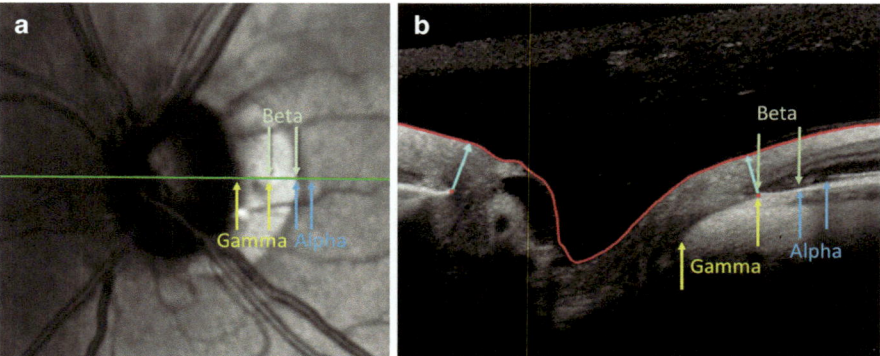

Fig. 10.12 (**a**) Disc photograph of a patient with superonasal peripapillary retinoschisis. The patient had primary open angle glaucoma and moderate myopia. (**b**) Retinal nerve fiber layer profile and thickness plot of optical coherence tomography image shows abnormal elevation of the RNFL. Note thinning of the RNFL in the temporal-inferior sector

Fig. 10.13 (**a**) Peripapillary atrophy zones in the infrared image. Note that the β- and γ-zones cannot be distinguished on the IR images. (**b**) The OCT optic nerve head scan demonstrates the peripapillary α-zone (Bruch's membrane-RPE complex is present with irregularities of the retinal pigment epithelium), β-zone (Bruch's membrane present with no retinal pigment epithelium) and γ-zone (no Bruch's membrane or retinal pigment epithelium)

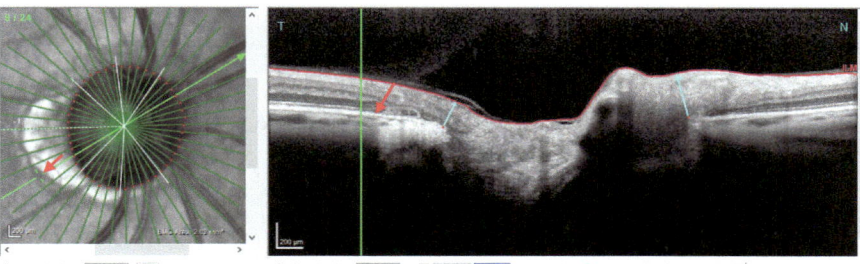

Fig. 10.14 The outer edge of the hyper-reflective area in β-zone peripapillary atrophy (PPA) corresponds to the retinal pigment epithelium ending (red arrows). Due to the temporal absence of RPE, more light can reach the underlying structures so they appear hyper-reflective on the infrared (IR) optical coherence tomography image. The Bruch's membrane ends at the same location as the choroid and the sclera. The Bruch's membrane opening is correctly identified at the inner edge of the β-zone PPA

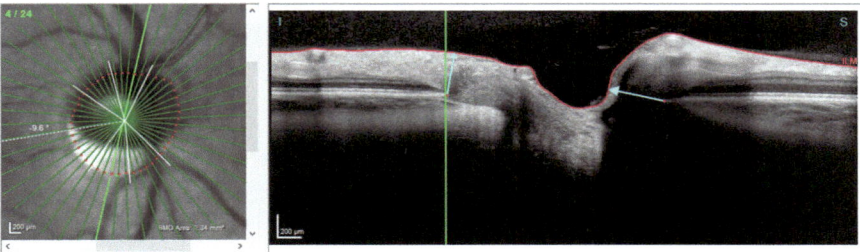

Fig. 10.15 Left, tilted optic nerve head with an infero-temporal myopic crescent (γ-zone peripapillary atrophy). As seen on the optical coherence tomography scan, the Bruch's membrane terminates before reaching the border tissue of Elschnig with significant thinning of the underlying choroid. Absence of the retinal pigment epithelium and thinned choroid enable a direct view onto the sclera seen as a white sharply demarcated zone on the infrared (IR) image. The Bruch's membrane opening is correctly detected at the outer edge of the hyper-reflectance area seen in the IR image

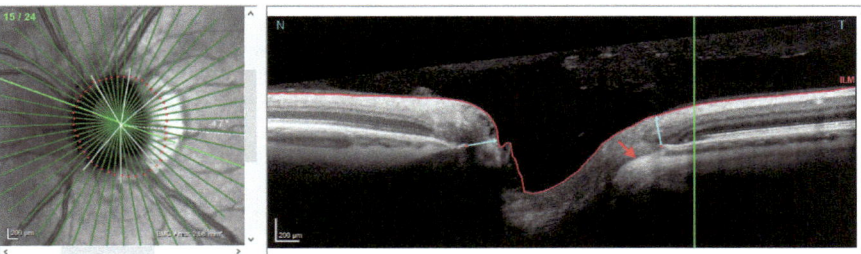

Fig. 10.16 A combination of peripapillary atrophy and temporal conus, for example in a tilted myopic disc, is possible. The outer edge of the hyper-reflective area on the infrared (IR) image corresponds to the retinal pigment epithelium (RPE) termination (green marker) while the inner edge matched an area of the border tissue of Elschnig (red arrow). The Bruch's membrane extends further than the RPE does. Therefore, the Bruch's membrane opening is located within the hyper-reflective area at the outer edge of γ-zone or rather at the inner edge of β-zone

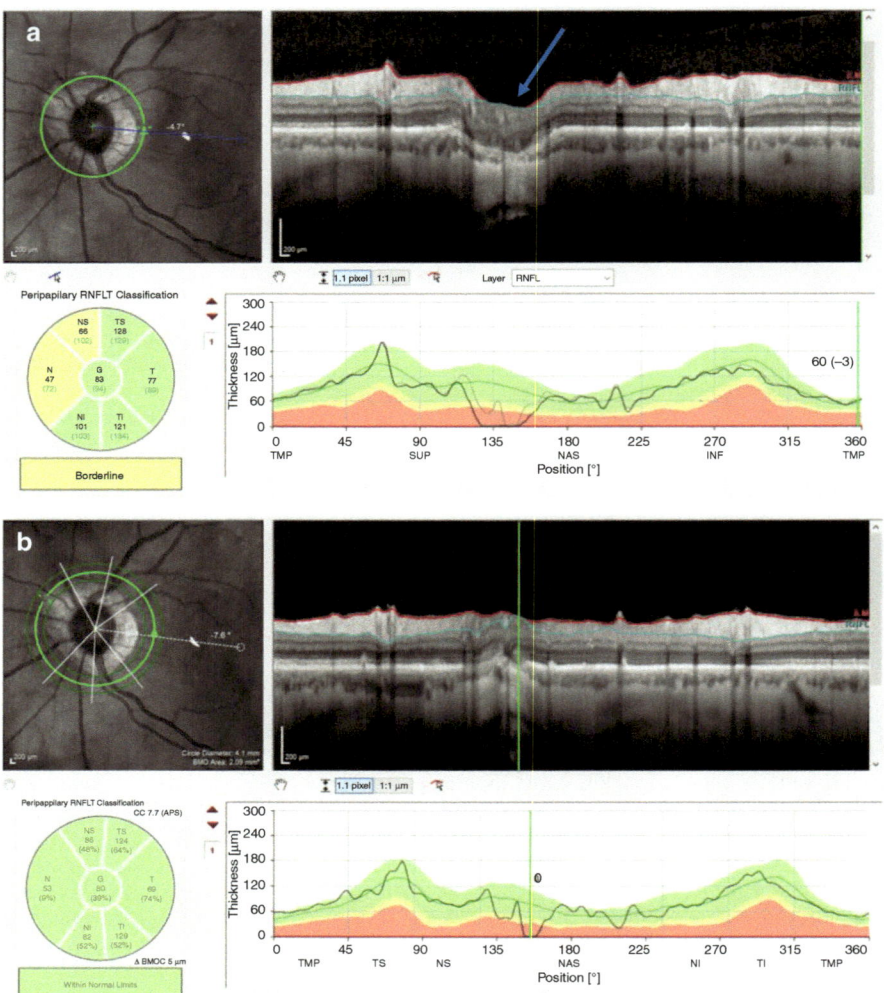

Fig. 10.17 (**a**) Peripapillary atrophy may cause localized segmentation error (blue arrow). (**b**) Changing the scan circle size to 4.1 mm decreased the extent of the area showing the segmentation error and demonstrated that the retinal nerve fiber layer (RNFL) thickness is mostly within normal limits in all the sectors. (**c**) The RNFL is within normal limits with circle scan size of 4.7 mm. (**d**) Minimum rim width analysis of the same eye revealed that neuroretinal rim thickness is within normal limits circumferentially and globally

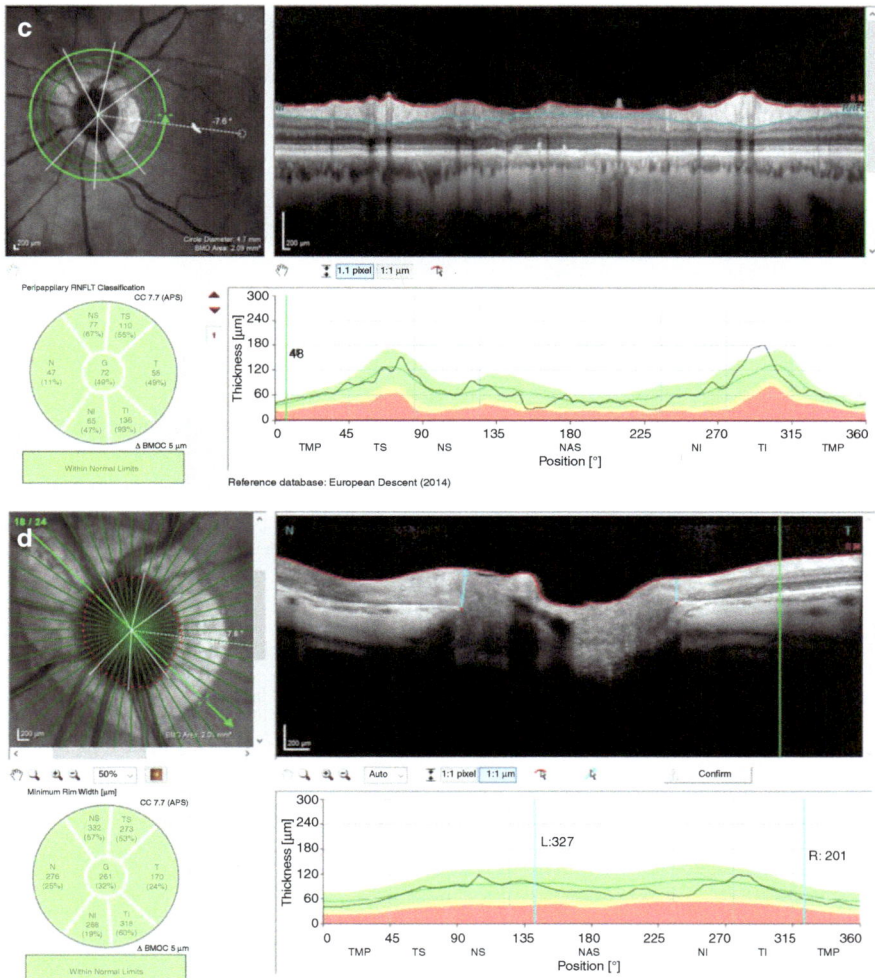

Fig. 10.17 (continued)

10.3.4 Macular Area

As the normative database of current OCT devices largely consists of data collected from normal eyes with no or low myopia, interpreting the RNFL thickness deviation maps in highly myopic eyes is commonly fraught with difficulties. Therefore, measuring the RGC cell bodies and their neural processes in the macula instead of the peripapillary axons could be a viable alternative (Fig. 10.18). The ganglion cell layer (GCL) or ganglion cell complex (GCC) can be segmented and measured in

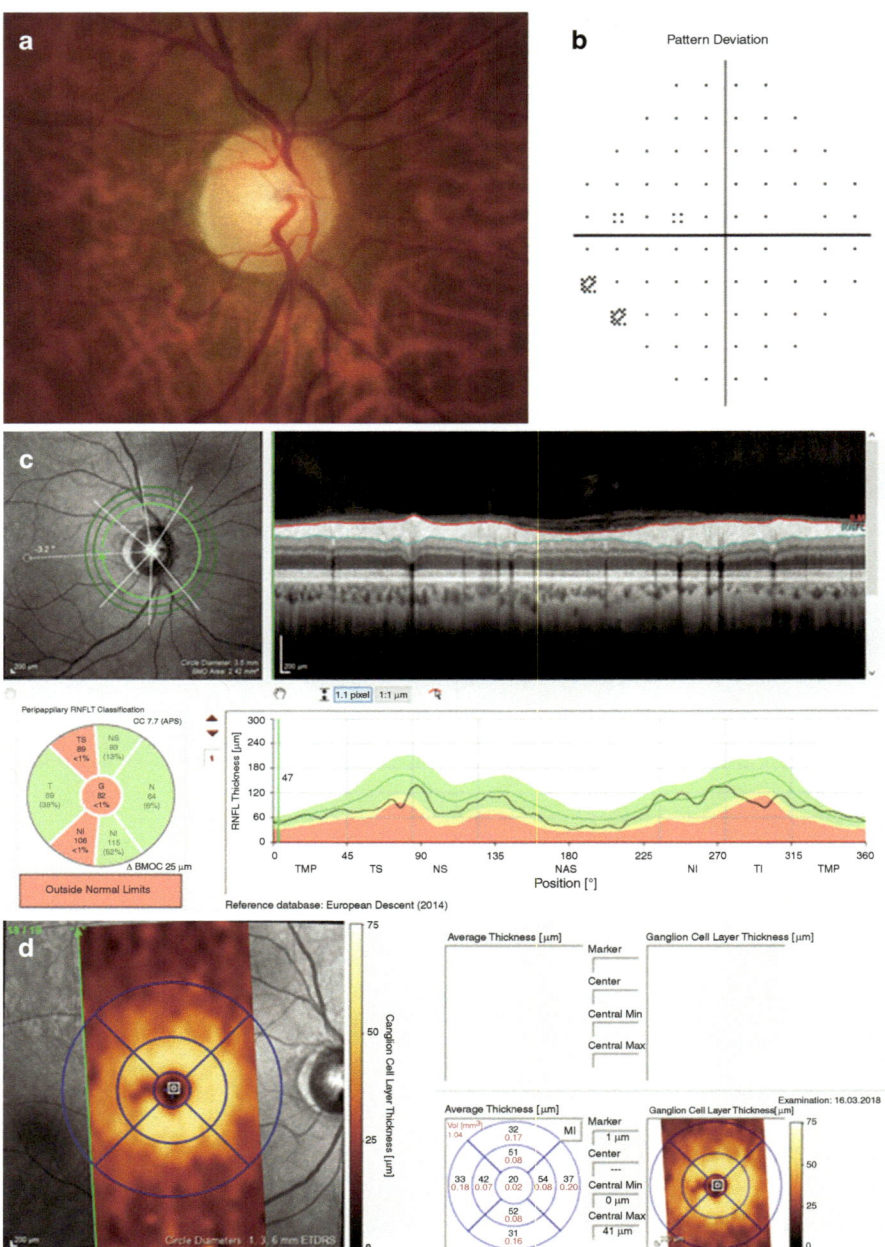

Fig. 10.18 (a) A young male patient with ocular hypertension and moderate myopia (−3.25 diopters spherical equivalent) in the right eye. The optic disc appeared healthy on exam. (b) The central 24-2 visual field test was within normal limits. (c) Retinal nerve fiber layer analysis showed thinning in the temporal superior and temporal inferior sectors both classified as outside normal limits. (d) The ganglion cell layer thickness map did not show any loss compatible with glaucoma and average thickness values on the ETDRS grid were symmetrical between the superior and inferior hemispheres. (e) The minimum rim width analysis results were within normal limits

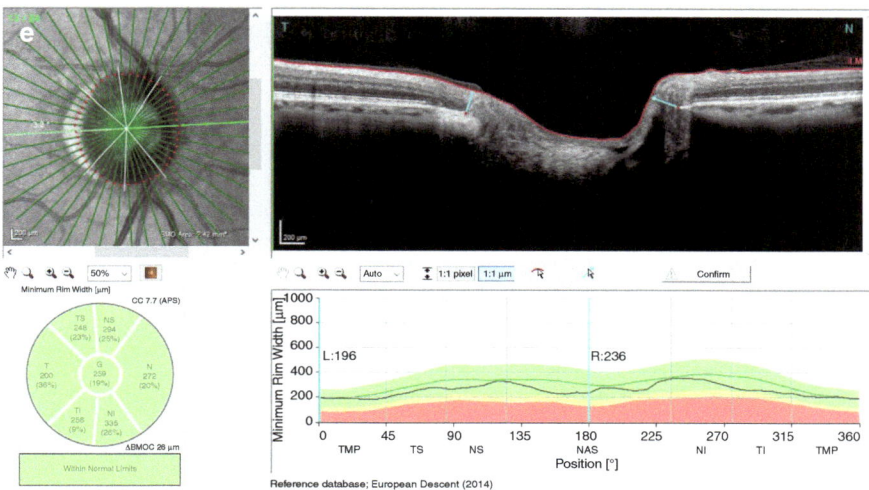

Fig. 10.18 (continued)

highly myopic eyes, but further longitudinal, large-scale studies are needed to validate its translation into clinical practice.

Several studies reported that the GCC parameters of SD-OCT attained higher diagnostic power than both ONH parameters and peripapillary RNFL measurements for detection of glaucoma concomitant with high myopia [35–37]. These studies concluded that assessment of GCC parameters is a useful technique complementary to peripapillary RNFL thickness assessment for clinically evaluating concomitant glaucoma and high myopia. Akashi and associates reported significant differences in the diagnostic performances of the peripapillary RNFL thickness measurements for detection of glaucoma in highly myopic eyes with early VF loss when highly myopic normal eyes were used as the control group compared to a nonhighly myopic normal group regardless of the OCT device used [38]. Highly myopic normal eyes showed higher receiver operating characteristic curves (AUCs) for the temporal quadrant circumpapillary RNFL thickness but lower AUCs for the superior and inferior RNFL thicknesses compared with nonhighly myopic normal eyes. In contrast, when the GCC thickness was used for this purpose, the difference was not statistically significant. However, use of macular RNFL thickness led to high false positive detection rate in high myopia.

Application of a myopic normative database for ganglion cell inner plexiform layer (GCIPL) thickness has been reported to significantly improve detection of glaucoma in myopic eyes [34]. Seo and associates investigated the effect of myopia and optic disc size on the GCIPL and RNFL thickness profiles obtained with Cirrus HD-OCT. RNFL and GCIPL thickness profiles were affected by the refractive error and optic disc size. They recommend RNFL and GCIPL analysis in the evaluation of glaucoma should always be interpreted with reference to the refractive status and optic disc size [39].

10.4 Key Points

- The clinician should look for signs of segmentation errors and artifacts on the OCT images and always examine the raw images. Significant defects seen on the OCT frequently correspond with defects on the VF.
- Instead of relying on the color coding of OCT results to indicate abnormality, monitoring the RNFL and ONH parameters with OCT *over time* in myopic eyes may be helpful, since these parameters would not be expected to change in normal myopic patients but would do so in a progressive optic neuropathy such as glaucoma. In other words, the clinician should focus on comparing the patient to himself or herself rather than the general population. Examination of the RNFL raw images over time can be helpful.
- Before making a clinical decision, the family history, ethnicity, severity of myopia, central corneal thickness, corneal hysteresis, and the IOPs of the patient also need to be considered.
- The clinician should gather as much information and data as he or she can, including ONH photographs, VFs, and OCT images of the ONH (BMO-MRW), RNFL, and macula, and should put more emphasis on his or her clinical impression in myopic eyes.

References

1. Shim SH, Sung KR, Kim JM, Kim HT, Jeong J, Kim CY, Lee MY, Park KH. Korean ophthalmological society. The prevalence of open-angle glaucoma by age in myopia: the Korea National Health and nutrition examination survey. Curr Eye Res. 2017;42:65–71.
2. Chon B, Qiu M, Lin SC. Myopia and glaucoma in the south Korean population. Invest Ophthalmol Vis Sci. 2013;54:6570–7.
3. Mitchell P, Hourihan F, Sandbach J, Wang JJ. The relationship between glaucoma and myopia: the blue mountains eye study. Ophthalmology. 1999;106:2010–5.
4. Xu L, Li Y, Wang S, Wang Y, Wang Y, Jonas JB. Characteristics of highly myopic eyes: the Beijing eye study. Ophthalmology. 2007;114:121–6.
5. Melo GB, Libera RD, Barbosa AS, Pereira LM, Doi LM, Melo LA Jr. Comparison of optic disk and retinal nerve fiber layer thickness in nonglaucomatous and glaucomatous patients with high myopia. Am J Ophthalmol. 2006;142:858–60.
6. You QS, Peng XY, Xu L, Chen CX, Wang YX, Jonas JB. Myopic maculopathy imaged by optical coherence tomography: the Beijing eye study. Ophthalmology. 2014;121:220–4.
7. Leung CK, Mohamed S, Leung KS, Cheung CY, Chan SL, Cheng DK, Lee AK, Leung GY, Rao SK, Lam DS. Retinal nerve fiber layer measurements in myopia: an optical coherence tomography study. Invest Ophthalmol Vis Sci. 2006;47:5171–6.
8. Wong YZ, Lam AK. The roles of cornea and axial length in corneal hysteresis among emmetropes and high myopes: a pilot study. Curr Eye Res. 2015;40:282–9.
9. Jiang Z, Shen M, Mao G, Chen D, Wang J, Qu J, Lu F. Association between corneal biomechanical properties and myopia in Chinese subjects. Eye (Lond). 2011;25:1083–9.
10. Shen M, Fan F, Xue A, Wang J, Zhou X, Lu F. Biomechanical properties of the cornea in high myopia. Vis Res. 2008;48:2167–71.
11. Kim TW, Kim M, Weinreb RN, Woo SJ, Park KH, Hwang JM. Optic disc change with incipient myopia of childhood. Ophthalmology. 2012;119:21–6.

12. Jonas JB, Gusek GC, Naumann GO. Optic disk morphometry in high myopia. Graefes Arch Clin Exp Ophthalmol. 1988;226:587–90.
13. Witmer MT, Margo CE, Drucker M. Tilted optic disks. Surv Ophthalmol. 2010;55:403–28.
14. Jonas JB, Xu L. Histological changes of high axial myopia. Eye (Lond). 2014;28:113–7.
15. Morgan WH, Yu DY, Alder VA, Cringle SJ, Cooper RL, House PH, Constable IJ. The correlation between cerebrospinal fluid pressure and retrolaminar tissue pressure. Invest Ophthalmol Vis Sci. 1998;39:1419–28.
16. Tezel G, Trinkaus K, Wax MB. Alterations in the morphology of lamina cribrosa pores in glaucomatous eyes. Br J Ophthalmol. 2004;88:251–6.
17. Tay E, Seah SK, Chan SP, Lim AT, Chew SJ, Foster PJ, Aung T. Optic disk ovality as an index of tilt and its relationship to myopia and perimetry. Am J Ophthalmol. 2005;139:247–52.
18. Jonas JB. Optic disk size correlated with refractive error. Am J Ophthalmol. 2005;139:346–8.
19. Jonas JB, Nguyen XN, Gusek GC, Naumann GO. Parapapillary chorioretinal atrophy in normal and glaucoma eyes. I. Morphometric data. Invest Ophthalmol Vis Sci. 1989;30:908–18.
20. Jonas JB, Budde WM, Panda-Jones S. Ophthalmoscopic evaluation of the optic nerve head. Surv Ophthalmol. 1999;43:293–320.
21. Jonas JB, Jonas SB, Jonas RA, Holbach L, Dai Y, Sun X, Panda-Jones S. Parapapillary atrophy: histological gamma zone and delta zone. PLoS One. 2012;7(10):e47237.
22. Dichtl A, Jonas JB, Naumann GO. Histomorphometry of the optic disc in highly myopic eyes with absolute secondary angle closure glaucoma. Br J Ophthalmol. 1998;82:286–9.
23. Fantes FE, Anderson DR. Clinical histologic correlation of human peripapillary anatomy. Ophthalmology. 1989;96:20–5.
24. Dai Y, Jonas JB, Huang H, Wang M, Sun X. Microstructure of parapapillary atrophy: beta zone and gamma zone. Invest Ophthalmol Vis Sci. 2013;54:2013–8.
25. Ng DS, Cheung CY, Luk FO, Mohamed S, Brelen ME, Yam JC, Tsang CW, Lai TY. Advances of optical coherence tomography in myopia and pathologic myopia. Eye (Lond). 2016;30:901–16.
26. Hosseini H, Nassiri N, Azarbod P, Giaconi J, Chou T, Caprioli J, Nouri-Mahdavi K. Measurement of the optic disc vertical tilt angle with spectral-domain optical coherence tomography and influencing factors. Am J Ophthalmol. 2013;156:737–44.
27. Kimura Y, Akagi T, Hangai M, Takayama K, Hasegawa T, Suda K, Yoshikawa M, Yamada H, Nakanishi H, Unoki N, Ikeda HO, Yoshimura N. Lamina cribrosa defects and optic disc morphology in primary open angle glaucoma with high myopia. PLoS One. 2014;9(12):e115313. https://doi.org/10.1371/journal.pone.0115313. eCollection 2014
28. Kang SH, Hong SW, Im SK, Lee SH, Ahn MD. Effect of myopia on the thickness of the retinal nerve fiber layer measured by cirrus HD optical coherence tomography. Invest Ophthalmol Vis Sci. 2010;51:4075–83.
29. Lee KH, Kim CY, Kim NR. Variations of retinal nerve fiber layer thickness and ganglion cell-inner plexiform layer thickness according to the torsion direction of optic disc. Invest Ophthalmol Vis Sci. 2014;55:1048–55.
30. Bae SH, Kang SH, Feng CS, Park J, Jeong JH, Yi K. Influence of myopia on size of optic nerve head and retinal nerve fiber layer thickness measured by spectral domain optical coherence tomography. Korean J Ophthalmol. 2016;30:335–43.
31. Budenz DL, Anderson DR, Varma R, Schuman J, Cantor L, Savell J, Greenfield DS, Patella VM, Quigley HA, Tielsch J. Determinants of normal retinal nerve fiber layer thickness measured by stratus OCT. Ophthalmology. 2007;114:1046–52.
32. Nowroozizadeh S, Cirineo N, Amini N, Knipping S, Chang T, Chou T, Caprioli J, Nouri-Mahdavi K. Influence of correction of ocular magnification on spectral-domain OCT retinal nerve fiber layer measurement variability and performance. Invest Ophthalmol Vis Sci. 2014;55:3439–46.
33. Savini G, Barboni P, Parisi V, Carbonelli M. The influence of axial length on retinal nerve fibre layer thickness and optic-disc size measurements by spectral-domain OCT. Br J Ophthalmol. 2012;96:57–61.
34. Seol BR, Kim DM, Park KH, Jeoung JW. Assessment of optical coherence tomography color probability codes in myopic glaucoma eyes after applying a myopic normative database. Am J Ophthalmol. 2017;183:147–55.

35. Zhang C, Tatham AJ, Weinreb RN, Zangwill LM, Yang Z, Zhang JZ, Medeiros FA. Relationship between ganglion cell layer thickness and estimated retinal ganglion cell counts in the glaucomatous macula. Ophthalmology. 2014;121:2371–9.
36. Shoji T, Sato H, Ishida M, Takeuchi M, Chihara E. Assessment of glaucomatous changes in subjects with high myopia using spectral domain optical coherence tomography. Invest Ophthalmol Vis Sci. 2011;52:1098–102.
37. Kim NR, Lee ES, Seong GJ, Kang SY, Kim JH, Hong S, Kim CY. Comparing the ganglion cell complex and retinal nerve fibre layer measurements by Fourier domain OCT to detect glaucoma in high myopia. Br J Ophthalmol. 2011;95:1115–21.
38. Akashi A, Kanamori A, Ueda K, Inoue Y, Yamada Y, Nakamura M. The ability of SD-OCT to differentiate early glaucoma with high myopia from highly myopic controls and nonhighly myopic controls. Invest Ophthalmol Vis Sci. 2015;56:6573–80.
39. Seo S, Lee CE, Jeong JH, Park KH, Kim DM, Jeoung JW. Ganglion cell-inner plexiform layer and retinal nerve fiber layer thickness according to myopia and optic disc area: a quantitative and three-dimensional analysis. BMC Ophthalmol. 2017;17:22. https://doi.org/10.1186/s12886-017-0419-1.

Chapter 11
Anterior Segment Optical Coherence Tomography in Glaucoma

Atilla Bayer

11.1   History and Current Applications of Anterior Segment Optical Coherence Tomography in Ophthalmology

Optical coherence tomography (OCT) was initially developed for retinal imaging. In 1994 Izatt et al. used it for the first time for imaging of the anterior chamber structures. The prototype device was a slit-lamp mounted, 830-nm time-domain system [1]. The newer AS-OCT systems have rapidly become popular for assessment of the anterior chamber angle [2]. Currently, AS-OCT systems are classified according to the wavelength of the light source. Dedicated systems use 1310 nm wavelength and include Zeiss Visante (Carl Zeiss Meditec Inc., Dublin, CA), Heidelberg's SL-OCT (Heidelberg Engineering Inc., Heidelberg, Germany) and Tomey's CASIA (TOMEY Corp. Nagoya, Japan). On the other hand, systems converted from a retinal scanner use an 830-nm wavelength and include Spectralis OCT (Heidelberg Engineering Inc., Heidelberg, Germany), Cirrus HD-OCT (Carl Zeiss Meditec Inc., Dublin, CA), Optovue's RTVue (Optovue iVue; Optovue Inc., Fremont, CA) [3]. There are differences between these two groups of devices due to the different light sources. Shorter wavelength systems provide a higher axial resolution, but their imaging depth is limited. Longer-wavelength systems, on the other hand, provides deeper penetration by reducing the amount of scattering by the sclera and limbus, which allows visualization of the anterior chamber angle morphology in greater detail. Higher light intensities improve signal-to-noise ratio since most light entering the eye will be absorbed by the vitreous, protecting the retina from damage [4]. The stated axial resolution of Fourier or spectral domain AS-OCT systems ranges between 4 μm and 7 μm. The commercially available spectral domain AS-OCT systems include the following: RTVue SD-OCT, Cirrus HD-OCT,

A. Bayer
Department of Glaucoma, Dünyagöz Eye Hospital, Ankara, Turkey

Spectralis OCT, SOCT Copernicus (Optopol Technology, Zawiercie, Poland), and 3D OCT-3000 (Topcon Medical Systems, Oakland, NJ).

AS-OCT systems allow clinicians to document the anterior segment anatomy providing a cross-sectional view. After acquisition, the scanned images are processed by a customized software, which compensates for the transition of the index of refraction at the air-tear interface and the different indices in air, cornea and aqueous and account for the physical dimensions of the images [5]. Clinical applications of AS-OCT other than in the realm of glaucoma include tear meniscus measurement, ocular surface disease (e.g., pterygium, pinguecula, and scleromalacia), architectural analysis after cataract surgery, post-LASIK keratectasia, Descemet's membrane detachment, evaluation of corneal graft after keratoplasty, corneal deposits (corneal dystrophies and corneal verticillata), keratitis, and anterior segment tumors. Interactive measurement tools for cornea, sclera, anterior chamber angle and various abnormalities enable detailed investigation of the anterior segment structures and pathologies. It is preferable that testing is carried out before any ocular examination that can disturb the tear film such as use of a contact lens or applanation tonometry.

Current uses of AS-OCT in patients with established or suspected glaucoma include angle assessment, morphological analysis of the filtering blebs, corneal thickness, iris thickness, and anterior chamber depth and lens position. It is possible to use the ruler function to make interactive measurements of various anatomic and pathologic structures for diagnostic and research purposes. Anterior segment images can help in making decisions regarding laser treatment or choosing the most appropriate surgical approach. AS-OCT is therefore a useful adjunct in the diagnosis and management of glaucoma. With developments in the technology of three-dimensional AS-OCT [6] and increasing speed of scanning function, the future applications of this technology in glaucoma are promising.

11.2   Imaging the Anterior Chamber

11.2.1   Anterior Chamber Angle Evaluation

Evaluation of the anterior chamber angle during ophthalmic examination is crucial in determining the susceptibility of the angle to closure (Fig. 11.1). Although gonioscopy is the current gold standard for anterior chamber angle assessment, common flaws of this technique include artifacts caused by pressure on the cornea and the use of excessive amounts of light, both of which may affect the results. Findings of gonioscopy are subjective and semi-quantitative.

AS-OCT can measure the angle recess quantitatively. The use of infrared laser and real-time eye position monitoring during image acquisition permits the precise capture of angle morphology in the dark or under mesopic condition. With high scan speed, AS-OCT has the potential to provide valuable information regarding dynamic

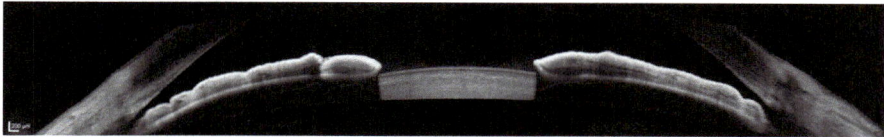

Fig. 11.1 AS-OCT of an eye with narrow angles as seen on anterior chamber angle images from Spectralis AS-OCT. Note the convex configuration of the iris and the small space between the root of the iris and the limbus

Fig. 11.2 Diagram illustrating several biometric descriptors of the anterior chamber angle, including AOD, ARA, SS-IR, IT, and ILCD. In this example, measurements are made 500 μm from scleral spur. *AOD* angle-opening distance, *ARA* angle recess area, *ILCD* iris-lens contact distance, *IT* iris thickness, *SS-IR* scleral spur-iris insertion distance

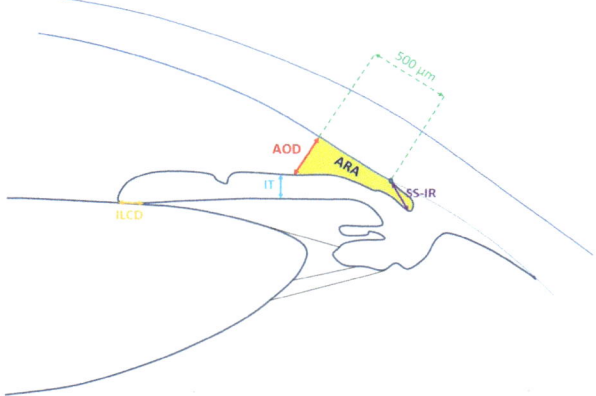

changes of the angle configuration under different lighting conditions. This is harder to accomplish with standard gonioscopy and ultrasound biomicroscopy (UBM). In addition, AS-OCT provides insight into the possible mechanism of the angle's narrowing or closure, including the possibility of plateau iris, lens-related mechanism and malignant glaucoma. One major limitation of AS-OCT compared to UBM is the fact that AS-OCTs do not provide any information from structures behind the iris as the laser light cannot pass beyond the iris. Many criteria developed for the assessment of the anterior segment with UBM [7–9] are applicable AS-OCT as well. The most important parameters during anterior chamber angle evaluation with AS-OCT are the angle opening distance (AOD), angle recess area (ARA), trabecular-iris angle (TIA), and trabecular-iris space area (TISA) at 500 or 750 μm from the scleral spur (Figs. 11.2 and 11.3). AOD is the distance from the cornea to iris at 500 or 750 μm from scleral spur. ARA is the area of triangle bordered by the anterior iris surface, corneal endothelium and a line perpendicular to the corneal endothelium going from a point from the iris surface to a point 500 or 750 μm anterior to the scleral spur. The ARA is theoretically, a better measurement parameter than the AOD since it takes into account the entire contour of the iris surface rather than measuring a single point on the iris as is the case with AOD. TIA is the angle formed from angle recess to points 500 or 750 μm from the scleral spur on trabecular meshwork and perpendicular on surface of iris. Iris thickness (IT) is usually measured at

Fig. 11.3 TISA is the trapezoid area between the iris and cornea delimited by a line perpendicular to the scleral spur and a second line perpendicular to the cornea 750 µm from the scleral spur

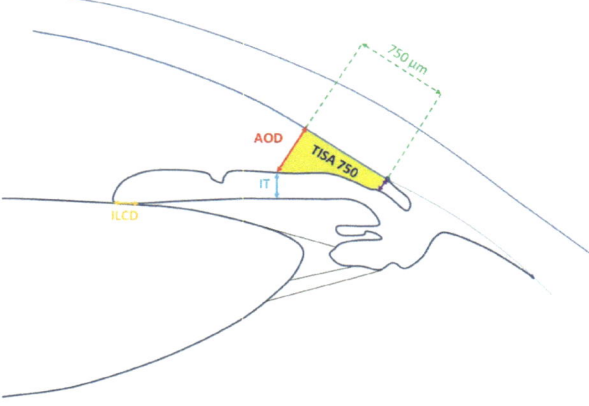

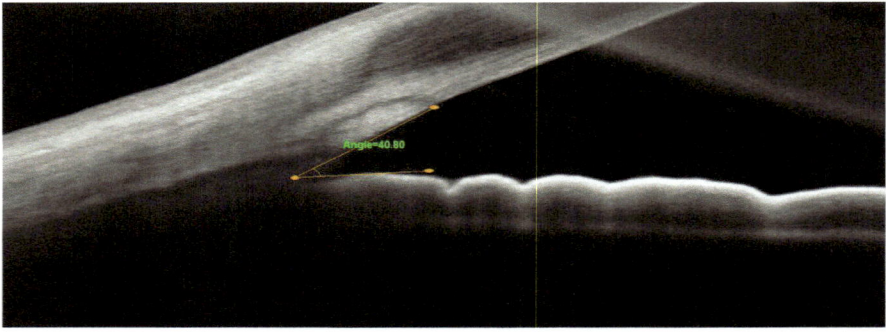

Fig. 11.4 Measurement of anterior chamber angle using RTVue AS-OCT. Here the scleral spur angle is 40.80° in an eye with healthy open angle

a location where a line perpendicular to cornea 500 µm from scleral spur crosses the iris. Iris-lens contact distance (ILCD) is the length of contact between the surfaces of lens and iris (Fig. 11.2). TISA is the trapezoid area between the iris and cornea delimited by a line perpendicular to the scleral spur and a second line perpendicular to the cornea 750 µm from the scleral spur [10]. This parameter is probably better related to the filtering function of the drainage system when compared with the ARA because the TISA excludes the non-filtering region behind the scleral spur (Fig. 11.3).

Commercially available AS-OCT devices have proprietary software for measurement of anterior chamber and angle parameters. An example of angle measurement of a healthy open angle with RTVue AS-OCT device is depicted at Fig. 11.4. Spectralis AS-OCT anterior chamber angle measurement of an eye with narrow angle is shown in Figs. 11.5 and 11.6. In Fig. 11.5, measurements are made 500 µm from scleral spur, whereas those in Fig. 11.6 are made at 750 µm distance from scleral spur. An example of angle measurement of a healthy eye with open angle from Cirrus HD AS-OCT device is shown in Fig. 11.7.

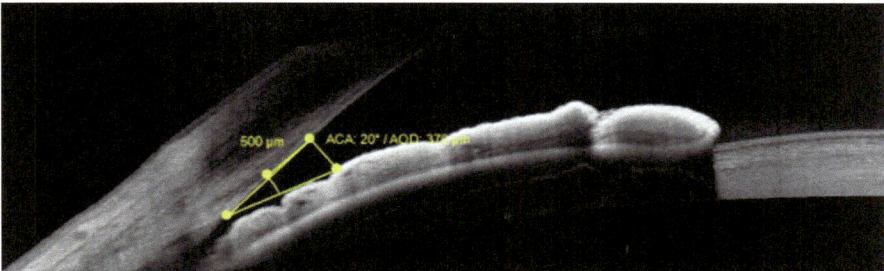

Fig. 11.5 Quantitative measurement of anterior chamber angle parameters using Spectralis AS-OCT in an eye with narrow angle. Here the measurements were made 500 μm from the scleral spur and ACA is 20°. *ACA* anterior chamber angle (in degrees), *AOD* angle opening distance

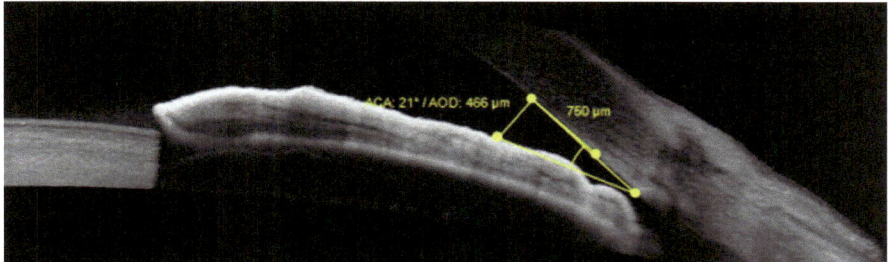

Fig. 11.6 Quantitative measurement of anterior chamber angle parameters with Spectralis AS-OCT in the same eye as Fig. 11.5. Here the measurements were made 750 μm from the scleral spur and ACA is 21°. *ACA* anterior chamber angle (in degrees), *AOD* angle opening distance

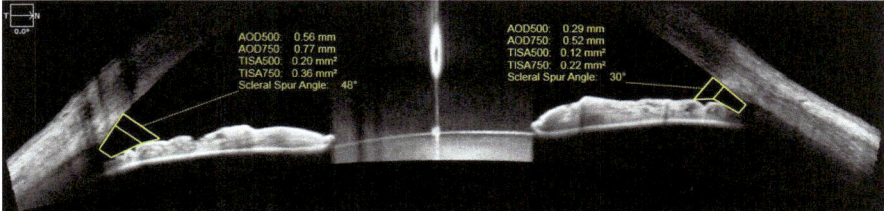

Fig. 11.7 Anterior chamber angle parameters in the nasal and temporal meridians derived from Cirrus HD AS-OCT in a healthy eye with open angles. Here the measurements were made 500 and 750 μm from the scleral spur

Most of the valuable parameters for quantitative measurements of the anterior chamber are based on the identification of the scleral spur. Sakata et al. found that, on Visante OCT images, the inter-observer agreement for detecting the scleral spur was moderate to substantial with a kappa value of 0.65 [5]. The distance between the repeat scleral spur localization points from the two sessions was within 10 μm in 83% of the 78 quadrants assessed and within 20 μm in 90%.

11.2.2 Anterior Segment Findings in Various Types of Glaucoma

In addition to quantitative measurement of the angle recess, AS-OCT can provide information about other angle components such as the Schlemm's canal (Fig. 11.8), and shed light on the possible mechanism of angle narrowing or closure including primary angle closure (PAC), plateau iris, lens-related mechanisms or glaucoma caused by aqueous misdirection. In PAC, the convex configuration of iris and angle narrowing from relative pupillary block can be detected in addition to the effect of laser peripheral iridotomy (Fig. 11.9). Widening of the angle following pilocarpine drop instillation (Fig. 11.10) or cataract surgery can also be demonstrated (Fig. 11.11). Plateau iris configuration can also be partially assessed with AS-OCT (Fig. 11.12); however, any ciliary body-mediated posterior pushing of the peripheral iris (such as plateau iris or iris cysts) cannot be diagnosed with this technology alone. UBM needs be used for evaluation of the ciliary processes.

One striking example of lens-related angle closure is microspherophakia. The definitive treatment in such cases is lensectomy although additional glaucoma surgery is needed in some cases (Fig. 11.13).

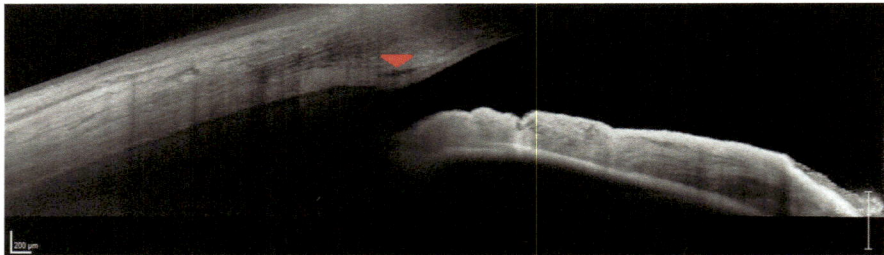

Fig. 11.8 Schlemm's canal (see arrowhead) is seen as a slit-shaped dark area on the inner part of the limbus

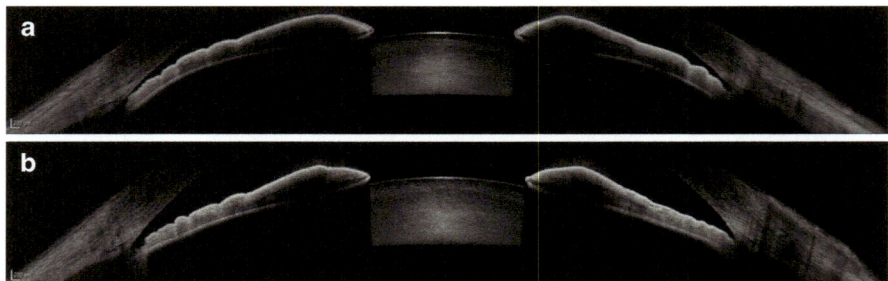

Fig. 11.9 (**a**) Low-magnification images of the anterior segment reveals convex iris configuration with narrow angles temporally and nasally in an eye with primary angle closure. (**b**) Following laser peripheral iridotomy, flattening of the iris and angle widening can be observed

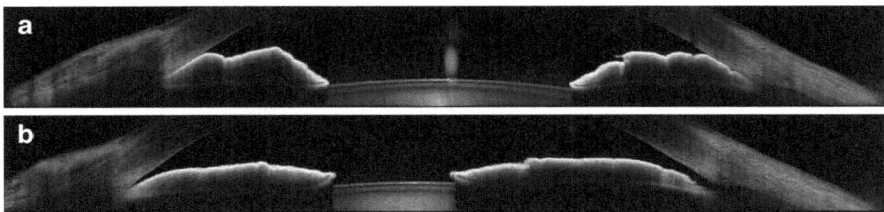

Fig. 11.10 (**a**) Low-magnification images of the anterior segment reveals convex iris configuration with closed angles temporally and nasally in an eye with primary angle closure. (**b**) Following pilocarpine administration, flattening of the iris and angle widening can be seen

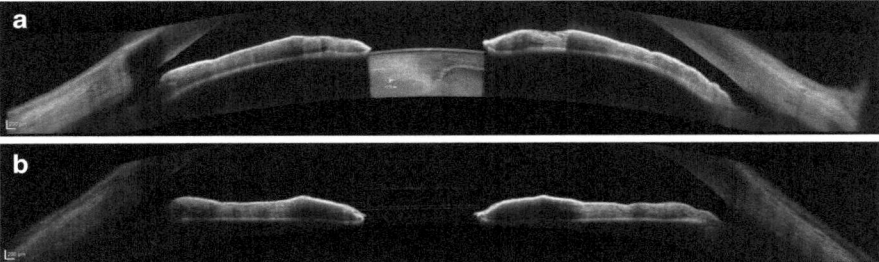

Fig. 11.11 (**a**) Low-magnification images of the anterior segment reveals convex iris configuration with narrow angles temporally and nasally in a hyperopic eye with visually significant cataract. (**b**) After cataract extraction and intraocular lens implantation, flattening of the iris and angle widening occurred

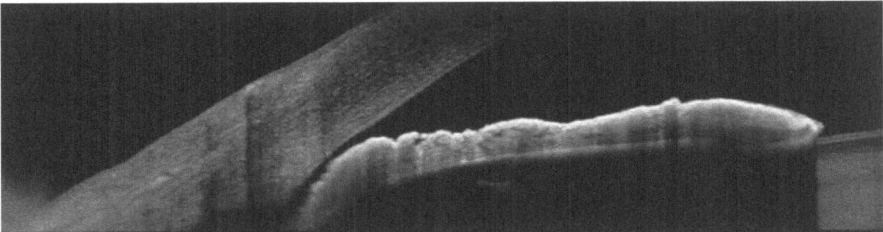

Fig. 11.12 An example of plateau iris configuration. The angle is narrow, central anterior chamber is deep and the peripheral iris appears to be propped up anteriorly while the rest of the iris has a flat configuration. There is a sharp bend in the most peripheral part of the iris

Another challenging entity is malignant glaucoma. In most cases, complete obliteration of the anterior chamber and elevated IOP are classical findings, but sometimes the manifestation of this disease can be subtle. AS-OCT can show angle closure, forward movement of the crystalline lens or IOL and flat anterior chamber, all of which resolve after proper management (Fig. 11.14).

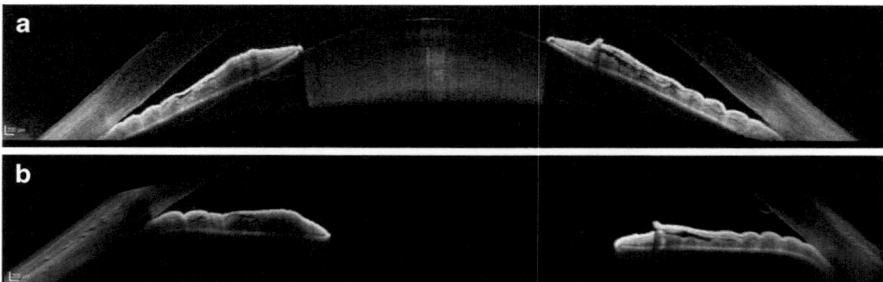

Fig. 11.13 (**a**) A patient with microspherophakia and angle closure glaucoma demonstrating significant lens-induced anterior bowing of iris. The anterior surface of the lens has a convex configuration due to microspherophakia. (**b**) The same patient after lens extraction displays chronic angle closure due to synechia formation although the iris is flat and anterior chamber is deep

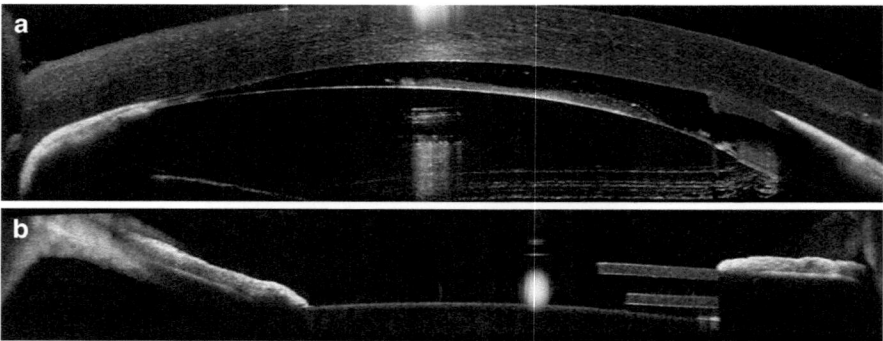

Fig. 11.14 (**a**) Malignant glaucoma in a pseudophakic eye following ciliary sulcus implantation of an Ahmed glaucoma valve. Note the flat anterior chamber and iris/corneal endothelial touch. On the right, the Ahmed valve tube can be seen between the iris and the intraocular lens which has partially prevented contact between the intraocular lens and the corneal endothelium. (**b**) After posterior vitrectomy combined with irido-zonulo-hyaloidotomy, the anterior chamber is formed, and the tube can be seen behind the iris

Iridoschisis is a disorder of the peripheral iris where superficial layers of the iris stroma undergo progressive separation. The anterior iris leaf may come into contact with the endothelium and angle closure glaucoma may ensue (Fig. 11.15).

Other disorders causing secondary angle closure such as IOL-related angle closure, neovascular glaucoma, post-vitrectomy silicone related glaucoma, iridocorneal endothelial syndrome and epithelial downgrowth lead to discernible findings in AS-OCT (Figs. 11.16, 11.17, 11.18, 11.19, 11.20, 11.21, and 11.22).

In addition to its utility in the imaging of narrow angles and angle closure, AS-OCT can provide unique views of some other disorders such as pigment

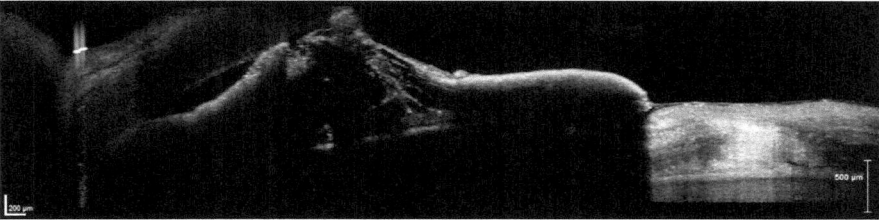

Fig. 11.15 AS-OCT of a patient with iridoschisis. There is synechiae between the anterior leaf of iris stroma and the corneal endothelium

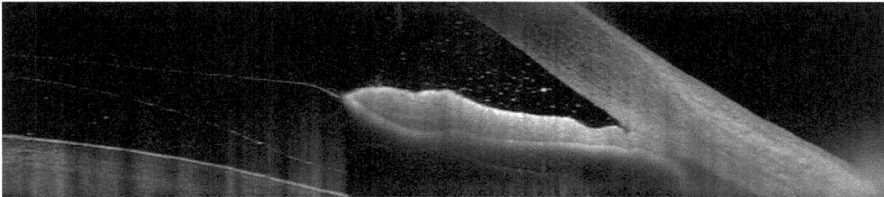

Fig. 11.16 AS-OCT of an eye with early postoperative IOP elevation following phakic posterior chamber intraocular lens implantation for high myopia. Anterior and posterior surfaces of the intraocular lens can be seen. There is a space between the posterior surface of the intraocular lens and the anterior lens capsule and the angle is closed

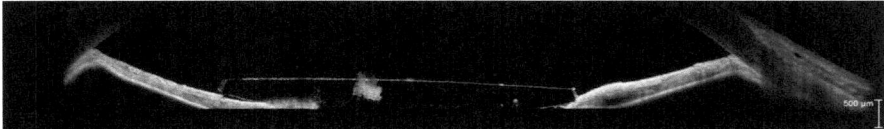

Fig. 11.17 Peripheral anterior synechiae, which are the sequelae of pupillary block caused by an anterior chamber intraocular lens. Although the pupillary block resolved following laser iridotomy, the peripheral anterior synechiae were permanent

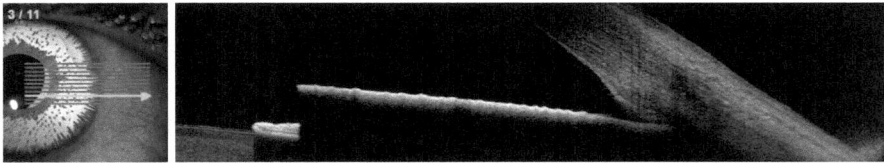

Fig. 11.18 This is a rare example of angle closure related to an artificial iris implant which was implanted in a healthy eye for cosmetic purposes. The pupillary border and anterior surface of the crystalline lens can be seen under the implant

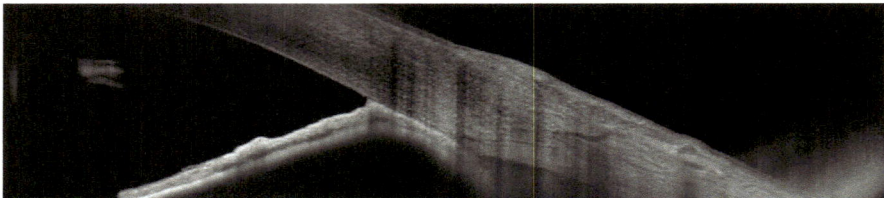

Fig. 11.19 AS-OCT of an eye with neovascular glaucoma. Note the high peripheral anterior synechiae. After a sharp peripheral bend, the iris has a flat configuration

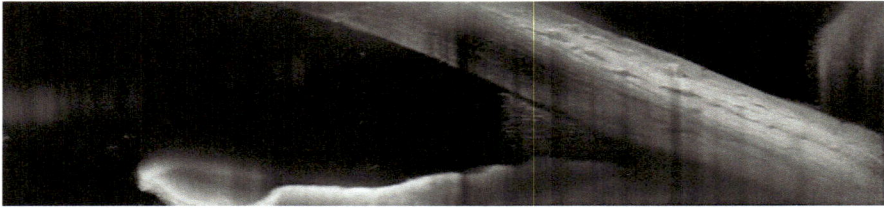

Fig. 11.20 AS-OCT of an eye with elevated pressures after vitreoretinal surgery. On gonioscopic examination, an inverse hypopyon was observed due to emulsified silicone particles. A section from the superior angle shows silicone particles filling the angle

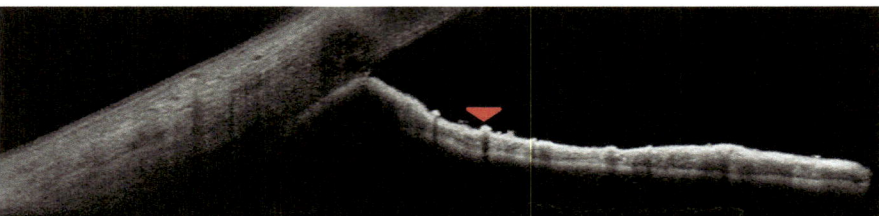

Fig. 11.21 AS-OCT of the angle in an eye with Cogan Reese syndrome. High peripheral anterior synechiae and dense nodular lesions of the iris (see arrowhead) can be seen

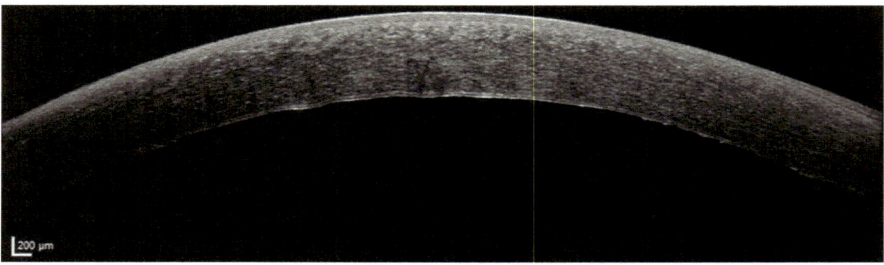

Fig. 11.22 A patient with glaucoma secondary to epithelial downgrowth after large incision cataract surgery. Note the railroad track appearance and irregularities in the corneal endothelium due to growth of the epithelial layer, which can be seen with AS-OCT

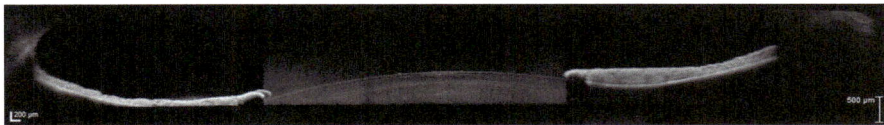

Fig. 11.23 Concave iris contour in a patient with pigment dispersion syndrome. The patient also had megalocornea and thinning of the iris

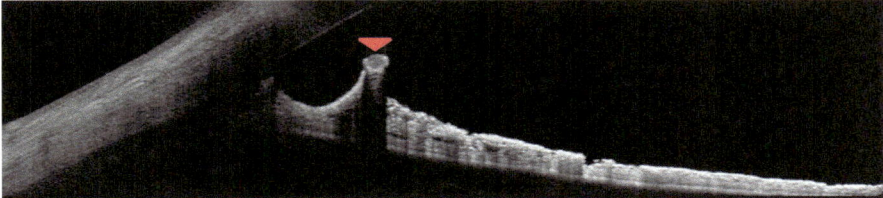

Fig. 11.24 AS-OCT image of an eye with Axenfeld-Rieger's anomaly. Note the detached Schwalbe's line to which the peripheral iris had adhesions (see arrowhead)

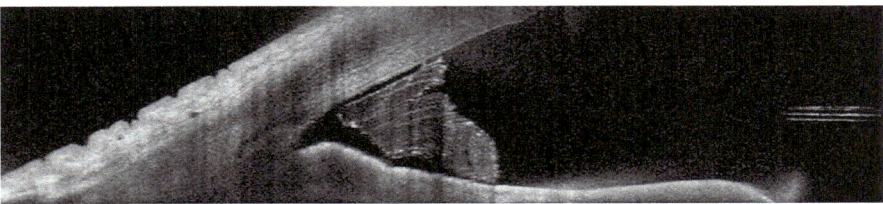

Fig. 11.25 This eye had an elevated IOP and corneal edema in the inferior half of the cornea following uneventful cataract surgery. The diagnosis of retained lens particle in the inferior angle was confirmed with AS-OCT

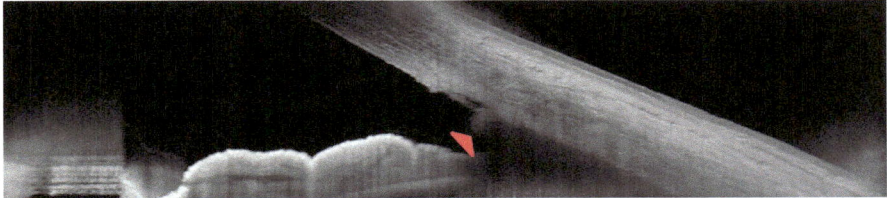

Fig. 11.26 AS-OCT image of a patient with trabecular meshwork tear following blunt trauma due to paintball. Note the posterior lip of the tear (see arrowhead)

dispersion syndrome, Axenfeld-Rieger's anomaly, lens particle induced glaucoma, and some types of traumatic glaucoma (Figs. 11.23, 11.24, 11.25, and 11.26). Rarely, iris or ciliary body cysts can be imaged through the iridectomy opening (Fig. 11.27).

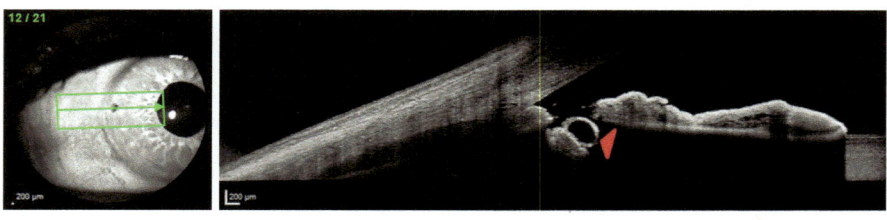

Fig. 11.27 This patient had a history of prior laser peripheral iridotomy with a diagnosis of primary angle closure. AS-OCT imaging through the iridotomy opening shows a ciliary body cyst (see arrowhead)

11.2.3 Anterior Chamber Depth and Anterior Chamber Volume

Shallow anterior chamber is a well-known risk factor for primary angle closure and therefore, anterior chamber depth (ACD) measurement has a crucial role in screening for glaucoma [11]. Using a prototype AS-OCT, Baikoff observed that the ACD increased over the early years of life, peaking at around 15–20 years, then slowly diminished until 80 years of age [12]. Anterior chamber volume (ACV) is also a useful parameter for detecting subjects at risk of developing PAC [13]. AS-OCT has been shown provide reliable ACV measurements [14]. Lei et al. observed that the ACV increased significantly from an average of 73.9 to 84.1 μL after laser iridotomy with the aid of Visante OCT device [15].

11.3 Imaging in Glaucoma Surgery

11.3.1 Surgical Planning and Imaging of Filtering Blebs

AS-OCT can be helpful for the planning and guidance of glaucoma surgery. As new glaucoma surgical techniques are emerging, the role of AS-OCT will likely continue to expand. AS-OCT has been reported to be superior to slit lamp exam for evaluation of bleb function and failure. As a non-contact imaging method, AS-OCT can be performed immediately after the surgery. Bleb types were classified by various authors depending on their characteristics at the AS-OCT images [16, 17]. Four different patterns of intra-bleb morphology, including diffuse filtering blebs, cystic blebs, encapsulated blebs and flat blebs have been identified and were closely related to slit-lamp appearance and bleb function [17]. Examples of these bleb types are shown in Figs. 11.28, 11.29, 11.30, 11.31, and 11.32. Tominaga et al. reported that mean IOP was significantly lower in eyes with low reflectivity bleb wall than in those with a highly reflective wall [18]. The thickness, height and apposition of the scleral flap to the scleral bed and patency of the internal ostium can be assessed using proper sections of AS-OCT. These images can potentially be used for

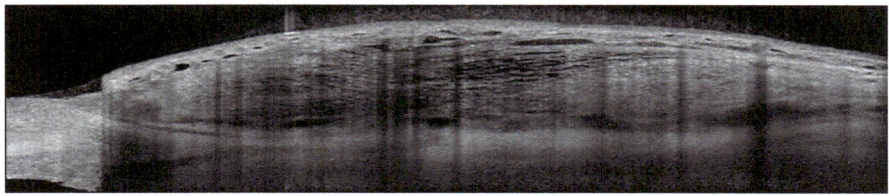

Fig. 11.28 A diffuse filtering bleb is characterized by the presence of subconjunctival fluid-filled spaces and low to moderate intrableb reflectivity

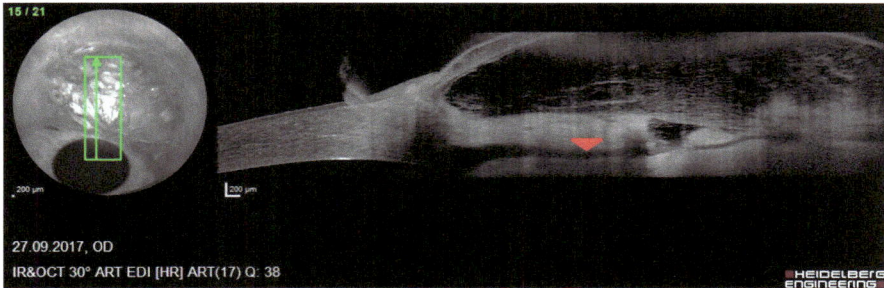

Fig. 11.29 A vertical AS-OCT section through a functioning bleb area demonstrates an open internal ostium, filtration pathway guarded by a scleral flap (see arrowhead), and a functioning elevated bleb

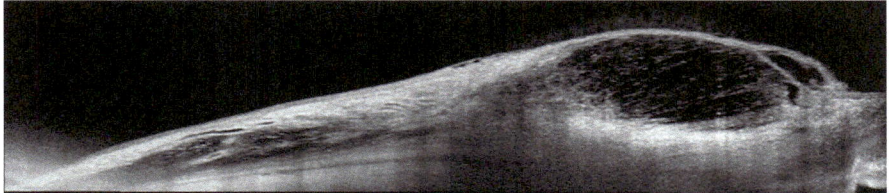

Fig. 11.30 A cystic bleb is composed of a large hyporeflective area filled with multiple fluid spaces of varying size and intensity. In this case, there is thickening of Tenon's capsule on the left side of the cystic area, which corresponded to the side of the bleb towards the fornix

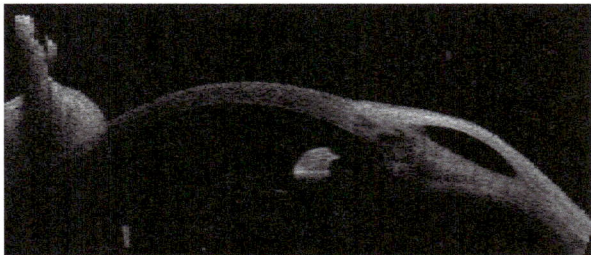

Fig. 11.31 AS-OCT image of an encapsulated bleb in which the encapsulated bleb is represented by a clear fluid-filled space surrounded by dense connective tissue with high signal reflectivity

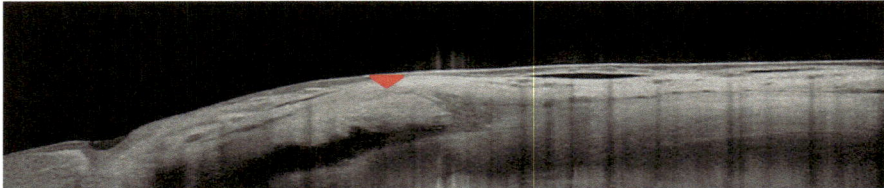

Fig. 11.32 There is no bleb elevation in an eye with flattened bleb and AS-OCT finding is characterized by high episcleral reflectivity. Although fluid can be observed under the scleral flap, episcleral fibrosis prevents flow of fluid under the conjunctiva (see arrowhead)

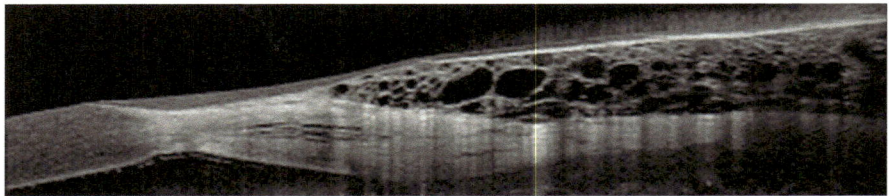

Fig. 11.33 Occasionally the bleb area may be full of silicone droplets in patients with postvitrectomy glaucoma after filtering surgery or in patients who had vitreoretinal surgery in the presence of a functioning bleb

Fig. 11.34 AS-OCT image of a glaucoma eye a few months after non-penetrating deep sclerectomy. Note the trabeculo-Descemet's membrane (see arrowhead), intrascleral lake and a flat bleb

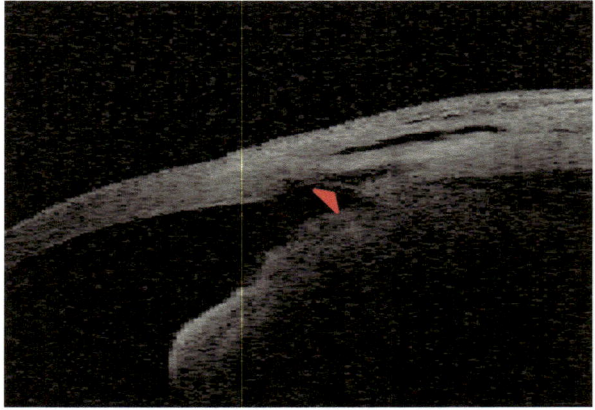

postoperative management such as suture lysis following filtration surgery [19]. Occasionally, silicone particles in the bleb area can be identified by AS-OCT (Fig. 11.33). Trabeculo-Descemet's membrane and intra-scleral lake can also be observed after non-penetrating surgery (Fig. 11.34). Figure 11.35 shows remnants of trabecular tissue as two stumps medial to Schlemm's canal in a patient after gonioscopy assisted transluminal trabeculotomy (GATT) surgery.

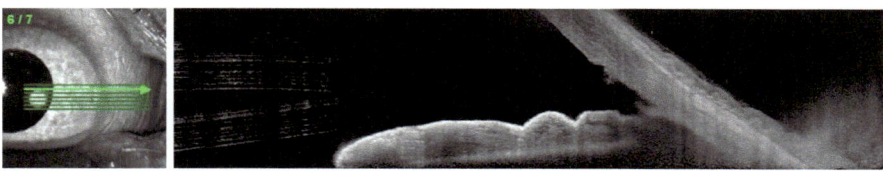

Fig. 11.35 AS-OCT of the nasal angle area of a pseudophakic patient after gonioscopy assisted transluminal trabeculotomy (GATT) about two years ago. One can see stumps superiorly and inferiorly medial to Schlemm's canal, which are the remnants of trabecular meshwork tissue

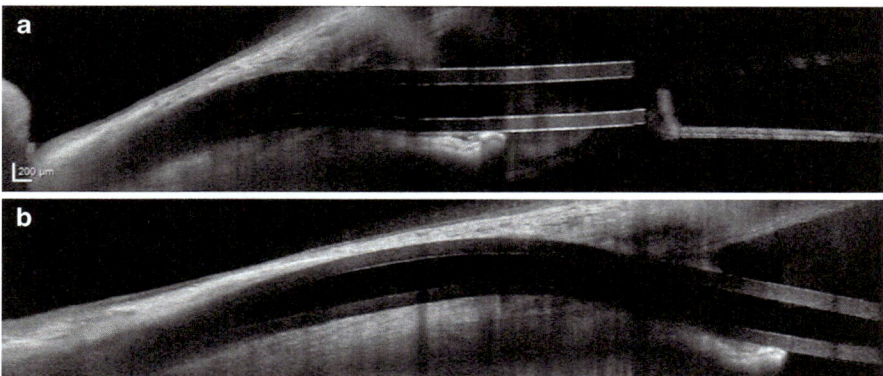

Fig. 11.36 (**a**) A well-positioned tube in the anterior chamber with open ostium. Since the patient had neovascular glaucoma related mydriasis, the iris leaflet is shorter than normal. (**b**) During its course outside the anterior chamber, the tube is well covered by conjunctiva and Tenon's capsule and there is no conjunctival erosion

11.3.2 Imaging of the Glaucoma Implants

The position, course and patency of aqueous drainage tubes can be ascertained with AS-OCT (Fig. 11.36). Proximity of the tube to the corneal endothelium can be visualized. Thickness of the tissue overlying the tube outside the anterior chamber, and presence of tube erosion can be assessed using proper sections. AS-OCT could be helpful for assessing tubes implanted into the ciliary sulcus.

Location and patency of other implants such as the Glaukos iStent implant (Glaukos Corporation, Laguna Hills, CA), and Xen Gel stent implant (AqueSys, CA, USA) can be evaluated by AS-OCT (Figs. 11.37, 11.38, and 11.39). Visualization of the distended Schlemm's canal postoperatively confirms that the suture tension has been achieved after canaloplasty. Other potential use of AS-OCT is imaging of the suprachoroidal space, thus permitting the evaluation of devices such as Cypass or gold supra-choroidal microshunt (Solx Gold Shunt;Solx, Inc., Waltham, MA).

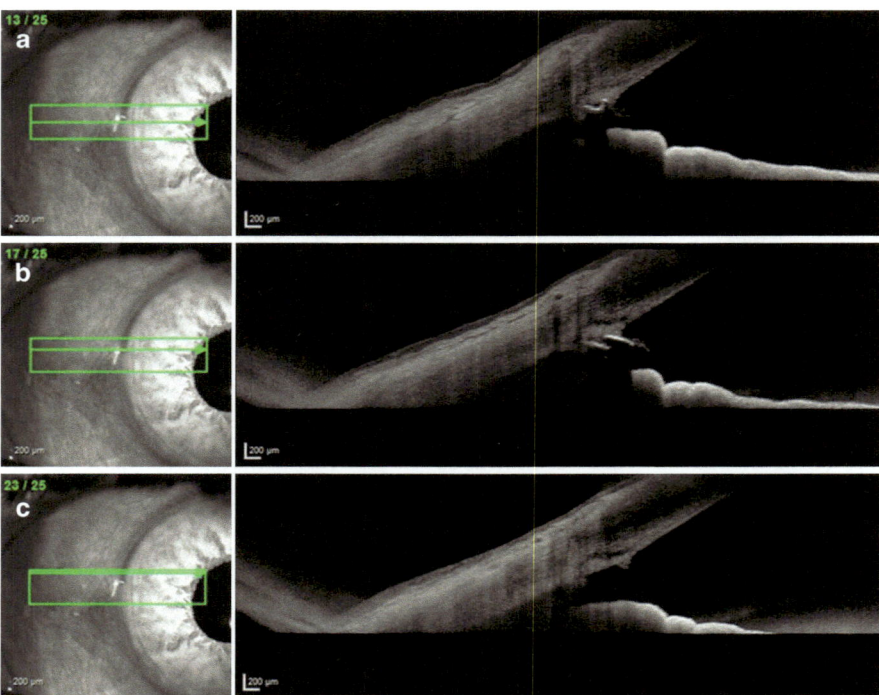

Fig. 11.37 Glaukos iStent (left eye version) implanted about 6 months before AS-OCT imaging. (**a**) The body or shaft of the improperly placed implant is seen in the angle but the Schlemm's canal, which was not stented can be seen superior to the implant. (**b**) The orifice of the snorkel part of the implant with its open lumen is in the anterior chamber angle. (**c**) In a cross-sectional image close to the implant, location of Schlemm's canal can be better assessed

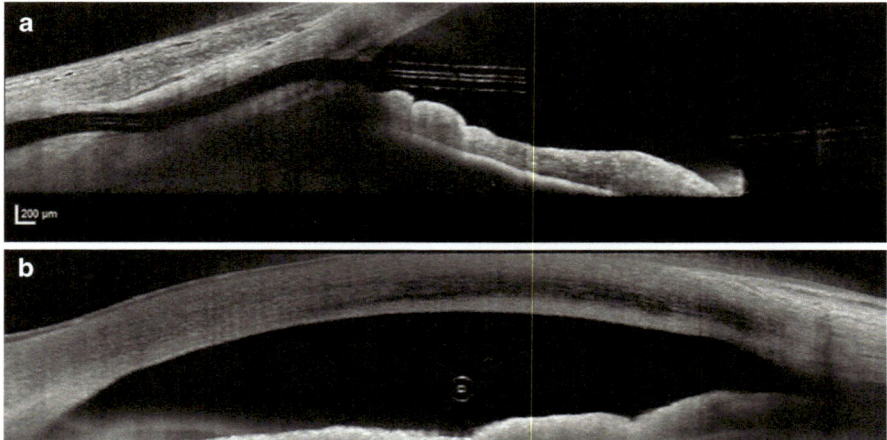

Fig. 11.38 (**a**) AS-OCT image of a Xen Gel stent. (**b**) Cross sectional image of the same implant. The implant is well positioned in the anterior chamber. On its course outside the anterior chamber, the tube is well covered by the sclera, conjunctiva and Tenon's capsule

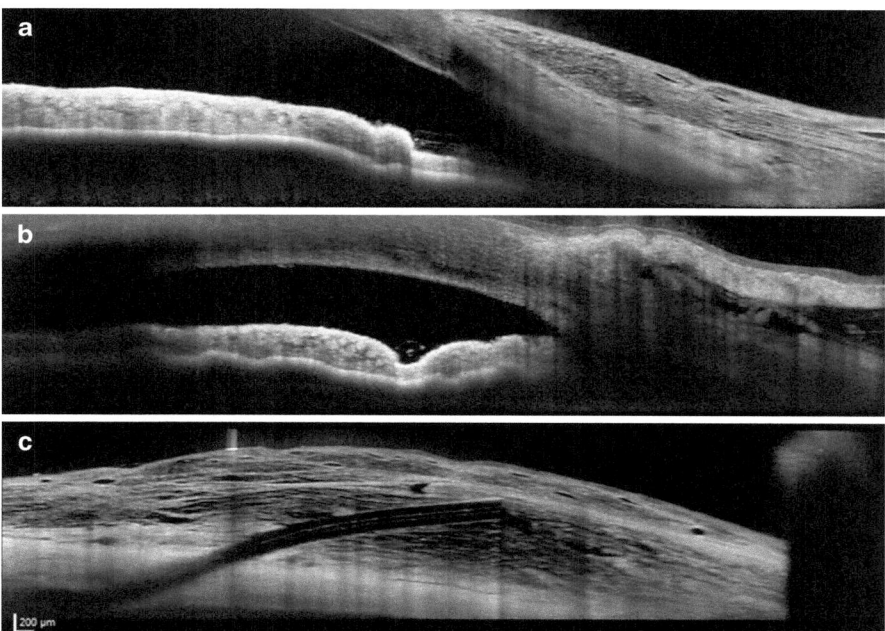

Fig. 11.39 (**a**) AS-OCT image of a Xen Gel stent. (**b**) Cross sectional image of the same implant. The implant is positioned deep in the anterior chamber and is partly been buried in the iris tissue. (**c**) Outside the anterior chamber, tube is well covered by the conjunctiva and Tenon's capsule. There is a diffuse filtering bleb characterized by the presence of subconjunctival fluid-filled spaces and low to moderate intrableb reflectivity

11.4   Pitfalls

Any technology including AS-OCT needs to be complemented with careful clinical examination by an experienced ophthalmologist. AS-OCT has several limitations, most notably its inability to image through pigmented tissue. Therefore, it is not possible to assess the ciliary body, lens zonules, posterior chamber and the anterior vitreous. Image acquisition requires a skilled technician and is prone to operator- and patient-related issues. Patient's cooperation is highly required during the examination of bleb or implant area, since the patient has to hold different gaze position for longer periods of time. Conjunctival or limbal vascular structures may affect the image quality as they can cause shadowing.

References

1. Izatt JA, Hee MR, Swanson EA, Lin CP, Huang D, Schuman JS, Puliafito CA, Fujimoto JG. Micrometer scale resolution imaging of the anterior eye in vivo with optical coherence tomography. Arch Ophthalmol. 1994;112:1584–9.

2. Radhakrishnan S, Rollins AM, Roth JE, Yazdanfar S, Westphal V, Bardenstein DS, Izatt JA. Real-time optical coherence tomography of the anterior segment at 1310 nm. Arch Ophthalmol. 2001;119:1179–85.
3. Huang D. Anterior segment optical coherence tomography. In: Proceedings of the American Academy of Ophthalmology annual meeting, NewOrleans, LA, 2013; p. 1–28.
4. Radhakrishnan S, Goldsmith J, Huang D, Westphal V, Dueker DK, Rollins AM, Izatt JA, Smith SD. Comparison of optical coherence tomography and ultrasound biomicroscopy for detection of narrow anterior chamber angles. Arch Ophthalmol. 2005;123:1053–9.
5. Sakata LM, Lavanya R, Friedman DS, Aung HT, Seah SK, Foster PJ, Aung T. Assessment of the scleral spur in anterior segment optical coherence tomography images. Arch Ophthalmol. 2008;126:181–5.
6. Yasuno Y, Yamanari M, Kawana K, Oshika T, Miura M. Investigation of post-glaucoma-surgery structures by 3D and polarization sensitive anterior eye segment optical coherence tomography. Opt Express. 2009;16:3980–96.
7. Pavlin CJ, Harasiewicz K, Foster FS. Ultrasound biomicroscopy of anterior segment structures in normal and glaucomatous eyes. Am J Ophthalmol. 1992;113:381–9.
8. Ishikawa H, Liebmann JM, Ritch R. Quantitative assessment of the anterior segment using ultrasound biomicroscopy. Curr Opin Ophthalmol. 2000;11:133–9.
9. Ramani KK, Mani B, Ronnie G, Joseph R, Lingam V. Gender variation in ocular biometry and ultrasound biomicroscopy of primary angle closure suspects and normal eyes. J Glaucoma. 2007;16:122–8.
10. Yao B, Wu L, Zhang C, Wang X. Ultrasound biomicroscopic features associated with angle closure in fellow eyes of acute primary angle closure after laser iridotomy. Ophthalmology. 2009;116:444–8.
11. Devereux JG, Foster PJ, Baasanhu J, Uranchimeg D, Lee PS, Erdenbeleig T, Machin D, Johnson GJ, Alsbirk PH. Anterior chamber depth measurement as a screening tool for primary angle-closure glaucoma in an East Asian population. Arch Ophthalmol. 2000;118:257–63.
12. Baikoff G, Jitsuo Jodai H, Bourgeon G. Measurement of the internal diameter and depth of the anterior chamber: IOLMaster versus anterior chamber optical coherence tomographer. J Cataract Refract Surg. 2005;31:1722–8.
13. Lee DA, Brubaker RF, Ilstrup DM. Anterior chamber dimensions in patients with narrow angles and angle-closure glaucoma. Arch Ophthalmol. 1984;102:46–50.
14. Wang N, Wang B, Zhai G, Lei K, Wang L, Congdon N. A method of measuring anterior chamber volume using the anterior segment optical coherence tomographer and specialized software. Am J Ophthalmol. 2007;143:879–81.
15. Lei K, Wang N, Wang L, Wang B. Morphological changes of the anterior segment after laser peripheral iridotomy in primary angle closure. Eye (Lond). 2009;23:345–50.
16. Ozcetin H. Glaucoma diagnoses, treatment, and types. 2nd rev. ed. Bursa: Nobel Medical Publishing; 2009. p. 669–76. ISBN:978-975-97187-1-5
17. Leung CK, Yick DW, Kwong YY, Li FC, Leung DY, Mohamed S, et al. Analysis of bleb morphology after trabeculectomy with Visante anterior segment optical coherence tomography. Br J Ophthalmol. 2007;91:340–4.
18. Tominaga A, Miki A, Yamazaki Y, Matsushita K, Otori Y. The assessment of the filtering bleb function with anterior segment optical coherence tomography. J Glaucoma. 2010;19:551–5.
19. Singh M, Aung T, Aquino MC, Chew PT. Utility of bleb imaging with anterior segment optical coherence tomography in clinical decision-making after trabeculectomy. J Glaucoma. 2009;18:492–5.

Part III
Optical Coherence Tomography and Progression

Chapter 12
Optical Coherence Tomography and Progression

Ahmet Akman

12.1 Progression in Glaucoma

Detecting progressive loss of retinal ganglion cells and their axons (RNFL) is the primary challenge for ophthalmologists caring for glaucoma. Timely diagnosis is the first step in preventing functional loss from glaucoma. Optical coherence tomography (OCT) provides clinicians with the opportunity to diagnose glaucoma at the earliest stages at this point [1]. Detection of progression is the next important step in decision making with regard to prevention of visual loss from glaucoma.

Glaucomatous progression can be evaluated structurally and functionally. This chapter concentrates on the structural progression and ability of spectral domain-OCT (SD-OCT) in monitoring structural changes in glaucoma. Structure and function relationship, which is also an essential part of glaucoma follow-up will be discussed in more detail in Chap. 16.

12.2 Detecting Structural and Functional Glaucoma Progression

Glaucoma is a slowly progressive disease, and the rate of progression could be variable among individuals. In addition, variability in diagnostic systems, age-related changes and lack of generally defined progression standards makes progression analysis very challenging with both structural and functional tests. Visual field (VF) analysis is the only universally accepted functional test used to establish disease progression. It is most useful in moderate to advanced stages of the disease. On the

A. Akman
Department of Ophthalmology, School of Medicine, Başkent University, Ankara, Turkey

© Springer International Publishing AG, part of Springer Nature 2018
A. Akman et al. (eds.), *Optical Coherence Tomography in Glaucoma*,
https://doi.org/10.1007/978-3-319-94905-5_12

Table 12.1 Advantages of OCT progression analysis in glaucoma

Objective and fast method
High reproducibility with low test-retest variability
Able to evaluate RNFL, macular thickness measures and optic nerve head changes at the same time
Structural progression often precedes functional progression in early glaucoma
Can detect progression at pre-perimetric stage

other hand, it is commonly accepted that structural progression frequently precedes functional progression [2–4]. Serial evaluation of stereoscopic optic disc photographs was the main approach for detecting structural progression for many years. With the advent of digital imaging methods like scanning laser polarimetry and confocal scanning laser systems, objective and quantitative evaluation of structural progression became possible [5–7]. OCT has replaced these systems during the last decade and has become a gold standard for detecting early glaucomatous damage and structural progression. Table 12.1 summarizes the advantages of assessing structural progression with OCT in glaucoma.

12.3 Basic Concepts in Structural Progression Analysis

Structural progression analysis aims to compare changes in data obtained from serial OCT scans. To make reliable comparisons, data from each point must be compared with the same point by registering serial images that are acquired at different time points. To be able to compare data from registered scans, statistical approaches such as event and trend analyses have been implemented [8].

12.3.1 Image Registration

Image registration is a fundamental task in image processing used to align two or more images taken at different times so that corresponding features can easily be matched and compared over time [9]. Accurate registration is necessary for any medical imaging system that compares or integrates data acquired from different sessions or modalities over time. Image registration was not very accurate with time domain OCT images due to the limited number of the available A-scans. Because of the inadequate registration, demonstration of glaucomatous progression was less reliable for time domain-OCT (TD-OCT) systems. On the other hand, with the introduction of SD-OCT, with higher number of A-scans and higher resolution of images, precise registration of serial images is now possible.

12.3.2   Reproducibility

Good reproducibility with low test-retest variability is indispensable for a test to detect true progression. Good reproducibility has been demonstrated for RNFL and macular measurements with most of the commercial SD-OCT devices [10–14]. An excellent reproducibility is also needed for detecting very early progression while OCT measurements are still in normal range (see Sect. 12.5).

12.3.3   Defining Progression

Event and trend analyses are commonly used for evaluating functional progression in glaucoma. Guided Progression Analysis software of Humphrey Field Analyzer uses both the event and trend analyses approaches to detect VF progression. OCT systems also rely on similar statistical methods for detection of progression. Cirrus HD-OCT's Guided Progression Analysis (GPA) uses both event and trend analyses, while other OCT devices mainly use trend analyses in their progression analysis software. Both of these methods can be used for RNFL, macular and optic nerve head (ONH) parameters.

12.3.3.1   Event Analysis

Event analysis depends on identifying change from baseline that exceed limits of variability for a given outcome measure. For any parameter of interest, such as RNFL thickness, when the magnitude of change from baseline at a given follow-up session is beyond limits of test-retest variability, true change is considered to have occurred [15]. Event analysis can be applied to regional changes such as RNFL or macula sectors, or to global parameters like average RNFL thickness or rim measurements. Cirrus HD-OCT user manual version 8.1 states that "Guided Progression Analysis compares an observed change with its population based test-retest variability (Fig. 12.1). The test-retest variability was determined by performing an in-house repeatability and reproducibility study" [12].
   Leung et al. demonstrated that inter-visit reproducibility coefficient for average RNFL thickness measured by Cirrus HD-OCT was 4.86 μm [10]. One can conclude that, if a given eye is repeatedly scanned over time, one would expect to observe a decrease beyond 4.86 μm in average RNFL thickness less than 2.5% of the time; hence, a reduction of more than 4.86 μm in average RNFL thickness is considered a statistically significant change that has a false positive rate of 2.5% [10, 11]. Test-retest variability for Spectralis OCT average RNFL thickness is 4.95 μm [13, 14]. The same assumptions apply to Spectralis OCT and therefore, a reduction of

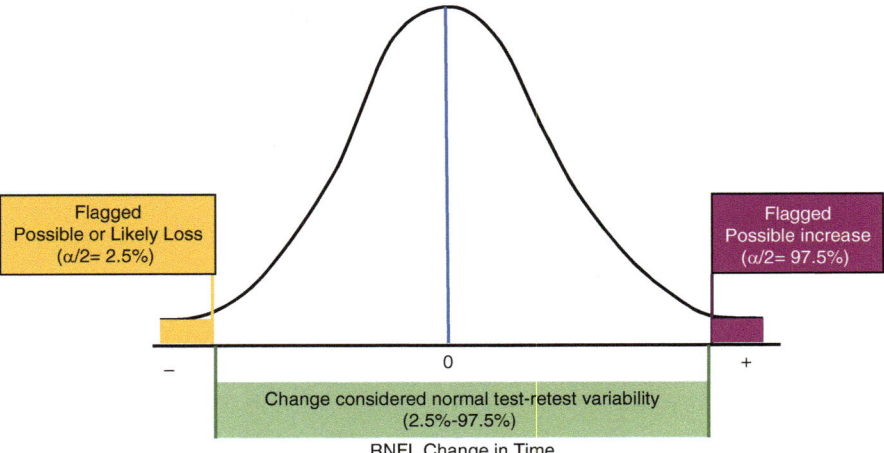

Fig. 12.1 Test-retest variability of Cirrus HD-OCT (modified from Cirrus HD-OCT manual Ver. 8.1 with permission from Carl Zeiss Meditec Inc.)

4.95 μm or more in average RNFL thickness would represent true progression in 97.5% of cases [13]. Other SD-OCT systems with comparable axial and lateral resolutions would be expected to have a magnitude of test-retest variability similar to Cirrus HD-OCT and Spectralis OCT. Based on the above information, one can potentially identify progression in glaucoma suspects by verifying a loss of 5 μm or more in average RNFL thickness on serial OCT scans. This change, if confirmed with a second test, can be randomly seen in less than 1% of the patients [16].

12.3.3.2   Trend Analysis

Trend analysis estimates rates of the change by carrying out regression analysis of the parameter of interest against time; it enables clinicians to estimate the future rates of functional loss assuming that the change will continue to be linear. A statistically significant negative slope (with $p < 0.05$) is defined as progression [15].

12.3.4   Age-Related Changes and Other Factors That Affect OCT Progression Analysis

A confounding factor for correct detection of progression is the influence of age-related changes in RNFL, macula and ONH. In most glaucoma patients, progression occurs very slowly over many years. During this time, aging can also result in changes in parameters used for identifying clinically significant progression. Such age-related attrition must be taken into account to prevent inappropriate treatment decisions.

Leung et al. studied the effect of age-related changes on detection of glaucoma progression with Cirrus HD-OCT in a group of eyes with a mean follow up of 46 months. Five parameters including, macular ganglion cell-inner plexiform layer (GCL + IPL), macular - inner retina (IR), macular - outer retina (OR), total macular thickness, and circumpapillary RNFL thickness was studied [17]. Progression was detected in 50%, 50%, 10%, 30% and 27% of the eyes for these parameters, respectively. After correction for age-related changes, these proportions decreased to 15%, 20%, 1%, 16%, and 27%. GCL + IPL was the most affected outcome as GCL + IPL values decrease sharply with age; in contrast, circumpapillary RNFL thickness measures are the least affected by aging [17]. In a similar study of RNFL and ONH parameters with Spectralis OCT, Vianna et al. concluded that the age-related changes in neuroretinal parameters could explain the deterioration observed in glaucoma patients under treatment [18]. In addition to age, baseline RNFL thickness can affect the rate of progression; eyes with thicker baseline RNFL are more prone to faster decline over time while the GCL + IPL rates of change were not affected by the baseline thickness [19].

12.4 OCT in Assessing Glaucoma Progression

Scanning laser polarimetry and confocal scanning laser-based systems were the first devices used to objectively detect structural progression in glaucoma [5–7]. OCT has replaced these devices in many clinics for monitoring glaucoma as it is widely available, has many technical advantages, and it can evaluate the ONH, RNFL and macular ganglion cell layer changes at the same time. Earlier studies using TD-OCT systems showed the utility of OCT in progression analysis [20, 21]. The SD-OCT systems have better resolution, faster scanning capabilities, higher reproducibility, more accurate image registration and improved computing power. All these advances have markedly improved the ability of OCT devices for detection of progression. Modern SD-OCT devices can identify progression before VF changes manifest [1]. Theoretically, the high reproducibility of the modern OCT systems allows detection of progressive RNFL loss while the RNFL thickness measurements are still in the normal range of the normative databases [22]. Hence, multiple steps of statistically significant change can be potentially demonstrated while the measurements are still in the normal (green) range.

12.4.1 RNFL Progression

RNFL parameters are the most studied measures for detection of progression. All OCT machines use the RNFL thickness values measured on the circumpapillary calculation circle, which is a 3.46 mm circular scan around the optic disc. Bruch's membrane opening (BMO) method is used for automatically determining the margins of the optic disc and for centration of the calculation circle. Although this is the most commonly studied approach for detection of structural progression, it may miss progression if the changes are outside or inside of this calculation circle [23]. A three-dimensional RNFL thickness map of the peripapillary region can demonstrate the RNFL changes inside and outside the calculation circle and may be superior for assessing glaucomatous progression; however, this has yet to be demonstrated. Although most commercial OCT systems scan the peripapillary region and construct RNFL thickness maps, only Cirrus-HD OCT enables using the data for RNFL progression analysis [23].

12.4.1.1 Circumpapillary RNFL Changes

Early studies exploring the utility of OCT for glaucoma progression analysis used the circumpapillary RNFL thickness measurements from Stratus OCT (Carl Zeiss Meditec) for assessing structural progression. In most of these studies, either the average RNFL thickness from the calculation ring or the quadrant/sector RNFL thickness averages were used. Wollstein et al. were the first to publish OCT progression analysis based on TD-OCT. In a group of eyes with a mean follow-up of 4.7 years, 22% of eyes progressed on OCT alone using a 20 μm reduction in average RNFL as the criterion for progression; this was in contrast to 9% of eyes according to VF mean deviation criteria, and 3% of eyes based on both VF and OCT criteria [24]. Mederios et al. classified 253 eyes as progressors and non-progressors using ONH stereo photographs and/or VFs and showed higher rates of average RNFL thinning for progressors compared with nonprogressors after a mean follow up of 4 years (−0.72 μ/year vs. −0.14 μ/year) [21]. Leung et al. reported a median loss of 3.3 μm/year in 116 eyes with negative trend on Stratus OCT GPA software after 5 years of follow-up [20]. As the OCT images were not registered on the Stratus OCT GPA software, scan circle misalignment was a common problem, resulting in measurement errors and issues with progression analyses.

SD-OCT systems overcame these problems by registering follow-up images to the baseline image. Eye tracking capabilities and automatic calculation circle placement based on the BMO has facilitated registration. In a study comparing SD-OCT (Cirrus HD-OCT) and TD-OCT (Stratus OCT), Leung et al. concluded that the Cirrus HD-OCT outperformed the Stratus OCT and detected more eyes with progression thanks to reduced measurement variability [25]. With the availability of SD-OCT and commercial progression analysis software on different OCT platforms, other studies have investigated the role of OCT in glaucoma progression.

Most studies categorized eyes as progressors and non-progressors based on disc stereo photographs, red-free RNFL photographs and/or VF data and compared the global or regional RNFL rates of change for progressors and non-progressors. In a study by Wessel et al., RNFL rates of progressive thinning was 2.1 μm/year in progressing glaucomatous eyes, 1.2 μm/year in non-progressing glaucomatous eyes and 0.60 μm/year in normal control eyes [26]. Detection of progression was based on ONH morphology in that study. Lee et al. studied 153 progressing and non-progressing glaucomatous eyes with localized RNFL defects. Rate of RNFL thinning was significantly greater in progressors [27]. Na and associates demonstrated that OCT-derived RNFL, macular volume and thickness, and ONH parameters deteriorated more rapidly in eyes progressing according to clinical criteria among 279 eyes followed for an average of 2.2 years [28]. Some other studies compared VF changes to OCT parameters for detection of progression. Seth and colleagues monitored 63 glaucoma suspects and 59 glaucoma patients over five years and concluded that structural change appeared to be more useful to detect progression in glaucoma suspects, while functional change was a better indicator as the disease progressed to advanced stages [29]. Zhang et al. found that OCT was more sensitive than VF for detection of progression in pre-perimetric glaucoma and early perimetric glaucoma in a group of 356 glaucoma suspect/pre-perimetric glaucoma eyes and 153 perimetric glaucoma eyes with a mean ($\pm$SD) follow-up time of 54 ± 16 months. In eyes with moderate to advanced glaucoma, GCC trend analysis was more helpful than RNFL trend analysis [30].

12.4.1.2 RNFL Thickness Map Changes

SD-OCT devices can scan the ONH region in a few seconds and can construct three-dimensional maps of the RNFL around the ONH with high precision. Most of the current commercial SD-OCT systems construct these maps, but only the Cirrus HD-OCT GPA algorithm performs change analysis on the 200 × 200 Optic Disc Cube (6 × 6 mm) [15]. Evaluating RNFL changes throughout the 6 × 6 mm (200 × 200 pixel) area around the ONH may detect progression better when compared to the 3.46 mm circumpapillary RNFL calculation circle. Please refer to the Chap. 13 for more detailed information about this approach. Leung et al. followed 186 eyes of 103 glaucoma patients for 44 months and found that the most common locations for progressive retinal thinning were at the inferior temporal region about 2 mm from the ONH center. This area is outside the radius of the arbitrary 1.73 mm calculation circle scan and may be missed on the TSNIT plots derived from the calculation circle [31].

Na et al. compared three RNFL strategies of the Cirrus HD-OCT GPA for detection of progression. They found that peripapillary thickness maps detected progression most frequently followed by RNFL thickness profiles and average RNFL thickness change [32]. Yu and colleagues analyzed progressive RNFL thinning with commercial GPA software (Cirrus HD-OCT) and a custom trend-based analyses (TPA) software. Two hundred forty eyes of 139 glaucoma patients were followed with Cirrus HD-OCT and VFs for at least 5 years. Eyes with progressive RNFL thinning based on TPA and GPA had a more than eight- and threefold increase in risk, respectively, for VF progression [33]. Lin et al. used trend analysis on RNFL thickness maps and reported that the peak and mean rates of RNFL thinning for the superpixels on the 200 × 200 Optic Disc Cube were associated with increased risk of VF progression [34]. This type of analysis, not yet commercially available, can display the topography of the rates of change, which could be a superior alternative to trend analysis solely based on circumpapillary RNFL calculation circle data.

12.4.2 Macular Thickness Progression

High resolution and fast scan capabilities of SD-OCT has made accurate segmentation of the individual retinal layers such as ganglion cell layer (GCL) possible. Macula has the highest concentration of retinal ganglion cells in the retina and measuring the thickness of the ganglion cell layer in the macula can contribute to glaucoma diagnosis. Different OCT systems use different macular outcomes for evaluating glaucoma diagnosis and progression. Cirrus HD-OCT uses GCL + IPL (ganglion cell layer + inner plexiform layer), RTVue OCT and Nidek OCT provide ganglion cell complex (GCC; mRNFL+GCL + IPL) measurements. Topcon OCT can produce different combination maps of these three layers. Spectralis OCT, on the other hand, provides the total macular thickness, although segmentation of all individual retina layers including mRNFL, GCL, and IPL is available.

Naghizadeh et al. showed that the GCC changes might better detect early structural progression in glaucoma than the ONH, RNFL and average GCC parameters of the RTVue OCT in one of the first studies published on the role of macular ganglion cell changes in detection of glaucoma progression [35].

Macula offers several advantages compared to RNFL measurements for detection of disease deterioration. GCL + IPL measurements have excellent long-term inter-visit reproducibility [36]. Also, in advanced glaucoma, GCL + IPL thickness remains above the measurement floor range longer compared to peripapillary RNFL thickness. This is an important advantage, as the measurement floor limits the role of RNFL based progression analysis in advanced glaucoma and the variability of VF starts increases with worsening glaucoma severity [37–39].

GPA for GCL + IPL became available commercially on Cirrus HD-OCT in 2015. Shin et al. classified 196 eyes of 123 eyes as progressors vs. nonprogressors according to VF criteria (mean follow up of 5 years) [40]. In eyes with mild glaucoma defined based on VF findings, both GCL + IPL and RNFL data demonstrated larger rates of change in the progressor group. On the other hand, only GCL + IPL rates of change were significant in moderate to advanced glaucoma eyes possibly due to RNFL thickness reaching to the measurement floor. Lee and associates followed 65 patients for a minimum of 3 years and categorized eyes as progressors and nonprogressors based on red-free RNFL photographs and VFs [41]. They reported that with all GCL + IPL parameters, rates of change were significantly faster in progressors on Cirrus HD-OCT's ganglion cell GPA trend analysis. Also, the rates of thinning of the temporal sector for the affected hemifields was significantly faster when compared to other sectors [41].

12.4.3 Optic Nerve Head Neuro–Retinal Rim Progression in Glaucoma

Changes in the ONH topography have been the main outcome to identify glaucoma progression till very recently and continues to be used clinically. Stereoscopic disc photography and scanning laser ophthalmoscopy (Heidelberg Retinal Tomograph) were typically used methods for this purpose. SD-OCT is now able to identify the BMO which is frequently used as a surrogate for disc area [42, 43]. More recently, a new structural outcome, BMO-based minimum rim width (MRW) has been proposed to objectively define the axonal complement of an eye at the level of the ONH [44]. Besides, lamina cribrosa (LC) can be imaged with SD-OCT and swept-source OCT, and changes in LC structure can be monitored longitudinally. Optic nerve head topography and neuroretinal rim change analysis is included in Cirrus HD-OCT GPA software, and new Glaucoma Module Premium Edition (GMPE) of the Spectralis OCT. The GMPE module provides detailed analysis of the ONH and neuroretinal rim. There are few published studies on the role of these analyses in glaucoma progression. Gardiner et al. showed that RNFL thickness measurements have a better longitudinal signal-to-noise ratio (SNR) than minimum rim width (MRW) and minimum rim area (MRA) measurements. They concluded that MRW and MRA may be more sensitive for early detection of glaucomatous damage but lower longitudinal SRN makes RNFL thickness a better parameter for monitoring change [45]. The BMO-MRW parameters have been shown to have a similar a measurement floor as those for the RNFL [47].

12.5   How Early Can We Demonstrate Progression

As described above, the low test-retest variability of OCT devices allows detection of RNFL progression, even at the pre-perimetric stage in some patients [22]. If average RNFL thickness is chosen as a single parameter, multiple steps of statistically significant change can be demonstrated while the patient is still in the normal (green) range.

As stated in Sect. 12.3.3.1, the inter-visit reproducibility coefficient of average RNFL thickness measured by Cirrus HD-OCT was about 5 μm in the studies by Leung et al. and Mwanza and colleagues [10, 11]. If one patient is repeatedly scanned over time, we expect to randomly see more than 5 μm decrease in average RNFL thickness less than 2.5% of the time, thus a reduction of 5 μm or more in the average RNFL thickness is a statistically significant change that has a false positive rate of 2.5% [10–12].

In other words, one can identify progression in glaucoma suspects by looking for 5 μm or more thinning in average RNFL thickness on serial OCT scans. Other OCT devices than Cirrus-HD OCT have similar test-retest variability [13, 14]. This amount of change, if confirmed with a second test, can be randomly seen in less than 1% of stable patients [16].

Figures 12.2, 12.3, and 12.4 summarize average RNFL thickness change over time If the average RNFL thickness measurement is used as the main outcome for identifying progression, a patient can lose nearly one-third of the RNFL thickness and can be still in the green range of the normative database for Cirrus HD-OCT (Fig. 12.2).

SD-OCT devices can allow the physician to measure multiple steps of statistically significant progression while the patient is still in the normal (green) range (Fig. 12.3). Therefore, an SD-OCT change from baseline could be an early detection strategy in glaucoma suspects (Figs. 12.4 and 12.5).

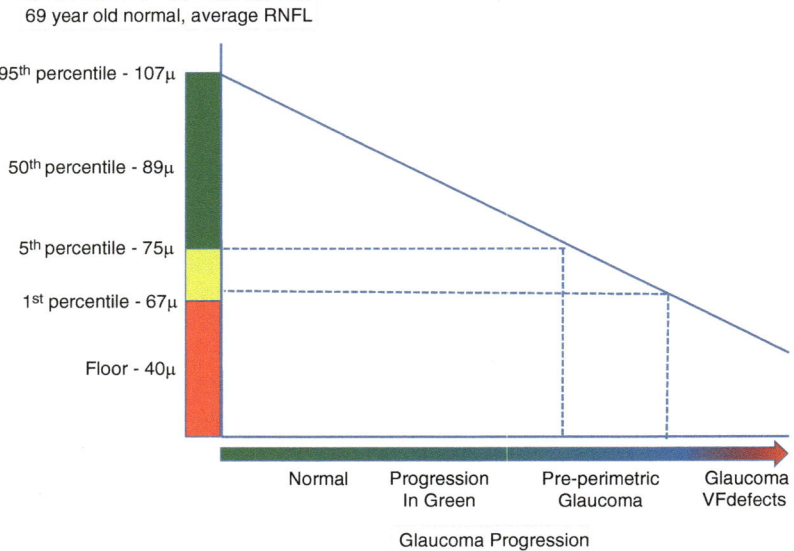

Fig. 12.2 A patient with normal RNFL thickness may lose nearly one-third of the average RNFL thickness before it is flagged as borderline by the software. Modified from presentation by Vincent Michael Patella with permission. Aurora Meeting, Berlin 2015, prepared by Patella M, Goni F, Bron A, Heijl H

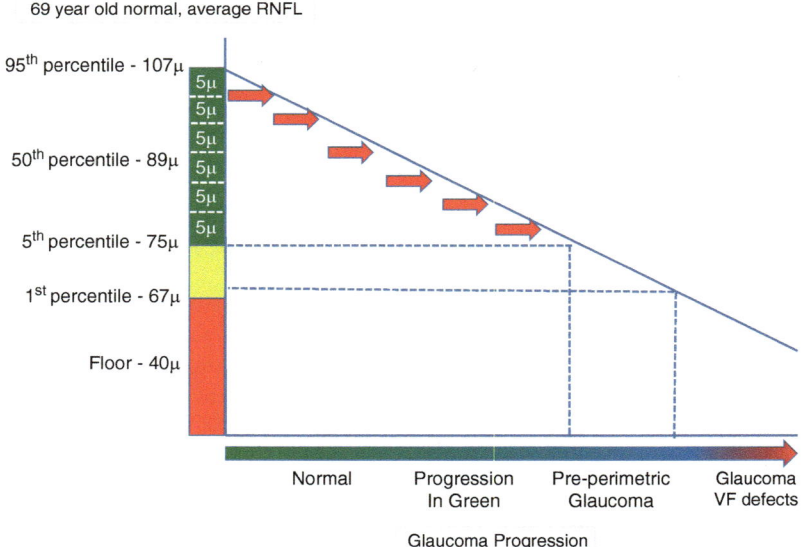

Fig. 12.3 Serial OCT scans and progression analysis software can show multiple steps of statistically significant change (red arrows). While losing RNFL and still in the normal thickness range of the normative database. Modified from presentation by Vincent Michael Patella with permission. Aurora Meeting, Berlin 2015, prepared by Patella M, Goni F, Bron A, Heijl H

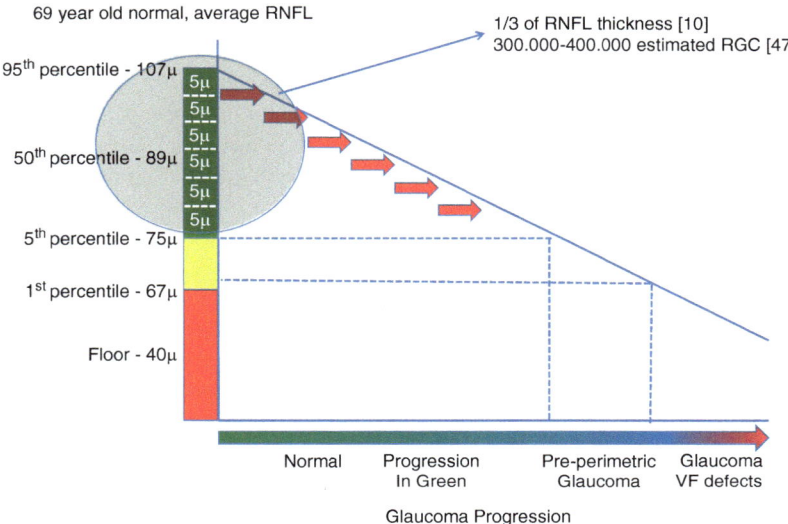

Fig. 12.4 Using serial OCT measurements, progression can be observed in multiple steps before the standard OCT report classifies an eye as borderline or out-of-normal range. A patient starting from 95th percentile average RNFL thickness and progressing to 5th percentile can lose 1/3 of RNFL thickness dynamic range or 300,000–400,000 estimated retinal ganglion cells [10, 46]. Modified from presentation by Vincent Michael Patella with permission. Aurora Meeting, Berlin 2015, prepared by Patella M, Goni F, Bron A, Heijl H

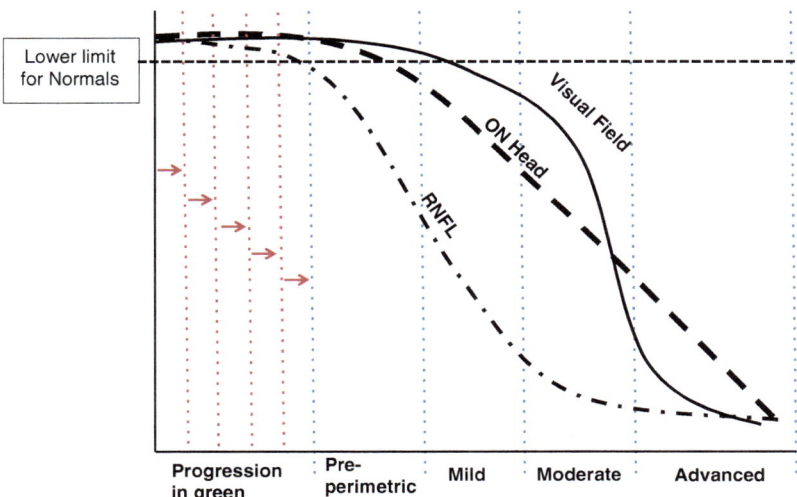

Fig. 12.5 RNFL thinning is one of the earliest signs of the glaucomatous damage and OCT progression analysis identifies multiple steps of statistically significant change while the patient is still in normal OCT RNFL thickness range (red arrows) (modified form original slide by Weinreb RN, Robert N. Shaffer Lecture at the 105th Annual Meeting of the American Academy of Ophthalmology, New Orleans, 2001, with permission from Robert N. Weinreb)

12.6   Limitations of OCT Progression Analysis

Identifying structural progression with OCT has some shortcomings. There is no multicentric randomized study concentrating on OCT progression data. Most of our data from randomized multi-centric studies like OHTS, EMGT are from the pre-OCT era. Second, none of the commercial progression analysis software of OCT manufacturers takes into account confounding variables like age-related changes or baseline RNFL thickness variations among individuals. Also, OCT quality may worsen over time due to progressing cataract, ocular surface problems or vitreous opacities. Removal of the cataract also introduces magnification related issues that are hard to account for. In addition, as disease severity advances, RNFL measurements become less useful for detection of progression as the RNFL thickness reaches the measurement floor. Structural assessments are particularly challenging in highly myopic patients regardless of whether detection of glaucoma or its progression is involved.

Regardless of potential limitations, OCT progression analysis is the one of most important advances for monitoring glaucoma and at this point, the only way one can identify progressive optic nerve damage in very early stages of glaucoma.

References

1. Kuang TM, Zhang C, Zangwill LM, Weinreb RN, Medeiros FA. Estimating lead time gained by optical coherence tomography in detecting glaucoma before development of visual field defects. Ophthalmology. 2015;122:2002–9.
2. Quigley HA, Addicks EM, Richard Green W. Optic nerve damage in human glaucoma III. Quantitative correlation of nerve fiber loss and visual field defect in glaucoma, ischemic neuropathy, papilledema, and toxic neuropathy. Arch Ophthalmol. 1982;100:135–46.
3. Hood DC, Kardon RH. A framework for comparing structural and functional measures of glaucomatous damage. Prog Retina Eye Res. 2007;26:688–710.
4. Sommer A, Katz J, Quigley HA, Miller NR, Robin AL, Richter RC, Witt KA. Clinically detectable nerve fiber atrophy precedes the onset of glaucomatous field loss. Arch Ophthalmol. 1991;109:77–83.
5. Kamal DS, Viswanathan AC, Garway-Heath DF, Hitchings RA, Poinoosawmy D, Bunce C. Detection of optic disc change with the Heidelberg retina tomograph before confirmed visual field change in ocular hypertensives converting to early glaucoma. Br J Ophthalmol. 1999;83:290–4.
6. Philippin H, Unsoeld A, Maier P, Walter S, Bach M, Funk J. Ten-year results: detection of long-term progressive optic disc changes with confocal laser tomography. Graefes Arch Clin Exp Ophthalmol. 2006;244:460–4.
7. Sehi M, Greenfield DS. Assessment of retinal nerve fiber layer using optical coherence tomography and scanning laser polarimetry in progressive glaucomatous optic neuropathy. Am J Ophthalmol. 2006;142:1056–9.
8. Weinreb RN, Garway-Heath D, Leung CK, Mederios FA, Crowston JG, editors. WGA Consensus series 8: progression. The Hague: Kugler; 2011.
9. Brown LG. A survey of image registration techniques. ACM Comput Surv. 1992;24:325–76.

10. Leung CK, Cheung CY, Weinreb RN, Qiu Q, Liu S, Li H, Xu G, Fan N, Huang L, Pang CP, Lam DS. Retinal nerve fiber layer imaging with spectral-domain optical coherence tomography: a variability and diagnostic performance study. Ophthalmology. 2009;116:1257–63.
11. Mwanza J, Chang R, Budenz D, et al. Reproducibility of peripapillary retinal nerve fiber layer thickness and optic nerve head parameters measured with Cirrus HD-OCT in glaucomatous eyes. Invest Ophthalmol Vis Sci. 2010;51:5724–30.
12. Horne MR, Callan T, Durbin M, Inter-Visit AT. Inter-instrument variability for CIRRUS HD-OCT peripapillary retinal nerve fiber layer thickness measurements. ARVO 2008 Abstracts. Invest Ophthalmol Vis Sci. 2008;49:4624.
13. Tan BB, Natividad M, Chua KC, Yip LW. Comparison of retinal nerve fiber layer measurement between 2 spectral domain OCT instruments. J Glaucoma. 2012;21:266–73.
14. Wu H, de Boer JF, Chen TC. Reproducibility of retinal nerve fiber layer thickness measurements using spectral domain optical coherence tomography. J Glaucoma. 2011;20:470–6.
15. Leung CK. Diagnosing glaucoma progression with optical coherence tomography. Curr Opin Ophthalmol. 2014;25:104–11.
16. Feuer WJ, Durbin MK. Performance of confirmation as a strategy to retain acceptable specificity and sensitivity when monitoring glaucoma over multiple visits. ARVO 2009 abstracts. Invest Ophthalmol Vis Sci. 2009;50:2250.
17. Leung CK, Ye C, Weinreb RN, et al. Impact of age-related change of retinal nerve fiber layer and macular thicknesses on evaluation of glaucoma progression. Ophthalmology. 2013;120:2485–92.
18. Vianna JR, Danthurebandara VM, Sharpe GP, Hutchison DM, Belliveau AC, Shuba LM, Nicolela MT, Chauhan BC. Importance of normal aging in estimating the rate of glaucomatous neuroretinal rim and retinal nerve fiber layer loss. Ophthalmology. 2015;122:2392–8.
19. Leung CK, Yu M, Weinreb RN, Liu S, Ye C, Liu L, He J, Lai GW, Li T, Lam DS. Retinal nerve fiber layer imaging with spectral-domain optical coherence tomography: a prospective analysis of age-related loss. Ophthalmology. 2012;119:731–7.
20. Leung CK, Cheung CY, Weinreb RN, Qiu K, Liu S, Li H, Xu G, Fan N, Pang CP, Tse KK, Lam DS. Evaluation of retinal nerve fiber layer progression in glaucoma: a study on optical coherence tomography guided progression analysis. Invest Ophthalmol Vis Sci. 2010;51:217–22.
21. Medeiros FA, Zangwill LM, Alencar LM, Bowd C, Sample PA, Susanna R Jr, Weinreb RN. Detection of glaucoma progression with stratus OCT retinal nerve fiber layer, optic nerve head, and macular thickness measurements. Invest Ophthalmol Vis Sci. 2009;50:5741–8.
22. Tatham AJ, Medeiros FA. Detecting structural progression in glaucoma with optical coherence tomography. Ophthalmology. 2017;124(Suppl):S57–65.
23. Leung CK, Yu M, Weinreb RN, Lai G, Xu G, Lam DS. Retinal nerve fiber layer imaging with spectral-domain optical coherence tomography: patterns of retinal nerve layer progression. Ophthalmology. 2012;119:1889–98.
24. Wollstein G, Schuman JS, Price LL, Aydin A, Stark PC, Hertzmark E, Lai E, Ishikawa H, Mattox C, Fujimoto JG, Paunescu LA. Optical coherence tomography longitudinal evaluation of retinal nerve fiber layer thickness in glaucoma. Arch Ophthalmol. 2005;123:464–70.
25. Leung CK, Chiu V, Weinreb RN, Liu S, Ye C, Yu M, Cheung CY, Lai G, Lam DS. Evaluation of retinal nerve fiber layer progression in glaucoma: a comparison between spectral-domain and time-domain optical coherence tomography. Ophthalmology. 2011;118:1558–62.
26. Wessel JM, Horn FK, Tornow RP, Schmid M, Mardin CY, Kruse FE, Juenemann AG, Laemmer R. Longitudinal analysis of progression in glaucoma using spectral-domain optical coherence tomography. Invest Ophthalmol Vis Sci. 2013;54:3613–20.
27. Lee EJ, Kim TW, Weinreb RN, Park KH, Kim SH, Kim DM. Trend-based analysis of retinal nerve fiber layer thickness measured by optical coherence tomography in eyes with localized nerve fiber layer defects. Invest Ophthalmol Vis Sci. 2011;52:1138–44.
28. Na JH, Sung KR, Lee JR, Lee KS, Baek S, Kim HK, Sohn YH. Detection of glaucomatous progression by spectral-domain optical coherence tomography. Ophthalmology. 2013;120:1388–95.

29. Seth NG, Kaushik S, Kaur S, Raj S, Pandav SS. 5-year disease progression of patients across the glaucoma spectrum assessed by structural and functional tools. Br J Ophthalmol. 2017;pii :bjophthalmol-2017-310731.
30. Zhang X, Dastiridou A, Francis BA, Tan O, Varma R, Greenfield DS, Schuman JS, Huang D, Advanced Imaging for Glaucoma Study Group. Comparison of glaucoma progression detection by optical coherence tomography and visual field. Am J Ophthalmol. 2017;184:63–74.
31. Leung CK, Yu M, Weinreb RN, Lai G, Xu G, Lam DS. Retinal nerve fiber layer imaging with spectral-domain optical coherence tomography: patterns of retinal nerve fiber layer progression. Ophthalmology. 2012;119:1858–66.
32. Na JH, Sung KR, Baek S, Lee JY, Kim S. Progression of retinal nerve fiber layer thinning in glaucoma assessed by cirrus optical coherence tomography-guided progression analysis. Curr Eye Res. 2013;38:386–95.
33. Yu M, Lin C, Weinreb RN, Lai G, Chiu V, Leung CK. Risk of visual field progression in glaucoma patients with progressive retinal nerve fiber layer thinning: a 5-year prospective study. Ophthalmology. 2016;123:1201–10.
34. Lin C, Mak H, Yu M, Leung CK. Trend-based progression analysis for examination of the topography of rates of retinal nerve fiber layer thinning in glaucoma. JAMA Ophthalmol. 2017;135:189–95.
35. Naghizadeh F, Garas A, Vargha P, Holló G. Detection of early glaucomatous progression with different parameters of the RTVue optical coherence tomograph. J Glaucoma. 2014;23:195–8.
36. Kim KE, Yoo BW, Jeoung JW, Park KH. Long-term reproducibility of macular ganglion cell analysis in clinically stable glaucoma patients. Invest Ophthalmol Vis Sci. 2015;56:4857–64.
37. Bowd C, Zangwill LM, Weinreb RN, Mederios FA, Belghith A. Estimating optical coherence tomography structural measurement floors to improve detection of progression in advanced glaucoma. Am J Ophthalmol. 2017;175:37–44.
38. Artes PH, Iwase A, Ohno Y, Kitazawa Y, Chauhan BC. Properties of perimetric threshold estimates from full threshold, SITA standard, and SITA fast strategies. Invest Ophthalmol Vis Sci. 2002;43:2654–9.
39. Wall M, Woodward KR, Doyle CK, Artes PH. Repeatability of automated perimetry: a comparison between standard automated perimetry with stimulus size III and V, matrix, and motion perimetry. Invest Ophthalmol Vis Sci. 2009;50:974–9.
40. Shin JW, Sung KR, Lee GC, Durbin MK, Cheng D. Ganglion cell-inner plexiform layer change detected by optical coherence tomography indicates progression in advanced glaucoma. Ophthalmology. 2017;124:1466–74.
41. Lee WJ, Kim YK, Park KH, Jeoung JW. Trend-based analysis of ganglion cell-inner plexiform layer thickness changes on optical coherence tomography in glaucoma progression. Ophthalmology. 2017;124:1383–91.
42. Reis AS, O'Leary N, Yang H, Sharpe GP, Nicolela MT, Burgoyne CF, Chauhan BC. Influence of clinically invisible, but optical coherence tomography detected, optic disc margin anatomy on neuroretinal rim evaluation. Invest Ophthalmol Vis Sci. 2012;53:1852–60.
43. Strouthidis NG, Yang H, Reynaud JF, Grimm JL, Gardiner SK, Fortune B, Burgoyne CF. Comparison of clinical and spectral domain optical coherence tomography optic disc margin anatomy. Invest Ophthalmol Vis Sci. 2009;50:4709–18.
44. Chauhan BC, Burgoyne CF. From clinical examination of the optic disc to clinical assessment of the optic nerve head: a paradigm change. Am J Ophthalmol. 2013;156:218–27.
45. Gardiner SK, Boey PY, Yang H, Fortune B, Burgoyne CF, Demirel S. Structural measurements for monitoring change in glaucoma: comparing retinal nerve fiber layer thickness with minimum rim width and area. Invest Ophthalmol Vis Sci. 2015;56:6886–91.
46. Amini N, Daneshvar R, Sharifipour F, Romero P, Henry S, Caprioli J, Nouri-Mahdavi K. Structure-function relationships in perimetric glaucoma: comparison of minimum-rim width and retinal nerve fiber layer parameters. Invest Ophthalmol Vis Sci. 2017;58:4623–31.
47. Mederios FA, Zangwill LM, Bowd C, Mansouri K, Weinreb RN. The structure and function relationship in glaucoma: implications for detection of progression and measurement of rates of change. Invest Ophthalmol Vis Sci. 2012;53:6939–46.

Chapter 13
Cirrus HD-OCT's Guided Progression Analysis

Ahmet Akman

13.1 Progression Analysis Software

Optical coherence tomography (OCT) manufacturers use different strategies for establishing glaucoma progression. The Guided Progression Analysis (GPA) is the progression analysis software package of Humphrey Field Analyzer (HFA) (Carl Zeiss Meditec, Dublin, CA). Zeiss decided to use the same name for the statistical progression analysis software package of Stratus TD-OCT. When Cirrus HD-OCT replaced the Stratus OCT, GPA was also created for the Cirrus HD-OCT software. Similar to Humphrey Field Analyzer's GPA, Cirrus HD-OCT provides both event and trend analyses for detecting glaucoma progression. Currently, it is the only commercial OCT software package capable of performing event and trend analysis both for retinal nerve fiber layer (RNFL) calculation circle measurements, peripapillary RNFL thickness maps, macular ganglion cell thickness maps, and optic nerve head (ONH) parameters.

13.2 Basic Concepts of Cirrus HD-OCT's GPA

Cirrus HD-OCT's GPA has two components, one for the RNFL and ONH area, and one for the macular region. As a rule, GPA's event analysis uses the first two scans as baseline data, and up to six subsequent scans are compared to the baseline images. The user can choose any available two scans as baseline images and look for progression after a specific date. One of the most important properties of the Cirrus' GPA is its independence from the normative database. GPA makes all the comparisons between the mean of the two baseline images and follow-up scans of the

A. Akman
Department of Ophthalmology, School of Medicine, Başkent University, Ankara, Turkey

© Springer International Publishing AG, part of Springer Nature 2018
A. Akman et al. (eds.), *Optical Coherence Tomography in Glaucoma*,
https://doi.org/10.1007/978-3-319-94905-5_13

individual patient, so the results in GPA are not related to any data derived from the normative database. Independence from the normative database prevents errors related to the anatomical variations, refractive errors, race and age-related differences. Thus, the results are specific for that individual.

13.3   How to Read Cirrus HD-OCT's RNFL/ONH GPA Report?

Cirrus HD-OCT's GPA uses four different strategies for investigating the progression of glaucomatous damage in the peripapillary area. These consist of progression analyses for RNFL thickness map, RNFL thickness profile, average and inferior/superior hemifield RNFL thickness, and average cup-to-disc ratio. The first three strategies analyze RNFL changes, and the last one addresses ONH changes over time.

The RNFL thickness map progression analysis mainly concentrates on focal changes, whereas the RNFL thickness profile graph focuses on broader focal changes, and the average RNFL thickness progression graph searches for diffuse progression.

13.3.1   Sections of the Printout (Fig. 13.1)

1. **Patient Data**: Check the name and date of birth (DOB) of the patient
2. **Baseline and Follow-Up RNFL Thickness Maps**: The first four rows give the date, patient ID, registration method, signal strength (SS) and the average RNFL values of the calculation circle. The second part consists of serial RNFL thickness maps. These maps show the actual values measured throughout the ONH cube using the false color code A scheme explained in Sect. 5.3.1. RNFL measurements and color code A are not related to the normative database values; therefore, these represent the raw RNFL thickness data for the scanned eye. Imaging artifacts must be ruled out on the maps before evaluating the results. Gross changes in RNFL thickness can be observed on these maps.
3. **RNLF Thickness Change Maps (Event Analysis)**: These maps show the observed RNFL thickness deviations from the two baseline images. If there is no change exceeding test-retest variability for the specific scan compared to baseline, only the OCT image is provided. If the change is greater than the test-retest variability, the super-pixels (4 × 4 pixel = 1 superpixel) are flagged as "possible loss" in orange. If the same region shows similar or greater amount of thinning (beyond the test-retest variability) on the next scan again, the area is

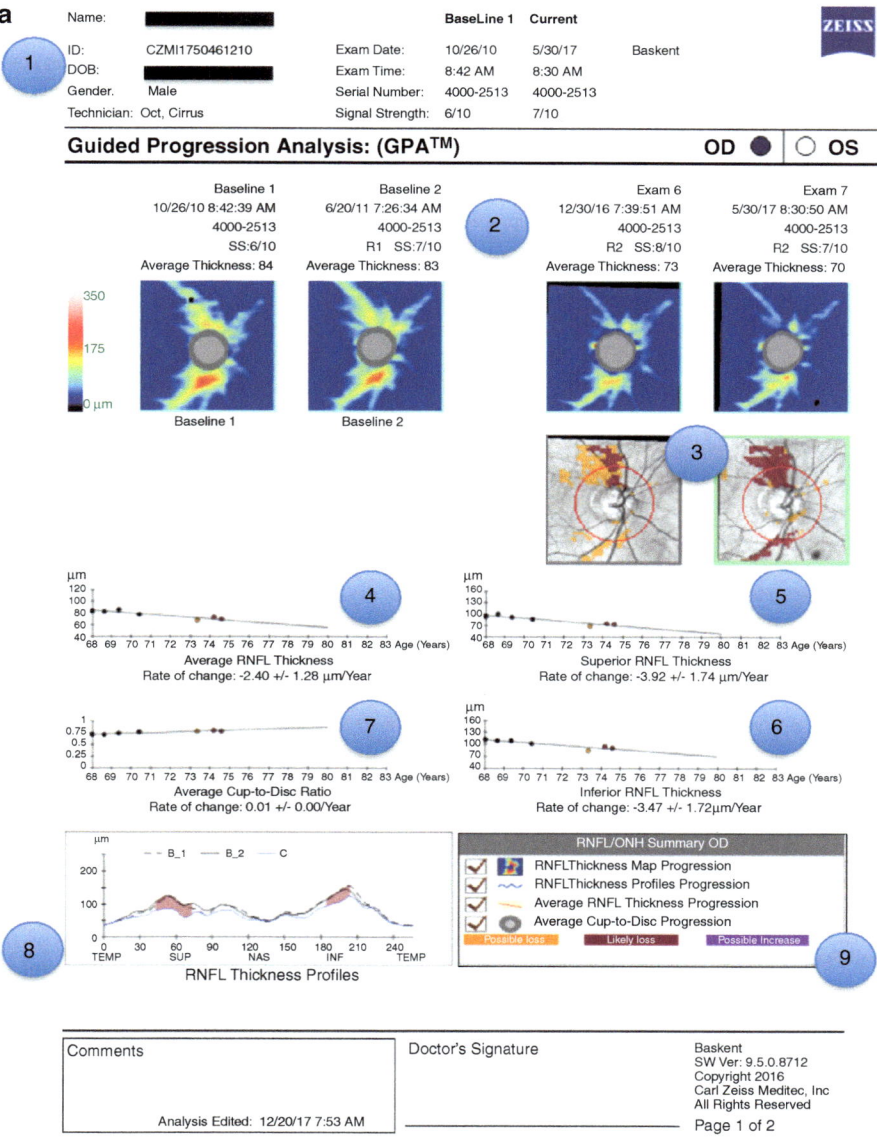

Fig. 13.1 (**a**) Page 1 and (**b**) Page 2 of the two page printout of the Cirrus HD-OCT's RNFL/ONH GPA Report. Sections of the printout are explained in the Sect. 13.3.1. The label numbers in blue circles correspond to the heading numbers used in Sect. 13.3.1

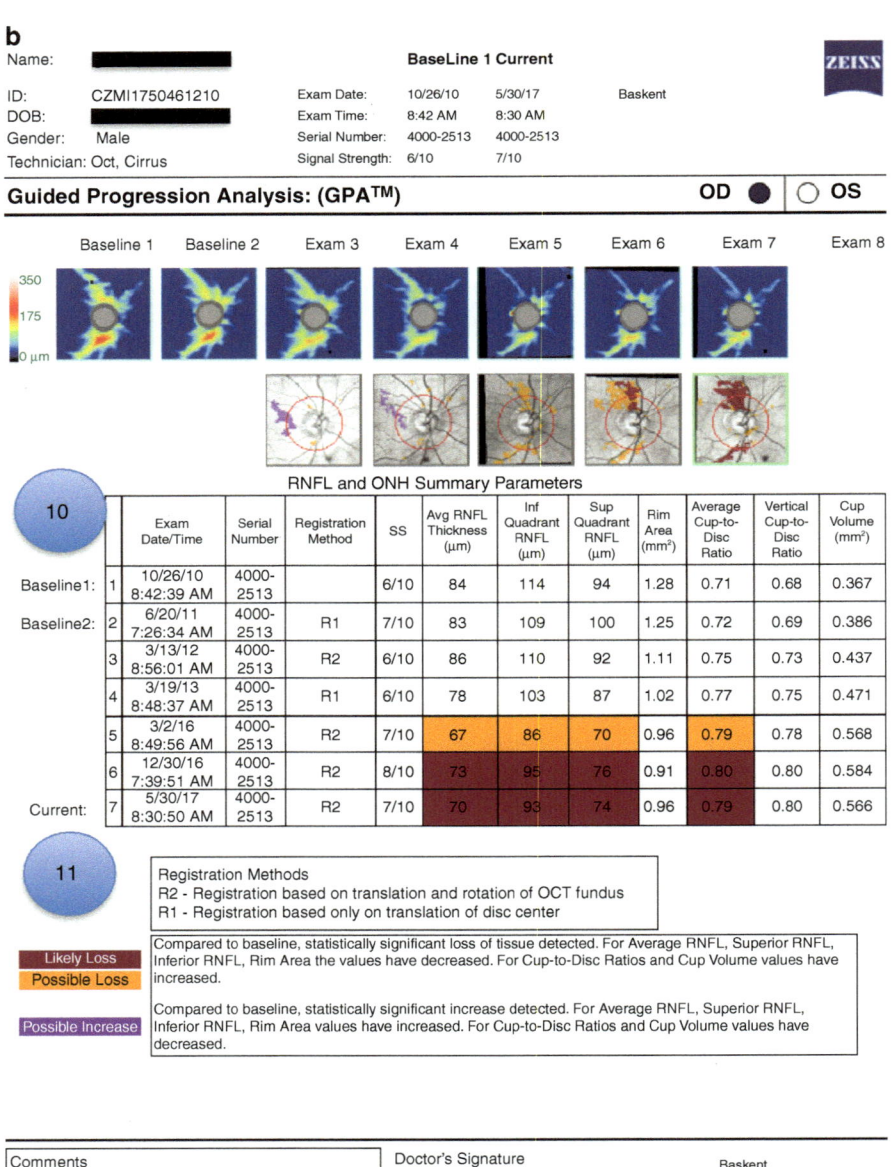

Fig. 13.1 (continued)

flagged as "likely loss" in red. Finally, if an area shows RNFL *thickening* beyond what is expected as test-retest variability, the area of interest is flagged as "possible increase" in lavender. This can result from retinal edema, vitreo-retinal traction, artifacts or random noise. The aforementioned flags are shown if the change is present in 20 or more adjacent superpixels. This change analysis is a type of event analysis as these maps use differences between the baseline images and follow-up scans to detect changes exceeding the test-retest variability regardless of how fast these changes occur.

4. **Average RNFL Thickness Change Plot (Trend Analysis)**: Average RNFL thickness values of the calculation circle are plotted as a function of time. Every single scan measurement is displayed as a small black circle if there is no change exceeding test-test variability. If there is thinning beyond the expected test-retest variability, the corresponding circle is colored in orange; if the following RNFL measurement remains significantly thinner compared to the baseline in the subsequent scan, the circle is colored in red. If there is both "likely loss" and a significant linear trend (p < 0.05), a linear regression line is drawn to calculate the rate of loss. The 95% confidence interval for the regression line is demonstrated as a shaded gray area around the regression line. The slope of the regression line is also presented as the rate of change in µm/year (± %95 confidence interval). The rate of change values is provided if there are at least four scans that span at least 2 years are available. Physicians evaluating these trend analyses need to keep in mind that the linear regression approach is affected by many factors and should not replace the clinical evaluation of the patient.

5. **Superior RNFL Thickness Change Plot (Trend Analysis)**: Superior quadrant RNFL calculation circle values are plotted as a function of time. The same presentation style used as for the **Average RNFL Thickness Change Plot**, described above.

6. **Inferior RNFL Thickness Change Plot (Trend Analysis)**: Inferior quadrant RNFL calculation circle values are plotted as a function of time. The same presentation style used as for the **Average RNFL Thickness Change Plot**, described above. In most patients with early glaucoma, the first signs of progression is observed in the inferior quadrants [1–3].

7. **Average Cup to Disc Ratio Change Plot (Trend Analysis)**: The average cup-to-disc ratio is plotted as a function of time. Again, the same presentation style used for the **Average RNFL Thickness Change Plot** is used. The regression line shows the trend over time and rate of change per year is presented under the graph.

8. **RNFL Thickness Profile Change Plot (Event Analysis)**: Three TSNIT profiles for the examined eye is plotted in overlapping style. B1 and B2 are two baseline scans and C represents the current scan. As all the scans in the GPA are

registered with each other, the same sectors of the calculation circle are overlaid with great precision. The changes are reported with the same color code used throughout the GPA with "likely loss" shown in orange, "possible loss" in red and "possible increase" in lavender. At least 14 adjacent A-scans, which correspond to 20 degrees of calculation circle, must show significant change to be reported. The area between the RNFL profiles that show the change is colored with the above-mentioned color codes.

9. **RNFL/ONH Summary**: This is the summary of the four analyses used in GPA. Three analyses are for detecting RNFL change and the last one is used for detecting ONH change. Each analysis has a checkbox, which is checked if significant change was observed. An orange checkmark represents "possible loss" meaning progression is detected in one follow-up scan, a red checkmark displays "likely loss" meaning progression is detected on two consecutive scans, and a lavender checkmark means "possible increase" in RNFL thickness.

10. **RNFL and ONH Summary Parameters Table**: This table in page 2 of the GPA report summarizes the data that were used to draw the plots in page 1 and an event analysis is performed on the measurements. The cells with values that demonstrate change beyond the test-retest variability when compared to the baseline are colored in orange representing "possible loss"; this means progression is detected on one follow-up scan only. Cells colored in red are considered to display "likely loss" meaning progression is detected on two or more consecutive scans; lavender color represents "possible increase".

11. **Legend**: The legend describes the available image registration modes, the color codes and the criteria for possible or likely loss and likely increase terminology. Two types of registrations are possible. R1 means images are registered based on translation of disc center, R2 means images are registered based on translation and rotation of the OCT fundus image.

13.4   How to Read Cirrus HD-OCT's Ganglion Cell GPA Report?

The most recent addition to the Zeiss Cirrus HD-OCT progression analysis software is the ganglion cell GPA which tracks changes in the thickness of macular ganglion cell and inner plexiform layers (GCL + IPL). The Ganglion Cell GPA uses two strategies similar to the RNFL/ONH GPA. Similar to the latter, two initial scans of adequate quality are used as the baseline images and the same registration methods (R1, R2, described previously) are used to compare the follow-up scans with the baseline ones. After registration, two strategies are used for monitoring progression. The first one is an event analysis that tracks changes in the GCL + IPL thickness map, which measures the GCL + IPL in an elliptical annulus centered on the fovea. The second one is a trend analysis that calculates the slope of change in GCL + IPL thickness measurements in the elliptical annulus. Again, the Ganglion Cell GPA makes all the comparisons between the baseline and follow up scan measurements of an individual patient, and therefore, the results of the ganglion cell GPA are not compared to the normative database. Macular ganglion cell GPA report uses the same approach used in RNFL/ONH GPA report; hence, the following sections repeats some of definitions from the previous pages.

13.4.1 Sections of the Printout (Fig 13.2)

1. **Patient Data**: Check the name and date of birth (DOB) of the patient
2. **Baseline and Follow Up Maps**: The first four rows provide the date, patient ID, registration method, SS and the average GCL + IPL values throughout the elliptical annulus. The second part consists of serial maps. These maps show the actual values measured inside the macular elliptical annulus using the false color code scheme explained in Sect. 5.3.1. As in the RNFL thickness map progression analysis, these are the raw thickness data for the scanned eye and color coding is independent of the normative database. Imaging artifacts need to be checked on these maps before evaluating the results. Gross changes in thickness values can be observed on these maps.
3. **Thickness Change Maps (Event Analysis)**: These maps demonstrate the observed deviations from the two baseline measurements. If the thickness change exceeds test-retest variability for the specific superpixels as compared to the baselines, those super-pixels are flagged in orange as "possible loss". If the same superpixels show thinning beyond the test-retest variability in the subsequent scan, those superpixels are flagged in red as "likely loss". Finally, if some super-pixels display thickening beyond the expected test-retest variability, they are flagged in lavender as "possible increase", which can result from macular edema, vitreo-macular traction, artifacts or simply measurement noise. The changing superpixels are flagged if the change is present in 20 or more adjacent superpixels.
4. **Average Thickness Change Plot (Trend Analysis)**: Average thickness values of the elliptical annulus are plotted as a function of time. Every single measurement is shown as a small black circle if there is the change compared to the baseline does not exceed test-retest variability. If there is thinning beyond test-retest variability, the circle for this scan is colored in orange, if the following GCL + IPL measurement continues to be significantly thinner than the baseline, the circle is colored as red. If there is both "likely loss" (on event analysis) and a significant linear trend ($p < 0.05$), a linear regression line is plotted to estimate the rate of loss. The confidence interval for the regression line is shaded as a gray area around the regression line. The slope of the regression line is also presented as rate of change μm/year (± %95 confidence interval). The rate of change is presented if there are at least four scans that span a minimum of 2 years.
5. **Total Superior Thickness Change Plot (Trend Analysis)**: The superior half of GCL + IPL measurements in the elliptical annulus are plotted as a function of

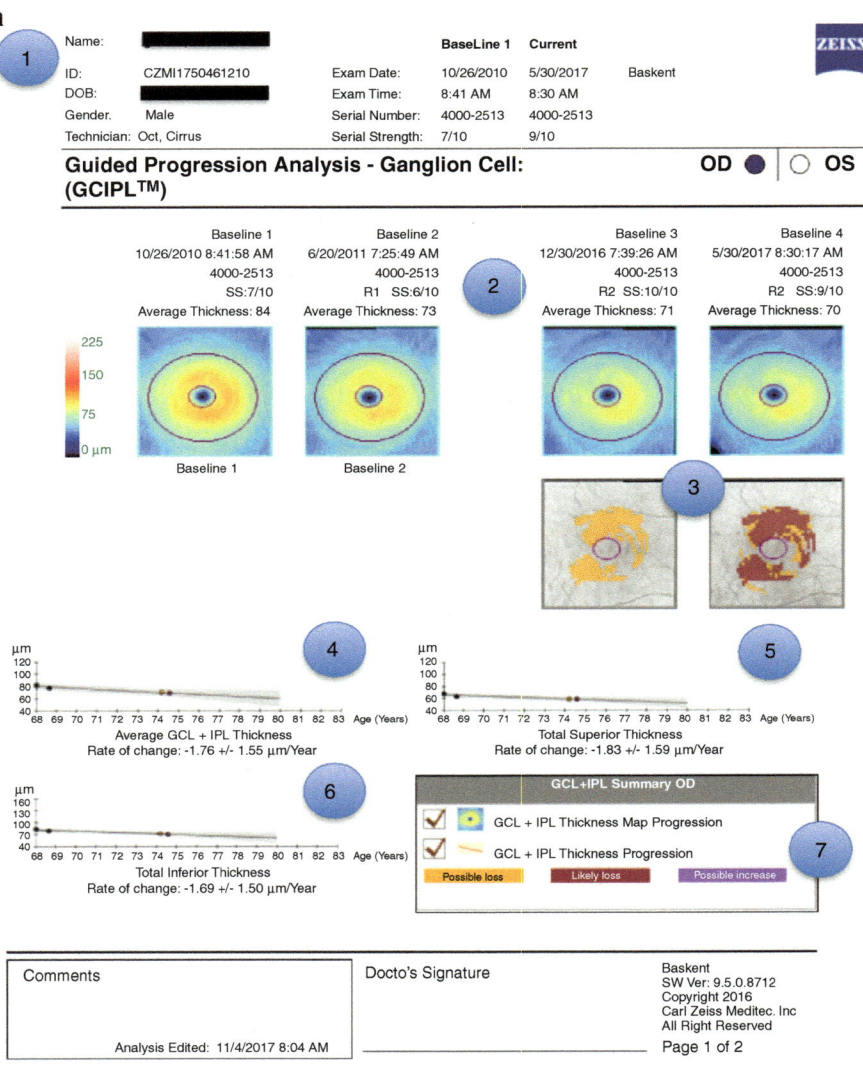

Fig. 13.2 (a) Page 1 and (b) Page 2 of the two page printout of the Cirrus HD-OCT's macular ganglion cell GPA Report. Sections of the printout are explained in the Sect. 13.4.1. The label numbers in blue circles corresponds to the heading numbers used in Sect. 13.4.1

b

Name:	███████████		BaseLine 1	Current		ZEISS
ID:	CZMI1750461210	Exam Date:	10/26/2010	5/30/2017	Baskent	
DOB:	███████████	Exam Time:	8:41 AM	8:30 AM		
Gender:	Male	Serial Number:	4000-2513	4000-2513		
Technician:	Oct, Cirrus	Serial Strength:	7/10	9/10		

Guided Progression Analysis - Ganglion Cell: (GCIPL™)

OD ● | ○ OS

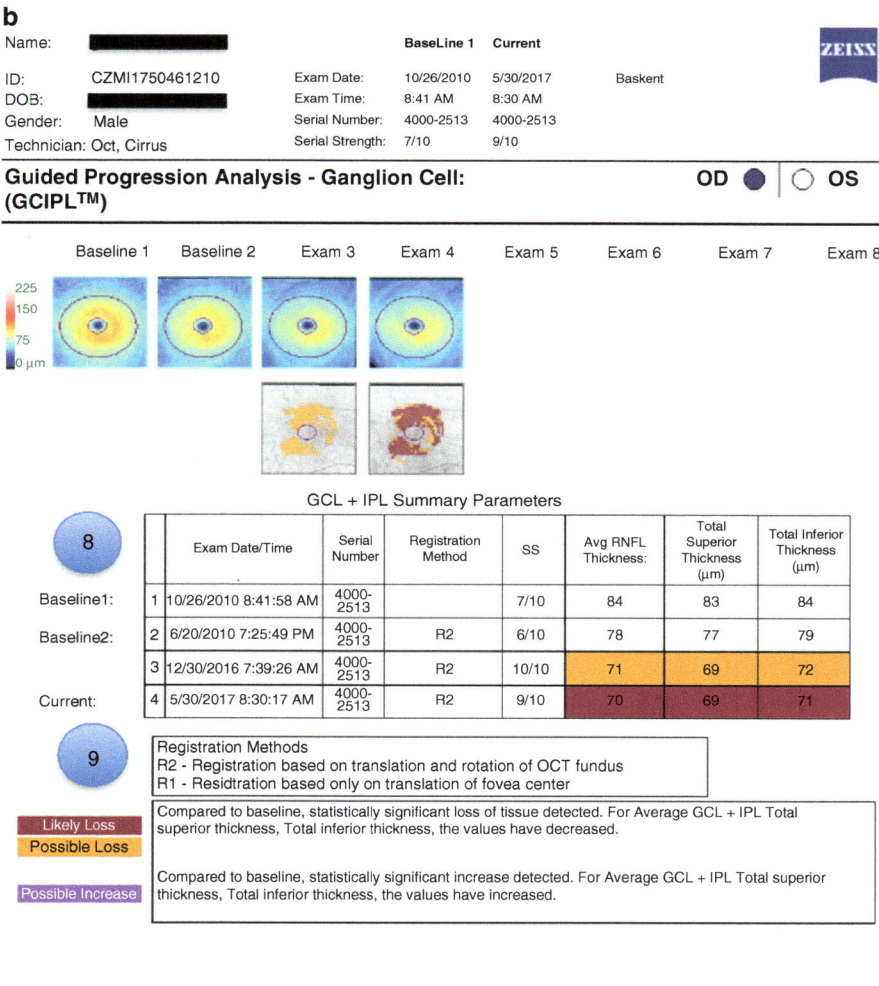

GCL + IPL Summary Parameters

		Exam Date/Time	Serial Number	Registration Method	SS	Avg RNFL Thickness:	Total Superior Thickness (µm)	Total Inferior Thickness (µm)
Baseline1:	1	10/26/2010 8:41:58 AM	4000-2513		7/10	84	83	84
Baseline2:	2	6/20/2010 7:25:49 PM	4000-2513	R2	6/10	78	77	79
	3	12/30/2016 7:39:26 AM	4000-2513	R2	10/10	71	69	72
Current:	4	5/30/2017 8:30:17 AM	4000-2513	R2	9/10	70	69	71

Registration Methods
R2 - Registration based on translation and rotation of OCT fundus
R1 - Residtration based only on translation of fovea center

Likely Loss
Possible Loss

Compared to baseline, statistically significant loss of tissue detected. For Average GCL + IPL Total superior thickness, Total inferior thickness, the values have decreased.

Possible Increase

Compared to baseline, statistically significant increase detected. For Average GCL + IPL Total superior thickness, Total inferior thickness, the values have increased.

Comments	Docto's Signature	Baskent SW Ver: 9.5.0.8712 Copyright 2016 Carl Zeiss Meditec. Inc All Right Reserved
Analysis Edited: 11/4/2017 8:04 AM		Page 2 of 2

Fig. 13.2 (continued)

time. The same presentation style used for **Average Thickness Change Plot**, described above, is also used here.

6. **Total Inferior Thickness Change Graph (Trend Analysis)**: The inferior half of GCL + IPL measurements in the elliptical annulus are plotted as a function of time. The same presentation style used for **Average Thickness Change Plot**, described above, is also used here. In most patients with early glaucoma, the first signs of progression is observed in the inferior temporal sector of the macula [4–6].

7. **Summary**: This is the summary of the two types of analyses used in ganglion cell GPA. These two analyses are the thickness progression map and thickness progression analysis. Each analysis has a checkbox, which is checked if significant change was observed. A orange check—"possible loss"—means progression is detected on one scan, a red check—"likely loss"—denotes that progression is detected on two consecutive scans, and a lavender check represents "possible increase".

8. **Summary Parameters Table**: This table on page 2 of the ganglion cell GPA report summarizes the data that were used to draw the plots on page 1 and an event analysis is performed on the measurements. The cells that contain values displaying change beyond the test-retest variability when compared to baseline values are colored in orange as "possible loss" meaning progression is detected on one scan, colored in red as "likely loss" denoting progression is detected on two consecutive scans and flagged in lavender if "possible increase" in thickness is detected.

9. **Legend**: The legend describes the available image registration modes, the color codes and the criteria for possible or likely loss and likely increase terminology.

13.5 Key Points

- It is important to remember that all the analyses on the above progression reports are based on measurements from individual patients compared over time. No information from the normative database is used in GPA.
- When evaluating the GPA reports, the first step is to check the patient ID and related clinical and demographic information. The next step involves checking the quality of the scans used in the progression analysis. This is done by first verifying the SS for each scan. Also, the scan quality needs to be monitored on the baseline and follow-up thickness maps so as to rule out artifacts.
- Finally, the registration protocol for each scan should be checked as R1 type registration can be affected by rotational artifacts more than R2 type.
- After the quality check, the event and trend analysis results and summary boxes should be assessed.

- If GPA detects progression, the results need to be evaluated for clinical relevance, as many factors other than the GPA results need to be considered with regard to treatment decisions.

References

1. Leung CK, Yu M, Weinreb RN, Lai G, Xu G, Lam DS. Retinal nerve fiber layer imaging with spectral-domain optical coherence tomography: patterns of retinal nerve fiber layer progression. Ophthalmology. 2012;119:1858–66.
2. Rao HL, Zangwill LM, Weinreb RN, Sample PA, Alencar LM, Medeiros FA. Comparison of different spectral domain optical coherence tomography scanning areas for glaucoma diagnosis. Ophthalmology. 2010;117:1692–9.
3. Dong ZM, Wollstein G, Schuman JS. Clinical utility of optical coherence tomography in glaucoma. Invest Ophthalmol Vis Sci. 2016;57:OCT556–67.
4. Tan O, Li G, Lu AT, Varma R, Huang D. Advanced Imaging for Glaucoma Study Group. Mapping of macular substructures with optical coherence tomography for glaucoma diagnosis. Ophthalmology. 2008;115:949–56.
5. Hood DC, Raza AS, de Moraes CG, Johnson CA, Liebmann JM, Ritch R. The nature of macular damage in glaucoma as revealed by averaging optical coherence tomography data. Transl Vis Sci Technol. 2012;1:3.
6. Kotera Y, Hangai M, Hirose F, Mori S, Yoshimura N. Three-dimensional imaging of macular inner structures in glaucoma by using spectral-domain optical coherence tomography. Invest Ophthalmol Vis Sci. 2011;52:1412–4.

Chapter 14
Spectralis OCT's Progression Analysis

Atilla Bayer

14.1 Introduction

Detecting progression of glaucoma is essential in both early and late stages of the disease. Evidence of progression will significantly influence the clinician's decision whether to start or modify glaucoma therapy. Spectral domain optical coherence tomography (SD-OCT), with its improved scanning speed, resolution, and reproducibility compared to time-domain OCT, has proved promising for earlier and more accurate detection of glaucomatous progression [1, 2]. Structural changes in glaucoma have been shown to be predictive of future functional loss and a decrease in the quality of life of the patients [3, 4]. Liu et al. have reported that almost half of the fellow eyes of patients with unilateral progression by conventional methods demonstrated statistically significant progression with Spectralis OCT [5]. In order not to miss these progressing eyes, the interpreter must be familiar with the properties and shortcomings of any given OCT device and its progression analysis software.

This chapter provides up to date information regarding understanding and evaluating the progression analysis approach used by the Spectralis OCT device (Heidelberg Engineering Inc., Heidelberg, Germany).

14.2 The Progression Analysis Suite

Spectralis OCT progression analysis is mainly based on the retinal nerve fiber layer (RNFL) measurement circle data. In order to improve the inter-test reproducibility of sequential scans, Spectralis OCT uses a dual-beam SD-OCT and a confocal

A. Bayer
Department of Glaucoma, Dünyagöz Eye Hospital, Ankara, Turkey

© Springer International Publishing AG, part of Springer Nature 2018
A. Akman et al. (eds.), *Optical Coherence Tomography in Glaucoma*,
https://doi.org/10.1007/978-3-319-94905-5_14

scanning laser ophthalmoscope, which work by emitting superluminescent diode light and an infrared scan to provide images of ocular microstructures simultaneously. A real-time eye tracking system couples confocal scanning laser ophthalmoscope and SD-OCT scanners to compensate for eye movements and to ensure that the same location is scanned over time, which is crucial for image registration. In addition, Spectralis OCT oversamples specific points on the scans and subsequently compares and combines them to reduce random noise, enhancing visualization of structures of interest. RNFL thickness measurements are obtained by averaging 16 consecutive circular scans of a 12° peripapillary circle (3.46 mm diameter) centered on the optic disc. After the reference image is identified by the operator, the system automatically registers the reference image scanning area and scans the same region during follow-up examinations.

14.2.1 RNFL Change Report

Spectralis SD-OCT device provides an "RNFL Change Report" that includes the baseline and follow-up scans for the global average and sectoral RNFL measurements and their classifications (Fig. 14.1). The software does not formally compare follow-up RNFL measurements with those at baseline or provide any p values.

1. **Patient and Test Information**: Displays general patient information such as patient name, patient ID, diagnosis, date of birth (DOB), examination date, gender and laterality. The examiner should verify the name and DOB of the patient, as the baseline results are compared to age matched data from the normative database.
2. **Baseline Display**: Baseline display providing infrared (IR) image, raw OCT scan, RNFL profile image, RNFL thickness profile, and classification chart.
3. **Baseline Test Date**: The date of the baseline test (Day/Month/Year format).
4. **Baseline Settings**: Settings used for the baseline image and quality score.
5. **Baseline RNFL Thickness Plot**: Baseline thickness values of the patient's scan around the optic disc from going through temporal, superior, nasal, inferior quadrants back to temporal quadrant (TSNIT).
6. **Follow-Up Displays**: Displays providing IR image, RNFL profile image, raw OCT scan, RNFL thickness profile, and classification chart of follow-up scans.
7. **Follow-Up Test Number and Date**: Follow-up test # and date.
8. **Follow-Up Settings**: Settings used for the follow-up images and quality scores.
9. **Follow-Up RNFL Thickness Plots**: Follow-up thickness values of the patient's scan around the optic disc on the TSNIT curve. If the RNFL thickness plot demonstrates thinning compared to the baseline, the area of change is flagged in red, whereas an increase in thickness is displayed in green.

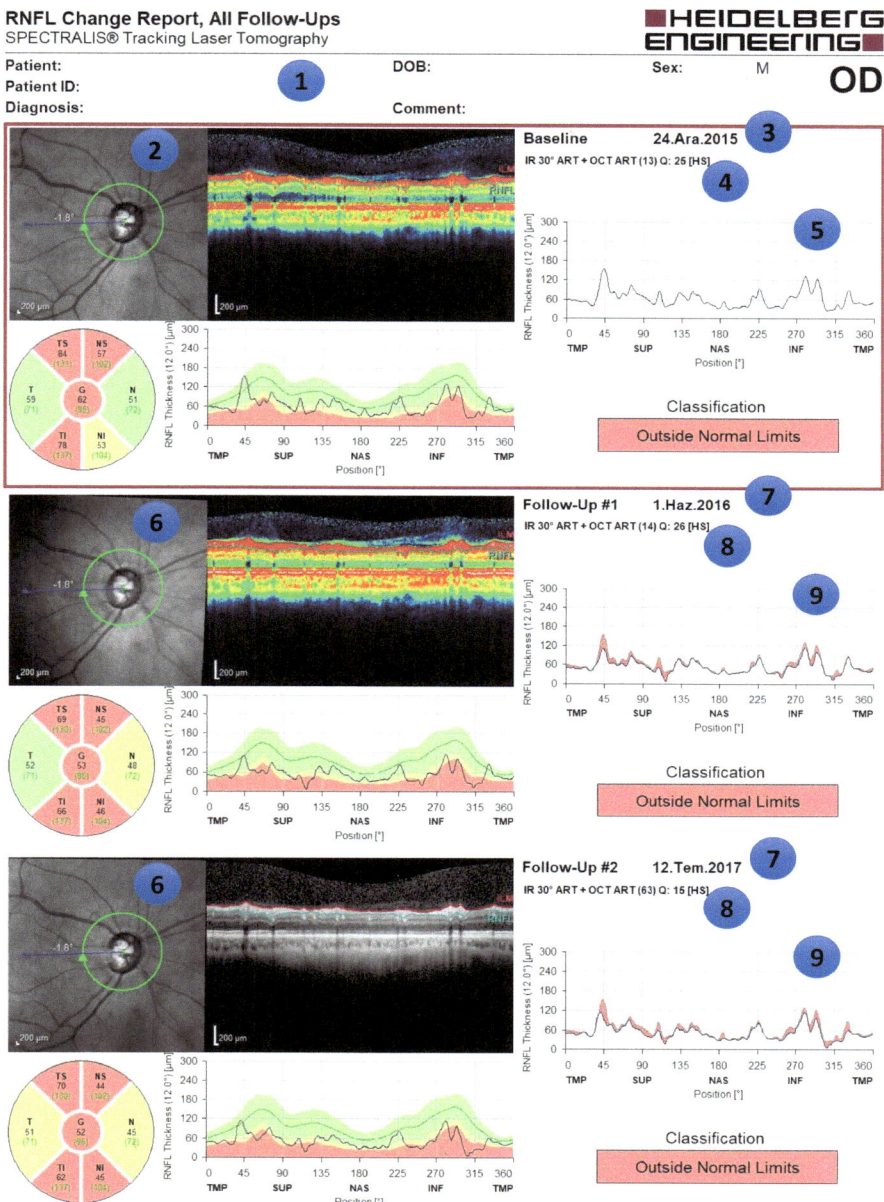

Fig. 14.1 The RNFL change report provided by Spectralis OCT. This report displays sequential scans of a patient with advanced glaucoma over a 2-year period with progressive thinning in most sectors

14.2.2   RNFL Trend Report

In the "RNFL Trend Report", the normalized RNFL thickness graph, global and sectoral RNFL thickness measurements on baseline and follow-up tests, and the differences of these values compared to the baseline measurements are presented (Fig. 14.2). This report does not formally compare the follow-up RNFL measurement to the baseline.

1. **Patient and Test Information**: Displays general patient information as patient name, patient ID, diagnosis, DOB, examination date, gender and laterality. The examiner has to check the name and DOB of the patient, as the results are compared to age-matched data from the normative database.
2. **Normalized RNFL Thickness Graph**: For the baseline and each follow-up examination (x-axis), normalized global RNFL thickness and sectoral RNFL thickness in the temporal, temporal superior, nasal superior, nasal, nasal inferior and temporal inferior sectors (y-axis) are displayed as a line graph. The thickness measurements are normalized compared to the average global or sectoral measurements of the normative database.
3. **Examination Date**: Baseline and follow-up examination dates.

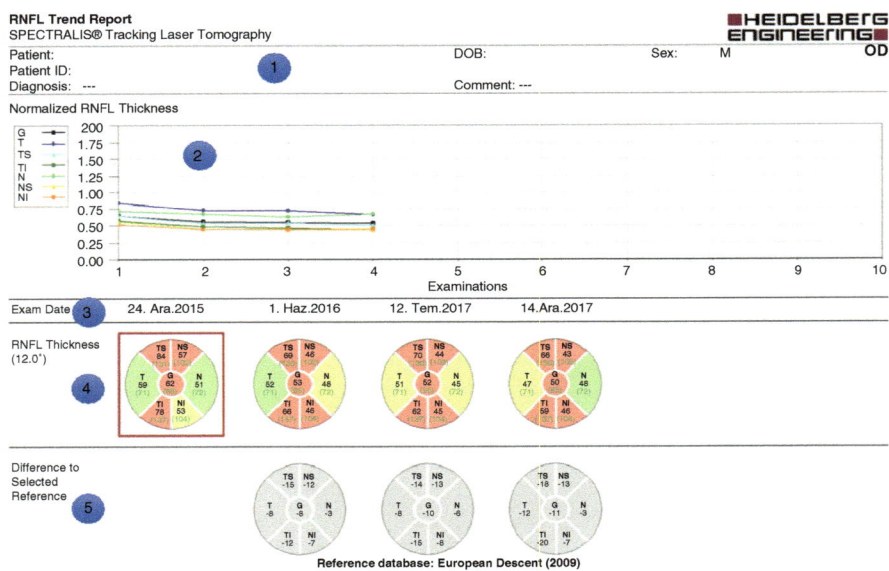

Fig. 14.2 The RNFL trend report of the patient in Fig. 14.1. The normalized RNFL thickness graph, global and sectoral RNFL thickness values of baseline and follow-up tests, and the differences between these values and the baseline measurements are shown. In (2), the thickness measurements are normalized compared to the average global or sectoral measurements of the normative database

4. **Classification Charts**: Global and sectoral RNFL thickness values of each examination are represented and classified as pie graphs. The baseline or reference test is outlined in red.
5. **Difference to Selected Reference Graphs**: Differences between the follow-up test values with the baseline measurements are shown for each sector as well as globally. Negative values denote progressive RNFL thinning whereas positive values indicate thickening of the RNFL.

14.2.3   RNFL Progression Trend Analysis Report

Spectralis OCT also provides a trend analysis for the RNFL thickness (Fig. 14.3). The slope of change is estimated based on regression of consecutive tests against time and compared to the normal age-related slope. This comparison is available for global and sectoral RNFL values. This test allows for assessment of change over time and whether the observed change would be considered statistically significant. The trend analysis graph displays the RNFL thickness at each time point overlaid on

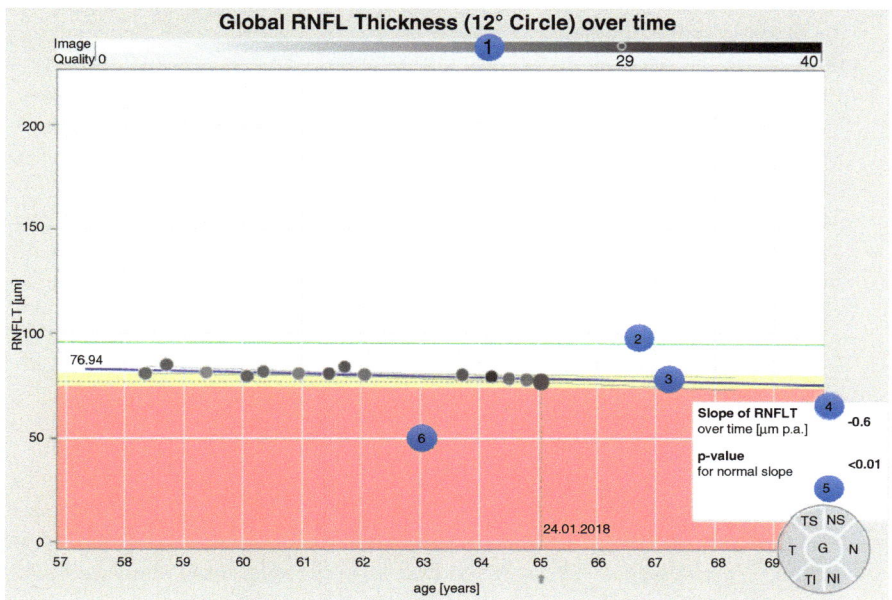

Fig. 14.3 Progression trend analysis report of a patient with slow progression over years with an annual loss of 0.6 μm/year. This patient had early glaucomatous damage on VFs at baseline. The regression line shows that, if treatment remains unchanged, this patient's classification for global RNFL thickness would be expected to become "outside normal limits" after about a decade

a color-coded normative database range. The blue linear regression line shows the estimated RNFL thickness change over time and an approximation of a 5-year trend. The green line indicates physiological thinning of the RNFL with age. The legend in the bottom right shows the rate of change in μm per year and the p value indicates whether this rate is significantly faster than normal aging. P values of <0.05 are considered statistically significant.

In the GMPE software, slope of progression is estimated over time and compared to normal age-related decay for the 3.5, 4.1, and 4.7 mm RNFL measurement circles. This comparison is also available for global and Garway-Heath sectoral values.

1. **Indicator for Quality of Examination**: Varies from grey (poor quality) to black (good quality). The intensity of gray color reflects the quality of a particular test.
2. **Plot of RNFL Thickness Decay Related to Normal Aging**: Normal aging related regression slope (green line).
3. **Plot of Progression Over Time**: The slope of progression is calculated from consecutive tests over time (blue regression line). It shows the estimated RNFL thickness change over time and an approximation of the five-year outcome.
4. **Slope of RNFL Over Time (μm/Year)**: Slope of progression is calculated over time as annual loss of thickness in μm.
5. **Significance for the RNFL Slope (p-Value)**: Indicates if the slope of progression is statistically significant. Slope of progression is estimated over time and compared to the regression slope for normal aging. This value is calculated for global and sectoral values. The legend in the bottom right displays the rate of change in μm per year, with the p value indicating whether this rate is significantly faster than normal aging (green line). P values of <0.05 are considered statistically significant and likely clinically relevant.
6. **Color-Coded Background**: The background is color-coded to demonstrate when a measurement falls within borderline abnormal or definitely abnormal range based on the classification chart percentile values defined in Chap. 6 for Spectralis OCT.

14.2.4   MRW Progression Trend Analysis Report

The Glaucoma Module Premium Edition (GMPE) software provides a progression trend analysis report for the minimum rim width (MRW) thickness (Fig. 14.4). Evaluation of this report is similar to the RNFL progression trend analysis report, except that the MRW values on the y-axis replace those of RNFL and the estimates of age-related decay were performed for the MRW normative data. The trend analysis provides the results for both Garway-Heath sectors as well as globally.

1. **Indicator for Quality of Examination**: Varies from grey (poor quality) to black (good quality). The intensity of gray color reflects the quality of a particular test.

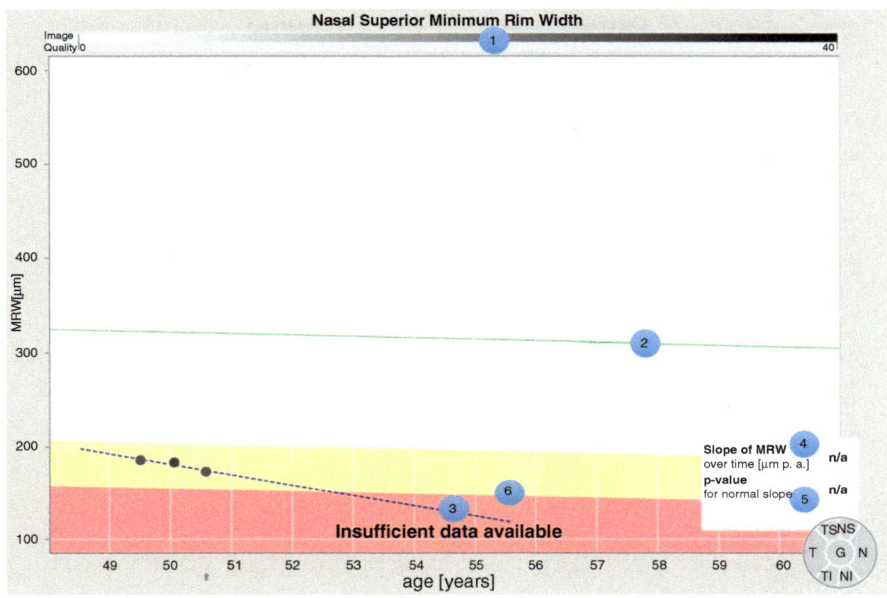

Fig. 14.4 Minimum rim width progression trend analysis report of the nasal superior sector of a patient with progression over years. This patient had moderate glaucomatous damage on VFs at baseline. The regression line shows that, if treatment remains unchanged, this patient's classification for Minimum Rim Width analysis for this sector would be expected to become "outside normal limits" after about 2 years

2. **Plot of MRW Decay Related to Normal Aging**: Normal aging related regression slope (green line).
3. **Plot of Progression Over Time**: The slope of progression is calculated from consecutive tests over time (blue regression line). It shows the estimated MRW change over time and an approximation of the 5-year outcome.
4. **Slope of MRW Over Time (μm/Year)**: Slope of progression is calculated over time as annual loss of thickness in μm.
5. **Significance for the MRW Slope (p-Value)**: Indicates if the slope of progression is statistically significant. Slope of progression is estimated over time and compared to the regression slope for normal aging. This value is calculated for global and sectoral values. The legend in the bottom right displays the rate of change in μm per year, with the p value indicating whether this rate is significantly faster than normal aging (green line). P values of <0.05 are considered statistically significant and likely clinically relevant. Since this patient has less than five tests, legend and p value are shown as n/a.
6. **Color-Coded Background**: The background is color-coded to demonstrate when a measurement falls within borderline abnormal or definitely abnormal range based on the classification chart percentile values defined in Chap. 6 for Spectralis OCT.

14.2.5   Posterior Pole Retinal Thickness Change Report

This report shows the change in the full thickness of the retina measured by the Posterior Pole Horizontal Algorithm (Fig. 14.5). A reduction in thickness is represented in red whereas increased thickness over time is flagged in green.

1. **Posterior Pole Thickness Map**: In each cell (superpixel) the averaged retinal thickness within that cell square is displayed. The warmer (the redder) the color of the thickness map, the thicker the measured retinal area. The compressed color scale on the right side of the map is used to localize even the smallest differences in retina thickness between adjacent areas.
2. **Horizontal Tomogram of the Macula**: This is important for two purposes. First, the interpreter must check whether the tomogram passes through the fovea. Next, it is helpful for excluding any macular pathology that can affect the test results. False color coding is used based on the reflectance of tissue layers with red representing the layer with the highest reflectance.
3. **Hemisphere Asymmetry Map and Posterior Pole Thickness Map of Reference Test**: The average retinal thickness in superpixels of one hemisphere is compared to the corresponding thickness in the opposite hemisphere. Superpixels that appear in various shades of gray in one hemisphere denote that the retinal thickness is reduced compared to those on the corresponding hemisphere. The intensity of gray scale reflects the magnitude of difference between corresponding hemispheric superpixels with a 30-μm difference displayed in black. The posterior pole thickness map is also included.

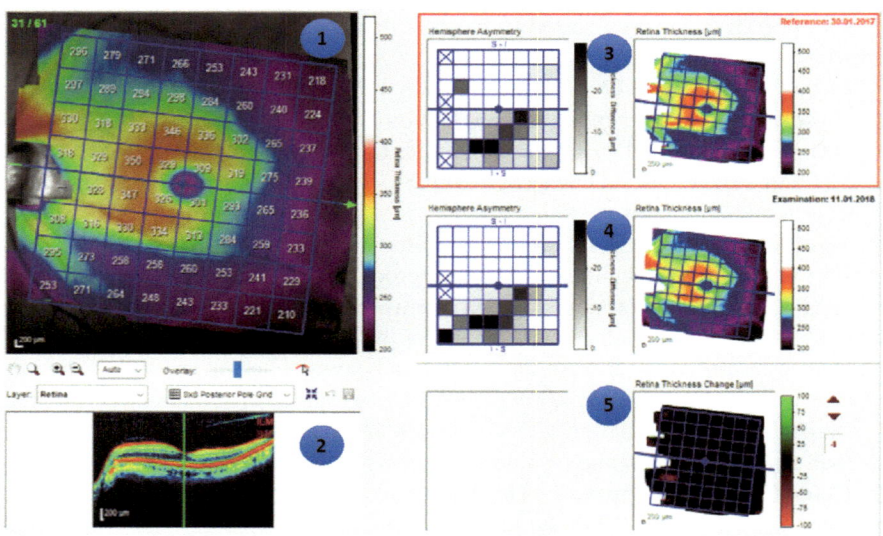

Fig. 14.5 The posterior pole retinal thickness change report of an eye with inferior thinning of the macular area in the left eye as shown in the hemisphere asymmetry map. Reference test and the follow-up test has about 1 year of interval. There is localized thinning in the inferior temporal area

4. **Hemisphere Asymmetry Map and Posterior Pole Thickness Map of Follow-Up Test**: Similar asymmetry and posterior pole thickness maps are provided for the follow-up test.
5. **Retinal Thickness Change Map**: A color-coded change map for the posterior pole retinal thickness is provided. The color scale on the right side of the map is used to define even the smallest differences in retinal thickness of the superpixels between the selected tests where increasing intensities of red represents increased thinning and green color represents thickening. Black color represents no change. This color scale is totally different from the false-color code used in the horizontal tomogram and the color-code used in the retinal thickness maps. Note that, in contrast to the retinal thickness maps, red color in the retina thickness change map denoted thinning.

14.3   Floor Effect, Dynamic Range and Rate of Progression

Although indispensable in early glaucoma, it is widely believed that SD-OCT measurements may not be as useful for monitoring RNFL thickness in advanced glaucoma because of a floor effect, after which thinning is much more difficult to ascertain [6]. This is one of the classical shortcomings of OCT RNFL progression analysis in advanced glaucoma. New studies on utility of macular ganglion cell change analysis have shown promising results for establishing evidence of progression in advanced glaucoma. In a recent study, Bowd et al. found that SD-OCT-measured ganglion cell-inner plexiform layer (GCL-IPL) thickness was the least likely parameter to reach the floor across most of the image area at baseline, suggesting that this parameter could be the most useful parameter investigated for detecting change in advanced glaucoma [7]. Belghith et al. showed that in very advanced glaucoma (MD $\leq$ −21 dB) eyes followed longitudinally for approximately 3.5 years, significant change in GCL-IPL thickness could be detected in 31% of eyes compared with 11% and 5% for minimum rim width (MRW) and RNFL thickness, respectively [8]. It might be still possible to monitor the less affected sectors of the RNFL rather than the global thickness in such advanced cases.

Bendschneider et al. reported that average RNFL thickness values from Spectralis OCT ranged from an average of 98 to 48 μm (dynamic range of 50 μm) in normal subjects [9]. Mwanza et al. has reported that the average RNFL thickness measured with Spectralis OCT reached the measurement floor at relative VF loss of −14.0 dB [10]. In their study, the dynamic range of Spectralis OCT device for RNFL measurements was highest for the inferior quadrant (76.9 μm), followed by the superior quadrant (66.0 μm) and global average (56.8 μm) with a simple linear regression change point analysis [10]. This finding may reflect a better ability for Spectralis OCT to detect RNFL thickness change in the superior and inferior regions as a result of the larger dynamic range of RNFL thickness measurements in these areas. When three commercially available devices were compared with regards to residual and dynamic range of global RNFL thickness in glaucoma eyes, the average VF change points and the corresponding residual thickness after which the RNFL stopped demonstrating further change were −22.2 dB and 57 μm (Cirrus), −25.3 dB and 49.2 μm (Spectralis), and − 24.6 dB and 64.7 μm (RTVue). The RNFL dynamic range derived from simple linear regression was wider on Spectralis OCT (52.6 μm) compared to the other two devices [10]. While expected RNFL loss from normal aging is approximately −0.2 to −0.50 μm/year [11–13], this rate can be largely different in progressing eyes. Previous reports have shown that rates of RNFL thickness change are predictive of future development of VF loss. Miki et al. found that glaucoma suspects who demonstrated VF loss over time had an average rate of RNFL change of −2.02 μm/year versus −0.82 μm/year in cases who did not develop VF loss [14]. In a study by Diniz-Filho et al., higher IOP was associated with faster rates of progressive RNFL loss over time as measured by Spectralis OCT. In eyes with progression, each 1 mmHg higher IOP was associated with an additional loss of 0.35 μm/year for the temporal superior sector and 0.31 μm/year for the temporal inferior sector. The association between IOP and rate of RNFL change was smaller for the temporal and nasal sectors [15].

14.4 Defining Progression with Spectralis OCT

Looking for signs of RNFL thinning is probably the most common way to watch for glaucomatous progression with OCT, but one has to be mindful of the potential caveats. Some inter-visit variability is inherent to all imaging modalities. Only when the magnitude of change is beyond the confines of variability, disease progression should be considered. The variability of the average or global RNFL thickness with Spectralis OCT is about 5 μm [16]. However, the inter-visit variability is much higher if focal change (such as change in a sector) is of concern. The superotemporal and the inferotemporal RNFL regions are most likely to demonstrate glaucomatous changes occur in early stages of the disease (Fig. 14.6). However, age-related decline also occurs most frequently in the same regions [11]. In cases where there is not enough certainty regarding RNFL thickness changes, it is often helpful to investigate other structural findings, including macular thickness. It is uncommon for an artifact to affect both the RNFL and the retinal thickness measurements; confirmation of corresponding changes on two or more structural and/or functional domains is a very important way to verify progression.

Although there are some studies about the usefulness of event-based analyses of change for the optic nerve head (ONH) or RNFL over time, trend-based analysis is more advantageous since it provides estimates of the rates of change for the parameter of interest. This permits the clinician to better assess how fast a patient is progressing. In a cohort study, Miki et al. showed, using a survival model, that a 1 μm/year faster rate of RNFL thickness loss corresponded to a 2.05 times higher risk of developing a VF defect [14]. They suggest that measuring the rate of Spectralis OCT RNFL loss may be a useful tool to help identify patients who are at a risk of developing VF loss. In another study, each 1 μm/year loss in binocular RNFL thickness with Spectralis OCT was associated with a change of 1.1 units/year in the National Eye Institute Visual Function Questionnaire (NEI VFQ) scores [17].

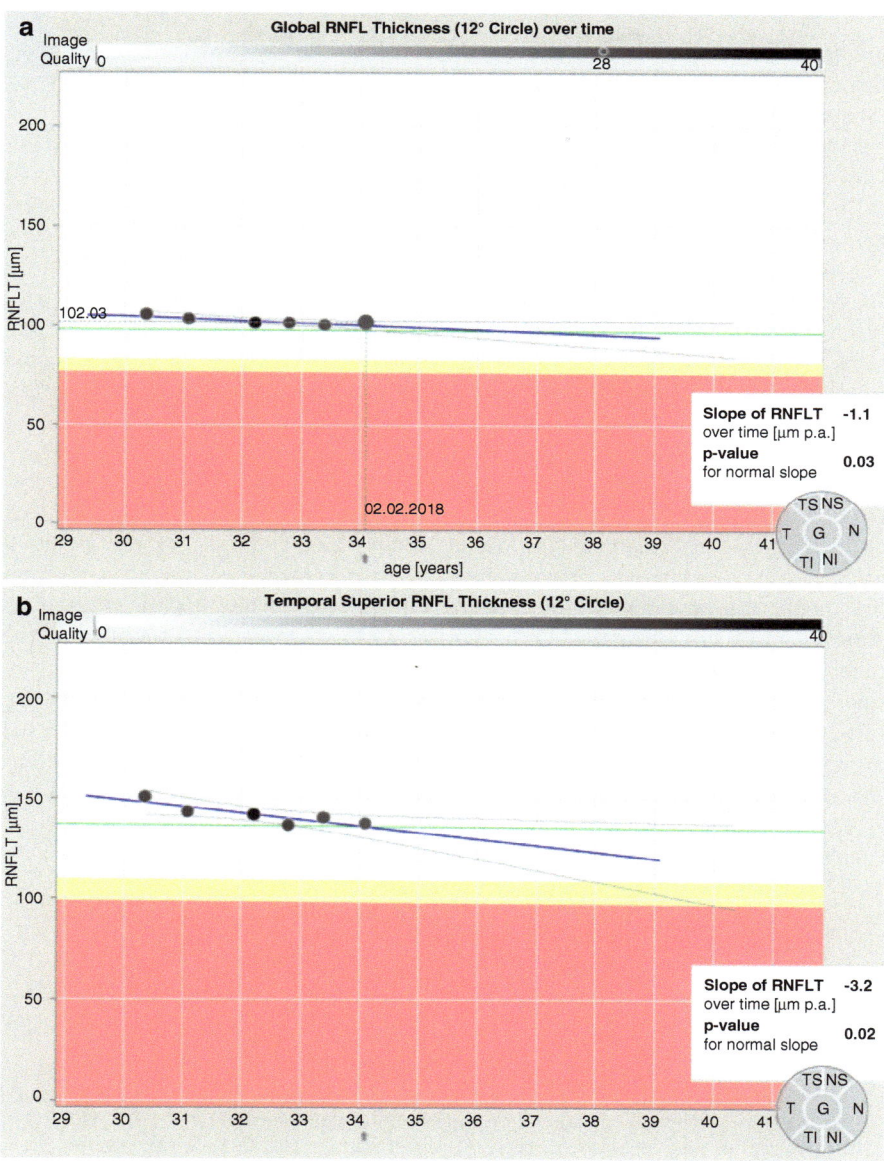

Fig. 14.6 (**a**) Progression Trend Analysis of the right eye of a young ocular hypertensive patient with statistically significant progressive thinning of the global average RNFL thickness over years. This patient has very slow slope for global average thickness (−1.1 μm/year) and approximation of a 5-year trend shows that the thickness will be within normal limits after 5 years. (**b**) Analysis of the temporal-superior sector of the same patient. Here the slope of progression is steeper with a loss of 3.2 μm/year. Approximation of regression line shows that he would be classified as "borderline" at the very least after a decade, if untreated. Note that this is a 34-years old patient and has a life expectancy of more than four decades

Since follow-up images are compared to the first or reference image during progression analysis, the first good-quality scan should be set as a reference immediately after acquisition. The recommended interval for OCT tests is usually six months although the optimal frequency is yet to be determined. A minimum of five measurements are needed before trend-based statistical analyses can be carried out with Spectralis OCT device. In the Glaucoma Module Premium Edition (GMPE) software, it is possible to calculate the rates of progression for RNFL thickness parameters from the 3.5, 4.1, and 4.7 mm circle scans.

One of the most important features of the progression analysis tool on Spectralis OCT is that it compares the measured values with the normative database and uses a colored background for the "borderline" and "outside normal limits" that represents the classification depending on the estimated percentiles. The normal aging related regression slope is provided, which enables the examiner to see the difference (if any) between the physiologic RNFL rate of change and the patient's rate of change calculated from available tests. This is possible for both the global average and sectoral (temporal, temporal superior, nasal superior, nasal, nasal inferior, temporal inferior) measurements. As with the trend analysis for the Visual Field Index on Humphrey Field Analyzer (Carl Zeiss Meditec Inc., Dublin, CA), extrapolation of the current trend based on the regression line for a specific eye provides information about the predicted RNFL thickness in 5 years. The Guided Progression Analysis (GPA) of Cirrus HD-OCT (Carl Zeiss Meditec Inc., Dublin, CA) on the other hand, compares only the follow-up tests of an individual patient to the baseline and does not relate these to the normative database. Neither does GPA take age related changes of the RNFL into consideration. GPA provides trend analysis for the average, superior quadrant, and inferior quadrant RNFL thickness values as well as the cup to disc ratio. In Spectralis OCT, on the other hand, RNFL trend analysis can be carried out for six sectors as well as for the global average value. Similar analyses are available for the Garway-Heath sectors in the GMPE software for both the RNFL and BMO-MRW thickness measurements.

References

1. Leung CK, Chiu V, Weinreb RN, Liu S, Ye C, Yu M, Cheung CY, Lai G, Lam DS. Evaluation of retinal nerve fiber layer progression in glaucoma: a comparison between spectral-domain and time-domain optical coherence tomography. Ophthalmology. 2011;118:1558–62.
2. van Velthoven ME, Faber DJ, Verbraak FD, van Leeuwen TG, de Smet MD. Recent developments in optical coherence tomography for imaging the retina. Prog Retin Eye Res. 2007;26:57–77.
3. Kuang TM, Zhang C, Zangwill LM, Weinreb RN, Medeiros FA. Estimating lead time gained by optical coherence tomography in detecting glaucoma before development of visual field defects. Ophthalmology. 2015t;122:2002–9.
4. Medeiros FA, Gracitelli CP, Boer ER, Weinreb RN, Zangwill LM, Rosen PN. Longitudinal changes in quality of life and rates of progressive visual field loss in glaucoma patients. Ophthalmology. 2015;122:293–301.

 5. Liu T, Tatham AJ, Gracitelli CP, Zangwill LM, Weinreb RN, Medeiros FA. Rates of retinal nerve fiber layer loss in contralateral eyes of glaucoma patients with unilateral progression by conventional methods. Ophthalmology. 2015;122:2243–51.
 6. Mwanza JC, Budenz DL, Warren JL, Webel AD, Reynolds CE, Barbosa DT, Lin S. Retinal nerve fibre layer thickness floor and corresponding functional loss in glaucoma. Br J Ophthalmol. 2015;99:732–7.
 7. Bowd C, Zangwill LM, Weinreb RN, Medeiros FA, Belghith A. Estimating optical coherence tomography structural measurement floors to improve detection of progression in advanced glaucoma. Am J Ophthalmol. 2017;175:37–44.
 8. Belghith A, Medeiros FA, Bowd C, Liebmann JM, Girkin CA, Weinreb RN, Zangwill LM. Structural change can be detected in advanced-glaucoma eyes. Invest Ophthalmol Vis Sci. 2016;57(9):OCT511–8.
 9. Bendschneider D, Tornow RP, Horn FK, Laemmer R, Roessler CW, Juenemann AG, Kruse FE, Mardin CY. Retinal nerve fiber layer thickness in normals measured by spectral domain OCT. J Glaucoma. 2010;19:475–82.
10. Mwanza JC, Kim HY, Budenz DL, Warren JL, Margolis M, Lawrence SD, Jani PD, Thompson GS, Lee RK. Residual and dynamic range of retinal nerve fiber layer thickness in glaucoma: comparison of three OCT platforms. Invest Ophthalmol Vis Sci. 2015;56:6344–51.
11. Vianna JR, Danthurebandara VM, Sharpe GP, Hutchison DM, Belliveau AC, Shuba LM, Nicolela MT, Chauhan BC. Importance of normal aging in estimating the rate of glaucomatous neuroretinal rim and retinal nerve fiber layer loss. Ophthalmology. 2015;122:2392–8.
12. Leung CK, Ye C, Weinreb RN, Yu M, Lai G, Lam DS. Impact of age-related change of retinal nerve fiber layer and macular thicknesses on evaluation of glaucoma progression. Ophthalmology. 2013;120:2485–92.
13. Leung CK, Cheung CY, Weinreb RN, Qiu K, Liu S, Li H, Xu G, Fan N, Pang CP, Tse KK, Lam DS. Evaluation of retinal nerve fiber layer progression in glaucoma: a study on optical coherence tomography guided progression analysis. Invest Ophthalmol Vis Sci. 2010;51:217–22.
14. Miki A, Medeiros FA, Weinreb RN, Jain S, He F, Sharpsten L, Khachatryan N, Hammel N, Liebmann JM, Girkin CA, Sample PA, Zangwill LM. Rates of retinal nerve fiber layer thinning in glaucoma suspect eyes. Ophthalmology. 2014;121:1350–8.
15. Diniz-Filho A, Abe RY, Zangwill LM, Gracitelli CP, Weinreb RN, Girkin CA, Liebmann JM, Medeiros FA. Association between intraocular pressure and rates of retinal nerve fiber layer loss measured by optical coherence tomography. Ophthalmology. 2016;123:2058–65.
16. Ghasia FF, El-Dairi M, Freedman SF, Rajani A, Asrani S. Reproducibility of spectral-domain optical coherence tomography measurements in adult and pediatric glaucoma. J Glaucoma. 2015;24:55–63.
17. Gracitelli CP, Abe RY, Tatham AJ, Rosen PN, Zangwill LM, Boer ER, Weinreb RN, Medeiros FA. Association between progressive retinal nerve fiber layer loss and longitudinal change in quality of life in glaucoma. JAMA Ophthalmol. 2015;133:384–90.

Chapter 15
Optical Coherence Tomography Progression Analysis: Sample Cases

Ahmet Akman

15.1 Case 1: OCT Progression in Pre-perimetric Glaucoma

This 75-year old male patient was diagnosed with ocular hypertension in 2006. He was followed until 2013 without treatment and his intraocular pressures varied between 21 and 24 mmHg in both eyes during this period. He was lost to follow-up in 2013 and re-examined in 2016 and found to have an IOP of 28 mmHg in the right eye and 26 mmHg in the left eye. Medical treatment was started and his intraocular pressure (IOP) decreased to 16 mmHg in the right eye and 15 mmHg in the left eye. Following are the Cirrus HD-OCT and visual field (VF) data including the progression analyses of the patient; OCT data begin from 2010 as the device became available in our clinic in 2010, VF data were available starting in 2006 (Figs. 15.1, 15.2, 15.3, 15.4, 15.5, 15.6, and 15.7).

A. Akman
Department of Ophthalmology, School of Medicine, Başkent University, Ankara, Turkey

© Springer International Publishing AG, part of Springer Nature 2018
A. Akman et al. (eds.), *Optical Coherence Tomography in Glaucoma*,
https://doi.org/10.1007/978-3-319-94905-5_15

278

A. Akman

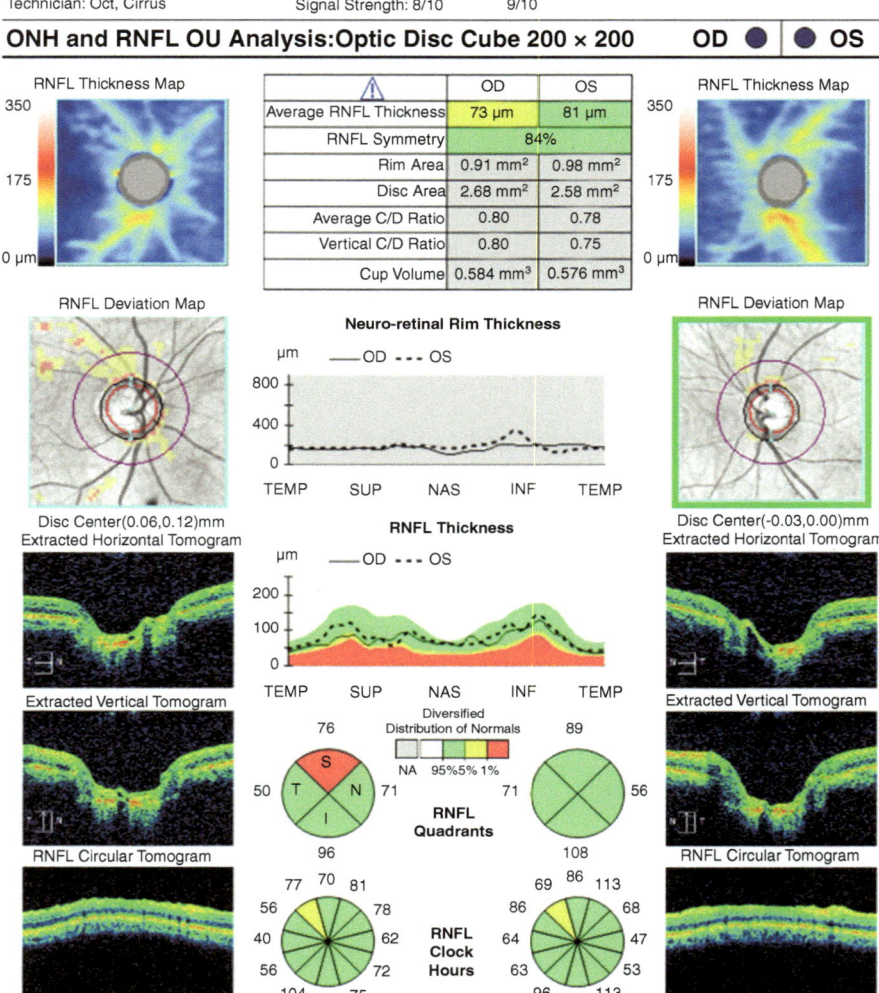

Fig. 15.1 Cirrus HD-OCT ONH and RNFL OU analysis of the patient in 2017. ONH analysis shows large discs with vertical cup-to-disc ratios of around 0.8 in both eyes. Normative data comparison is not possible as the large disc size (>2.5 mm²) is outside the limits of the normative database so ONH related parameters are shaded in gray. The RNFL analysis shows superior RNFL thinning in the right eye. Clock hour RNFL graph shows borderline changes in one clock hour for both eyes, whereas the superior quadrant is significantly abnormal at p < 1% level

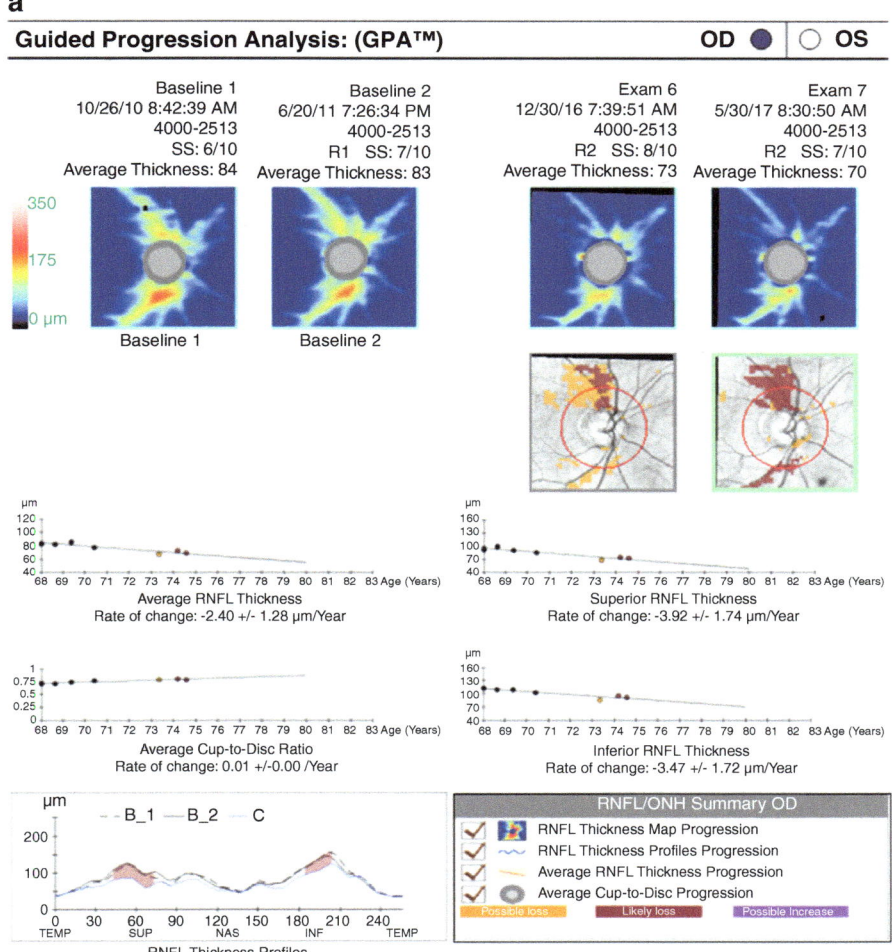

Fig. 15.2 Cirrus HD-OCT GPA, right eye. (**a**) The *RNFL/ONH Summary box* on the first page of the GPA report has red checks for all four progression analysis methods, *RNFL thickness map progression analysis* shows areas of "possible loss" in the 5th scan. RNFL thinning progressed to encompass a wider area in the sixth scan and persisted in the seventh scan leading to the flagging of these superpixels as "likely loss" in red. The *RNFL thickness profile progression graph* shows the current TSNIT plot is thinner in the superior and inferior quadrants compared to the baseline values. The areas with thinning beyond the test-retest variability are shown in red as "likely loss". The *average, inferior and superior RNFL thickness trend analyses* and *ONH average cup-to-disc ratio trend analysis* show progression and the orange and red dots displayed starting from the fifth scans. One can see the rate of progression under each plot and can extend the regression line for predicting future loss until the RNFL thickness reaches 40 μm. This is the floor level for RNFL thickness after which there is a high risk of significant VF loss and disability. The rate of change is −2.40 ± 1.28 μm/year for the average RNFL thickness. (**b**) In the second page, the *RNFL and ONH summary parameters* table shows all the values used in GPA. Measurements beyond the test-retest variability are also displayed in orange and red in this table. It is a good idea to check these values in addition to the plots on the first page to crosscheck the results and verify the chronology of change in the right eye

b

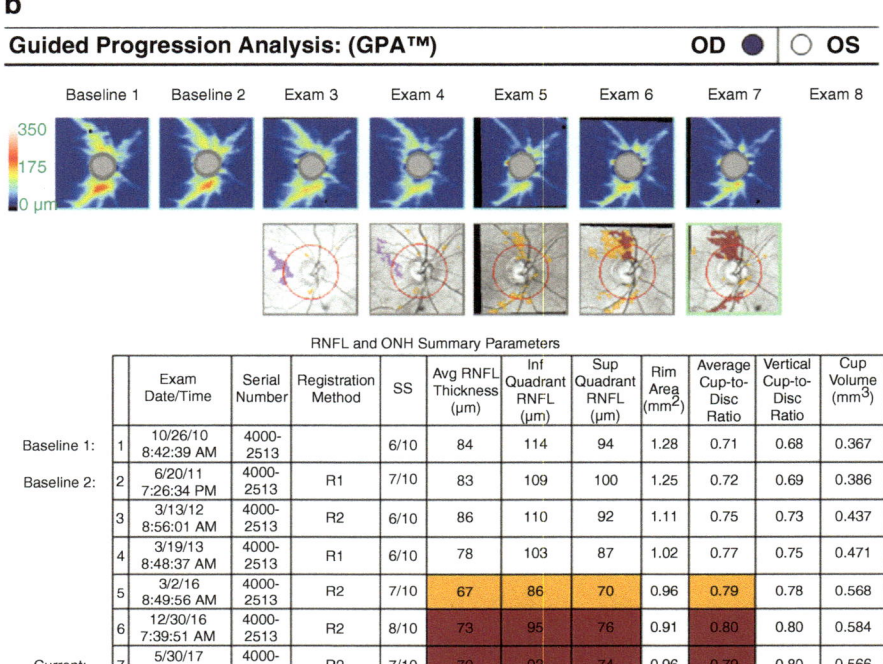

		Exam Date/Time	Serial Number	Registration Method	SS	Avg RNFL Thickness (μm)	Inf Quadrant RNFL (μm)	Sup Quadrant RNFL (μm)	Rim Area (mm²)	Average Cup-to-Disc Ratio	Vertical Cup-to-Disc Ratio	Cup Volume (mm³)
Baseline 1:	1	10/26/10 8:42:39 AM	4000-2513		6/10	84	114	94	1.28	0.71	0.68	0.367
Baseline 2:	2	6/20/11 7:26:34 PM	4000-2513	R1	7/10	83	109	100	1.25	0.72	0.69	0.386
	3	3/13/12 8:56:01 AM	4000-2513	R2	6/10	86	110	92	1.11	0.75	0.73	0.437
	4	3/19/13 8:48:37 AM	4000-2513	R1	6/10	78	103	87	1.02	0.77	0.75	0.471
	5	3/2/16 8:49:56 AM	4000-2513	R2	7/10	67	86	70	0.96	0.79	0.78	0.568
	6	12/30/16 7:39:51 AM	4000-2513	R2	8/10	73	95	76	0.91	0.80	0.80	0.584
Current:	7	5/30/17 8:30:50 AM	4000-2513	R2	7/10	70	93	74	0.96	0.79	0.80	0.566

Fig. 15.2 (continued)

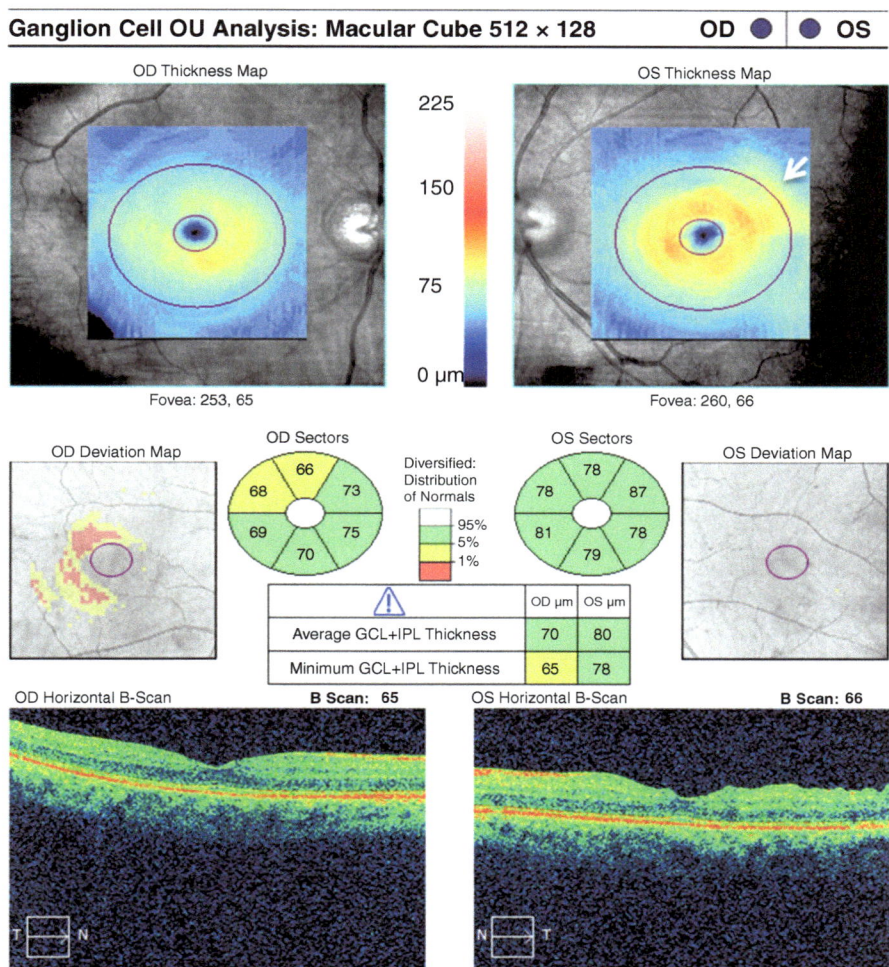

Fig. 15.3 Cirrus HD-OCT's macular ganglion cell analysis in 2017 shows borderline values for superior temporal sectors in the right eye and normal values for the left eye. The epiretinal membrane in the superior temporal quadrant of the macula in the left eye has caused some GCL + IPL thickening (white arrowhead)

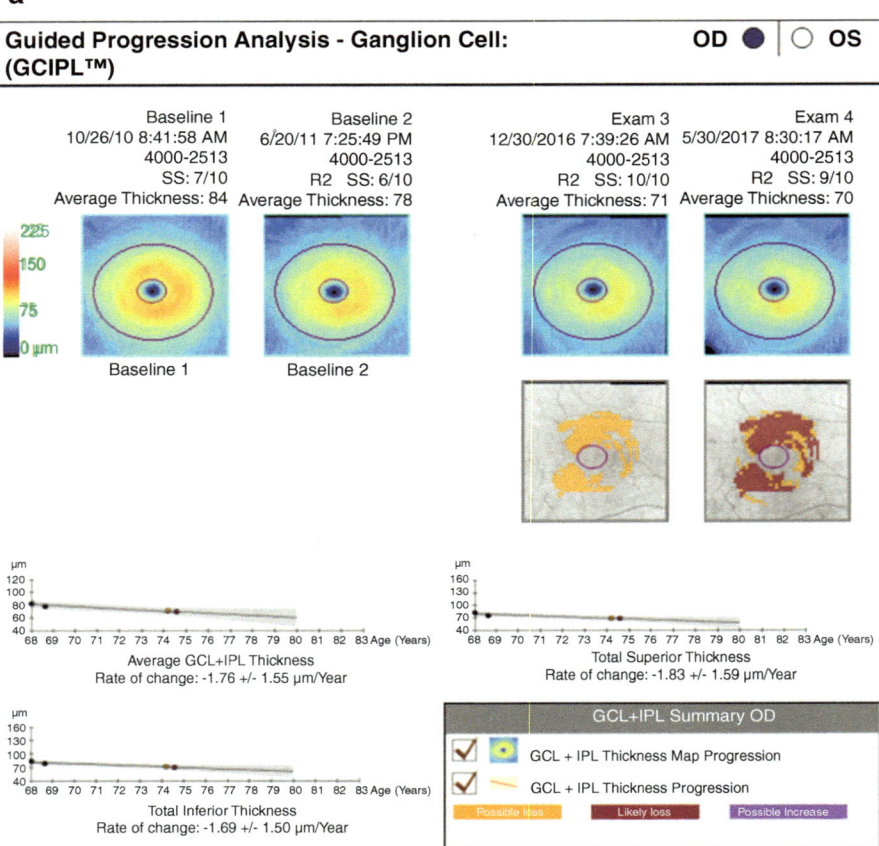

Fig. 15.4 Cirrus HD-OCT Ganglion Cell-GPA, right eye. (**a**) *GCL + IPL Summary box* on the first page of the GPA report has red checkmarks for both progression analysis methods. *GCL + IPL thickness map progression analysis* demonstrates superpixels that became significantly thinner as orange in the third exam. In the fourth exam, the superpixels that show persistent thinning for the second time are flagged in red and those that showed thinning for the first time are flagged in orange. During the follow-up period the average GCL + IPL thickness decreased from 84 to 70 μm. All three *GCL + IPL thickness trend analyses* show significant thinning for average, total superior and total inferior measurements. The rate of change for the average GCL + IPL thickness is −1.76 ± 1.55 μm/year. (**b**) On the second page, the *GCL + IPL summary parameters* table shows that progression is present for all three parameters

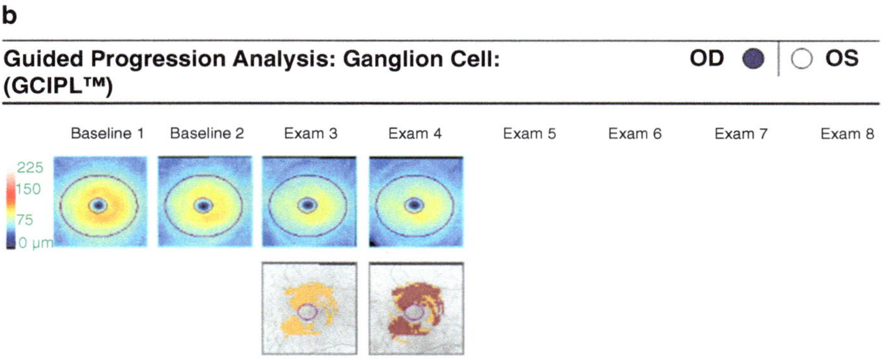
b
Guided Progression Analysis: Ganglion Cell: (GCIPL™)
OD
OS
Baseline 1
Baseline 2
Exam 3
Exam 4
Exam 5
Exam 6
Exam 7
Exam 8
225
150
75
0 µm

GCL + IPL Summary Parameters

		Exam Date/Time	Serial Number	Registration Method	SS	Average Thickness:	Total Superior Thickness (µm)	Total Inferior Thickness (µm)
Baseline 1:	1	10/26/2010 8:41:58 AM	4000-2513		7/10	84	83	84
Baseline 2:	2	6/20/2011 7:25:49 PM	4000-2513	R2	6/10	78	77	79
	3	12/30/2016 7:39:26 AM	4000-2513	R2	10/10	71	69	72
Current:	4	5/30/2017 8:30:17 AM	4000-2513	R2	9/10	70	69	71

Fig. 15.4 (continued)

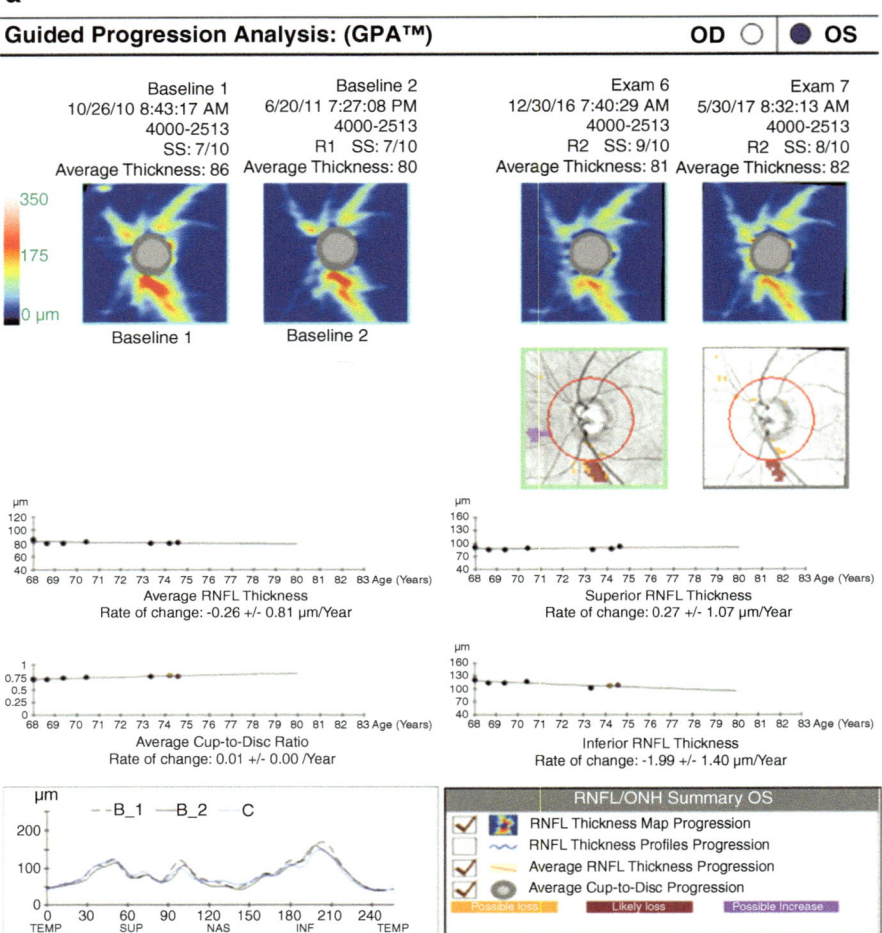

Fig. 15.5 Cirrus HD-OCT GPA, left eye. (**a**) *RNFL/ONH Summary box* in the first page of the GPA report shows red checkmarks for three progression analysis methods. *RNFL thickness map progression analysis* demonstrates an area of thinning in the inferior quadrant on the fifth scan. This region of thinning persisted on the sixth and seventh scans leading to the flagging of these superpixels in red denoting "likely loss". As described in the previous chapter, RNFL thickness maps can show progression earlier than the approach based on the calculation circle. In this eye, progression on the RNFL thickness map is present on the fifth scan, whereas the calculation circle based RNFL plots start to show progression on the sixth scan and the RNFL thickness profile progression remains negative even on the seventh scan. The *RNFL thickness profile progression graph* shows the current TSNIT graph is thinner in the inferior quadrant compared to the baseline. GPA requires the area of thinning to exceed a minimum of 20 degrees in order to flag progression. At this point, the magnitude of thinning has not met this requirement and no progression is indicated. The *inferior RNFL thickness plots* and *ONH average cup-to-disc ratio plot* display signs of progression and the dots for specific scans are in orange and red starting from the sixth scan. The rate of progression is indicated under each plot and one can use the regression line for predicting future loss. The *average* and *superior RNFL thickness plots* show no progression. (**b**) In the second page, the *RNFL and ONH summary* table shows all the parameters used in GPA. Parameters changing beyond the test-retest variability are also flagged in orange and red

b

Guided Progression Analysis: (GPA™)   OD ○ | ● OS

| | Baseline 1 | Baseline 2 | Exam 3 | Exam 4 | Exam 5 | Exam 6 | Exam 7 | Exam 8 |

RNFL and ONH Summary Parameters

		Exam Date/Time	Serial Number	Registration Method	SS	Avg RNFL Thickness (µm)	Inf Quadrant RNFL (µm)	Sup Quadrant RNFL (µm)	Rim Area (mm²)	Average Cup-to-Disc Ratio	Vertical Cup-to-Disc Ratio	Cup Volume (mm³)
Baseline 1:	1	10/26/10 8:43:17 AM	4000-2513		7/10	86	122	92	1.16	0.71	0.66	0.402
Baseline 2:	2	6/20/11 7:27:08 PM	4000-2513	R1	7/10	80	115	87	1.22	0.72	0.65	0.438
	3	3/13/12 8:57:02 AM	4000-2513	R2	6/10	81	115	87	1.07	0.74	0.69	0.458
	4	3/19/13 8:49:22 AM	4000-2513	R2	6/10	83	118	91	1.05	0.75	0.70	0.483
	5	3/2/16 8:50:42 AM	4000-2513	R2	7/10	81	103	87	0.99	0.77	0.73	0.555
	6	12/30/16 7:40:29 AM	4000-2513	R2	9/10	81	108	89	0.98	0.78	0.75	0.576
Current:	7	5/30/17 8:32:13 AM	4000-2513	R2	8/10	82	109	94	1.00	0.77	0.73	0.554

Fig. 15.5 (continued)

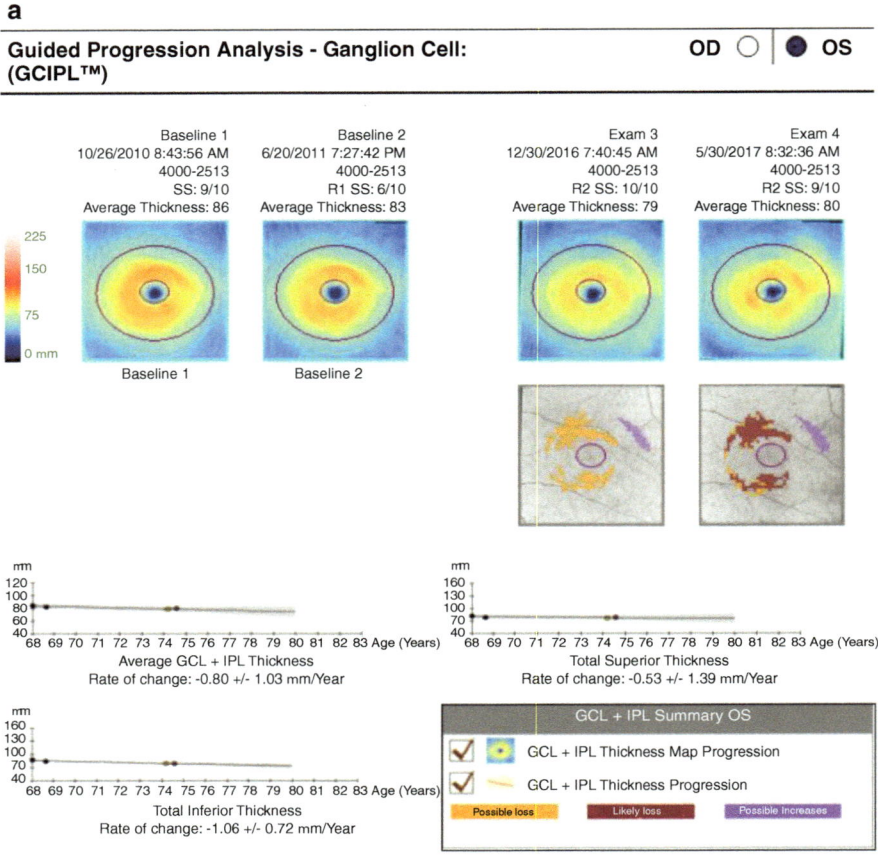

Fig. 15.6 Cirrus HD-OCT Ganglion Cell GPA, left eye. (**a**) Similar to the right eye, left eye also showed GCL + IPL thinning; *thickness map progression analysis* flagged these superpixels as described for the right eye. During the follow up period, the average GCL + IPL thickness decreased from 86 to 80 μm. All three *GCL + IPL thickness change plots* show significant thinning of the average, total superior and total inferior measurements. The rate of change for the average GCL + IPL thickness is −0.80 ± 1.03 μm/year. (**b**) *GCL + IPL Summary Parameters* table shows the results for the GCL + IPL thickness measurements. For all three parameters, "likely progression" can be observed

b

Guided Progression Analysis - Ganglion Cell: OD ○ | ● **OS**
(GCIPL™)

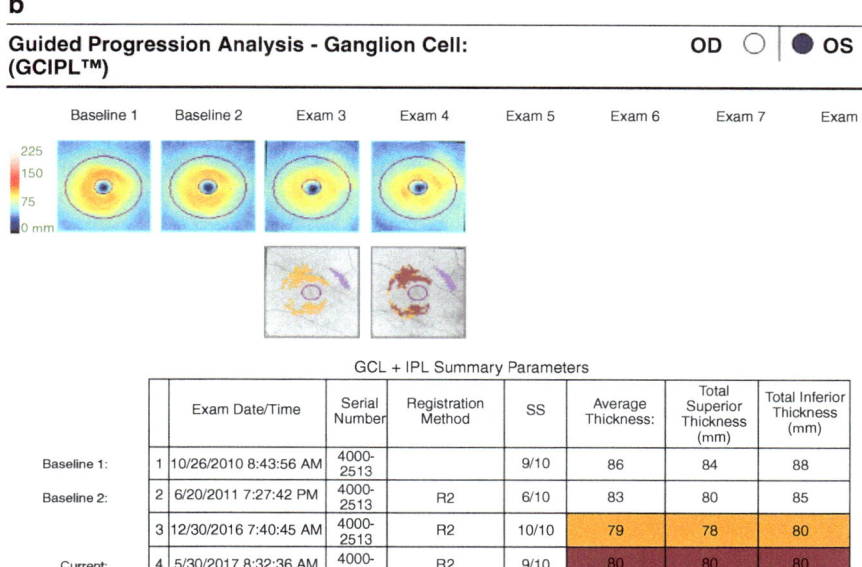

GCL + IPL Summary Parameters

		Exam Date/Time	Serial Number	Registration Method	SS	Average Thickness:	Total Superior Thickness (mm)	Total Inferior Thickness (mm)
Baseline 1:	1	10/26/2010 8:43:56 AM	4000-2513		9/10	86	84	88
Baseline 2:	2	6/20/2011 7:27:42 PM	4000-2513	R2	6/10	83	80	85
	3	12/30/2016 7:40:45 AM	4000-2513	R2	10/10	79	78	80
Current:	4	5/30/2017 8:32:36 AM	4000-2513	R2	9/10	80	80	80

Fig. 15.6   (continued)

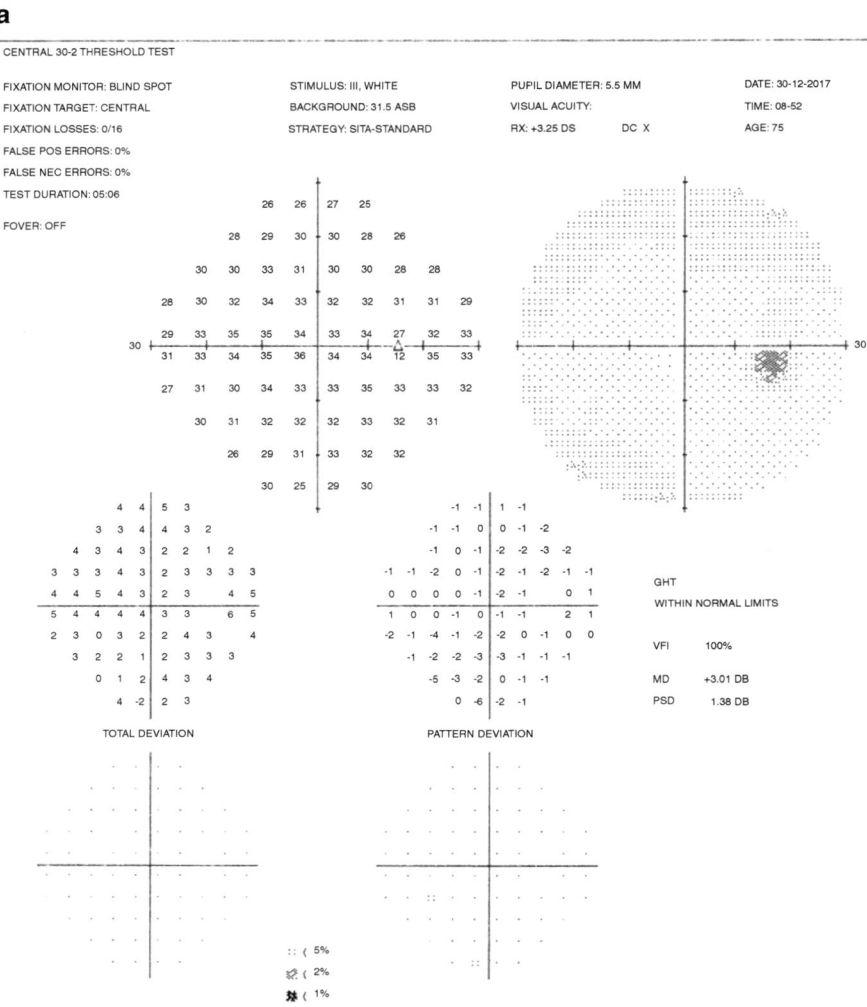

Fig. 15.7 Visual fields of the right and left eyes and Humphrey Field Analyzer (HFA) GPA reports. (**a** and **c**) Last VF printouts of both eyes in 2017 are within normal limits. (**b** and **d**) HFA GPA did not detect any progression between 2006 and 2017 in both eyes

b

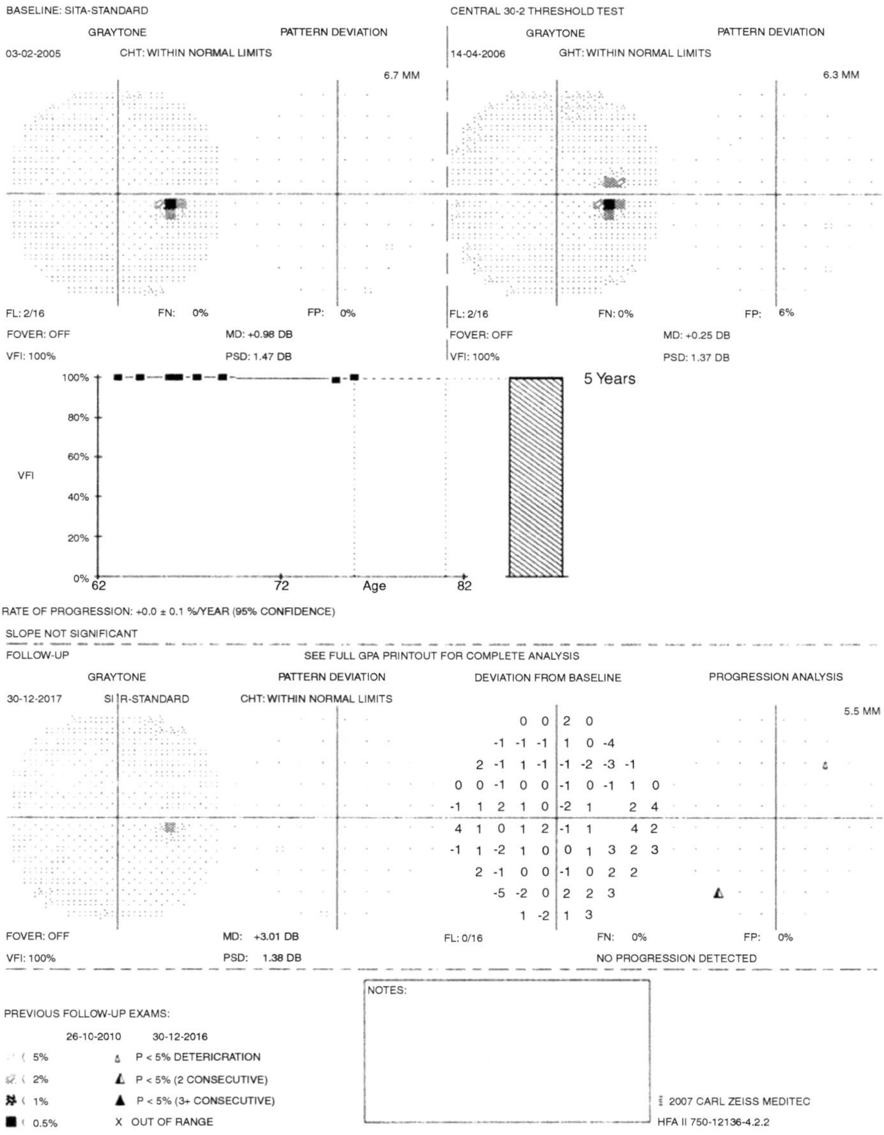

BASELINE: SITA-STANDARD   CENTRAL 30-2 THRESHOLD TEST

GRAYTONE   PATTERN DEVIATION   GRAYTONE   PATTERN DEVIATION

03-02-2005   CHT: WITHIN NORMAL LIMITS   14-04-2006   GHT: WITHIN NORMAL LIMITS

6.7 MM   6.3 MM

FL: 2/16   FN: 0%   FP: 0%   FL: 2/16   FN: 0%   FP: 6%
FOVER: OFF   MD: +0.98 DB   FOVER: OFF   MD: +0.25 DB
VFI: 100%   PSD: 1.47 DB   VFI: 100%   PSD: 1.37 DB

5 Years

VFI chart (100% down to 0%), Age axis 62, 72, 82

RATE OF PROGRESSION: +0.0 ± 0.1 %/YEAR (95% CONFIDENCE)

SLOPE NOT SIGNIFICANT

FOLLOW-UP   SEE FULL GPA PRINTOUT FOR COMPLETE ANALYSIS

GRAYTONE   PATTERN DEVIATION   DEVIATION FROM BASELINE   PROGRESSION ANALYSIS

30-12-2017   SITA-STANDARD   CHT: WITHIN NORMAL LIMITS   5.5 MM

          0   0 | 2   0
      -1 -1 -1 | 1   0 -4
    2 -1 1 -1 |-1 -2 -3 -1
  0   0 -1 0 0 |-1 0 -1 1 0
 -1   1 2 1 0 |-2 1   2 4
  4   1 0 1 2 |-1 1   4 2
 -1   1 -2 1 0 | 0 1 3 2 3
  2 -1 0 0 |-1 0 2 2
     -5 -2 0 | 2 2 3
       1 -2 | 1 3

FOVER: OFF   MD: +3.01 DB   FL: 0/16   FN: 0%   FP: 0%
VFI: 100%   PSD: 1.38 DB   NO PROGRESSION DETECTED

PREVIOUS FOLLOW-UP EXAMS:

          26-10-2010   30-12-2016

   5%   △   P < 5% DETERICRATION
   2%   ▲   P < 5% (2 CONSECUTIVE)
   1%   ▲   P < 5% (3+ CONSECUTIVE)   2007 CARL ZEISS MEDITEC
   0.5%   X   OUT OF RANGE   HFA II 750-12136-4.2.2

NOTES:

Fig. 15.7 (continued)

c

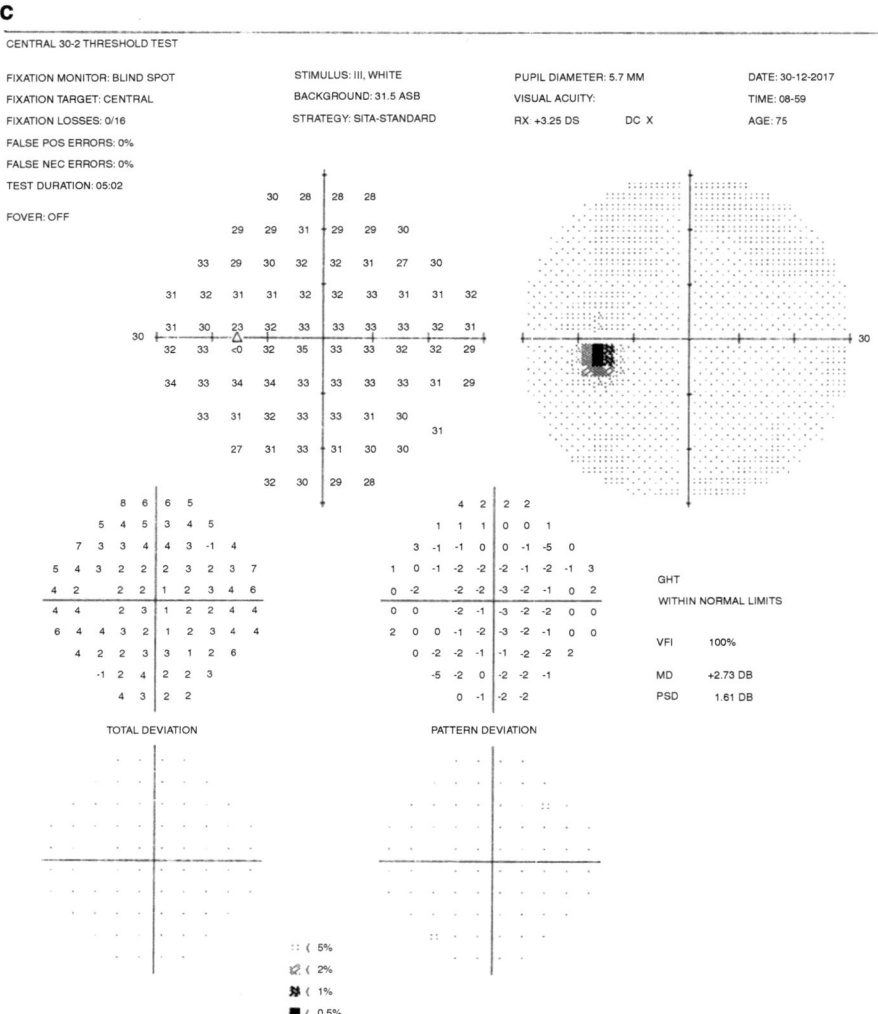

Fig. 15.7 (continued)

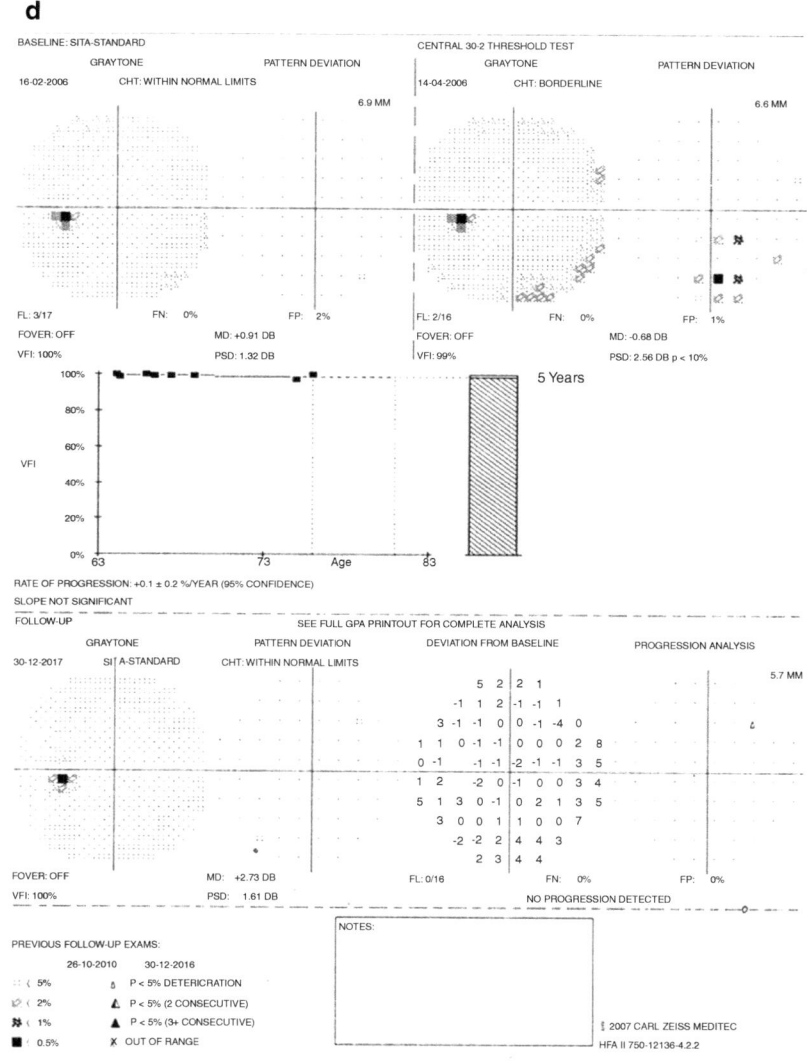

Fig. 15.7 (continued)

Conclusion: This case is an excellent example showing the importance of OCT progression analysis in detecting early glaucomatous progression, which is evident nearly in all GPA event and trend analyses of peripapillary RNFL and macular ganglion cells. On the other hand, the last peripapillary and macular OCT scans show only marginal damage. VF tests in 2017 are still within the normal range, and VF progression analysis does not show any progressive damage. OCT progression analysis enables the clinician to identify eyes that are progressing structurally, and treatment modifications can be made accordingly to prevent further structural and functional damage.

15.2 Case 2: Early OCT Progression and Setting a New Baseline After Treatment Changes

A 65-year old female was diagnosed as glaucoma suspect in 2010. Her IOP was 32 mmHg in both eyes. Medical treatment was started and she was followed till 2013 on travoprost and brinzolamide/timolol combination. Her IOPs remained around 23 mmHg in the right eye and 18 mmHg in the left eye during the three-year follow-up period. Following are the OCT reports of the patient between 2010 and 2013 (Figs. 15.8 and 15.9).

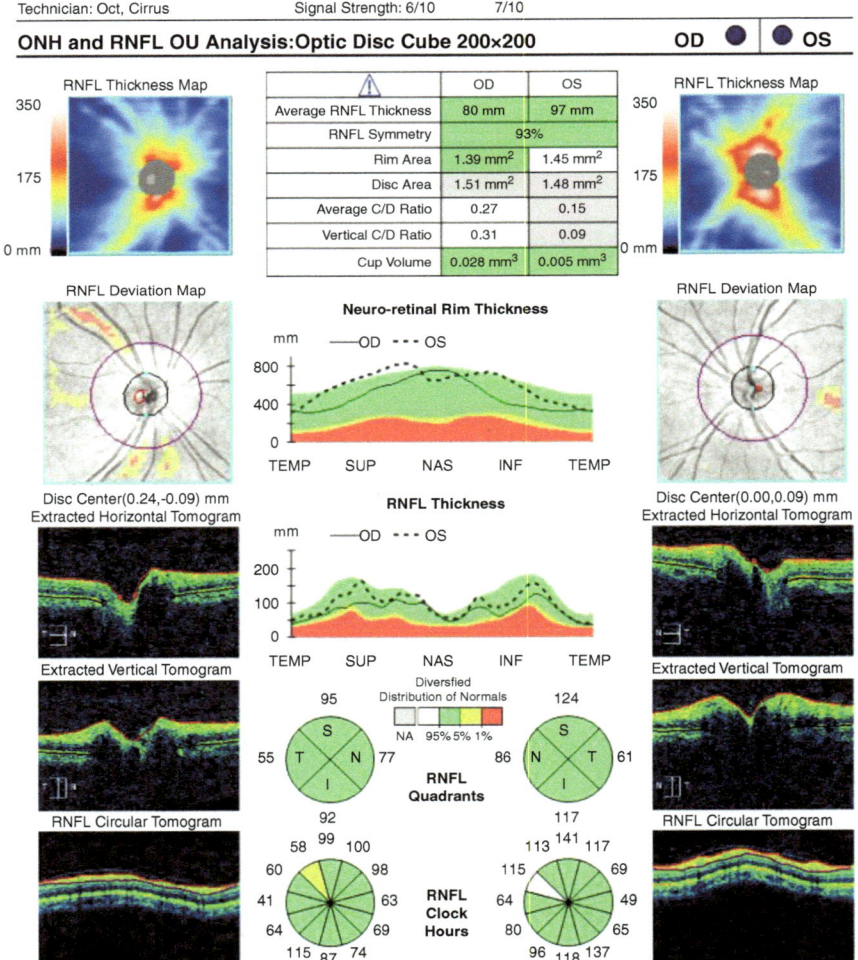

Fig. 15.8 Cirrus HD-OCT scan of the patient in 2013. Only a few hints of glaucomatous damage are present on this OCT report. In the right eye, an area of borderline RNFL thickness is present at the 11 o'clock sector. The OCT scan of the left eye is within normal limits. Average RNFL thickness values of both eyes are also within normal limits although the TSNIT curves show some asymmetry with some loss in the right eye

a

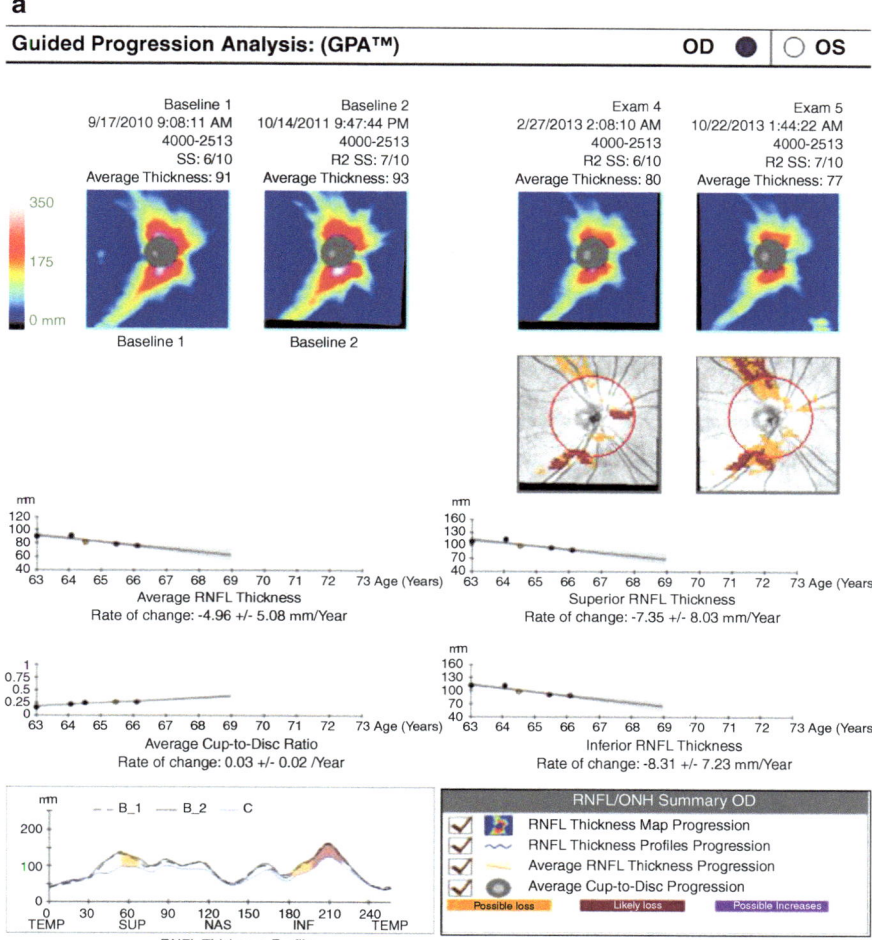

Fig. 15.9 Cirrus HD-OCT GPA (2010–2013), right eye. (**a**) *RNFL/ONH Summary box* on the first page of the GPA report has red check marks for all four progression analysis methods. *RNFL thickness map progression analysis* shows RNFL thinning both in the inferior and superior quadrants; GPA flags these superpixels as "orange—possible loss" if the thinning is present only in one scan and as "red—likely loss" if the thinning persists in the next scans. *RNFL thickness profile progression plot* shows the current TSNIT graph is significantly thinner than the baseline scans and areas with significant progression are colored in orange and red. The trend analysis based *RNFL thickness plots* detected statistically significant and fast progression with fitting of linear regression lines and yearly loss values. The *average cup-to-disc ratio progression* rate is also statistically significant. (**b**) *RNFL and ONH summary parameters* table in page two demonstrates progression of all RNFL thickness values and average cup-to-disc ratio. Average RNFL thickness of the right eye decreased to 80 μm from 91 μm in three years. Although average RNFL thickness value of 80 μm is still in the normal (green) range of the normative database, 11 μm of average RNFL thickness loss is more than two times of the test-retest variability of Cirrus HD-OCT, and GPA detected this change as true progression

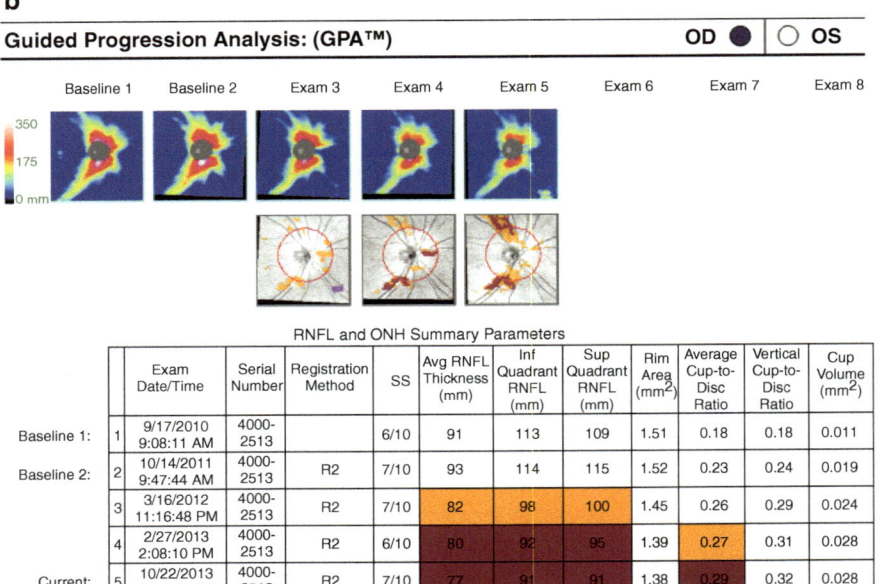

Fig. 15.9 (continued)

This is a good example that shows the power of OCT progression analysis in which multiple steps of statistically significant progression can be detected while the OCT parameters such as average RNFL thickness are still in the green zone. VF tests are completely within normal limits at this stage. Because of this fast progression rate and poor IOP control with medications, a trabeculectomy was performed in the right eye. After surgery IOP decreased to 10 mmHg and remained under 12 mmHg till last follow-up (Figs. 15.10 and 15.11).

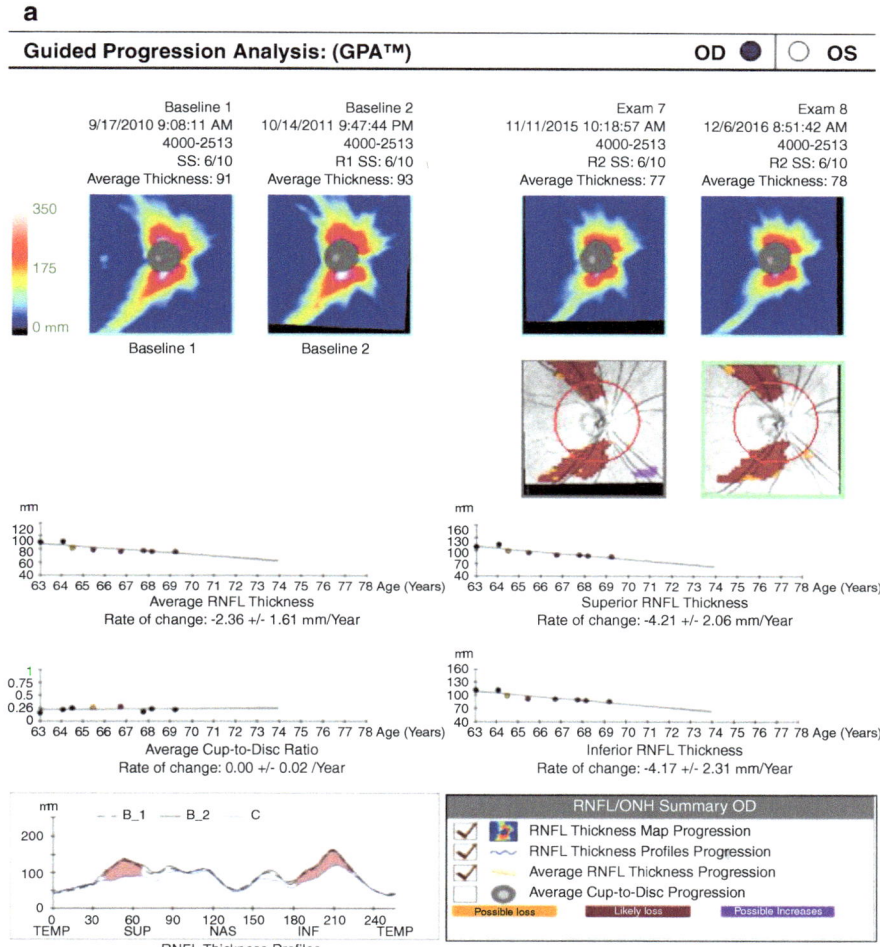

Fig. 15.10 Cirrus HD-OCT GPA, right eye (2010–2016). (**a, b**) After better control of IOP control with trabeculectomy in 2014, progression stopped and RNFL thickness values were stabilized; however, as the baselines exams from 2010 are used, GPA still shows progression for all parameters. When an important change in treatment is made, like surgery or starting new medications, new baseline images may need to be established in order to better observe the effectiveness of the new treatment. See the next figure with baselines set to 2013 and 2014

b

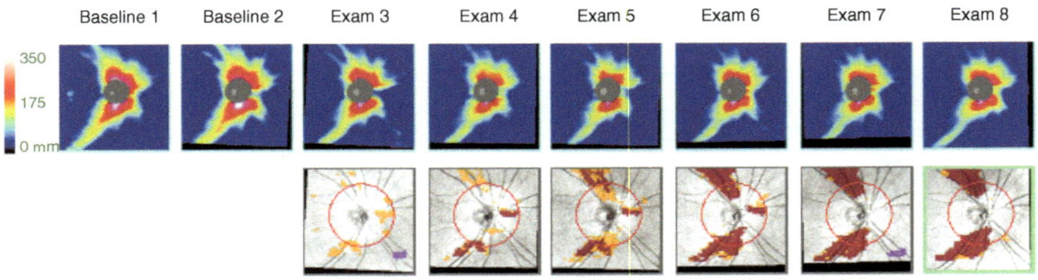

Fig. 15.10 (continued)

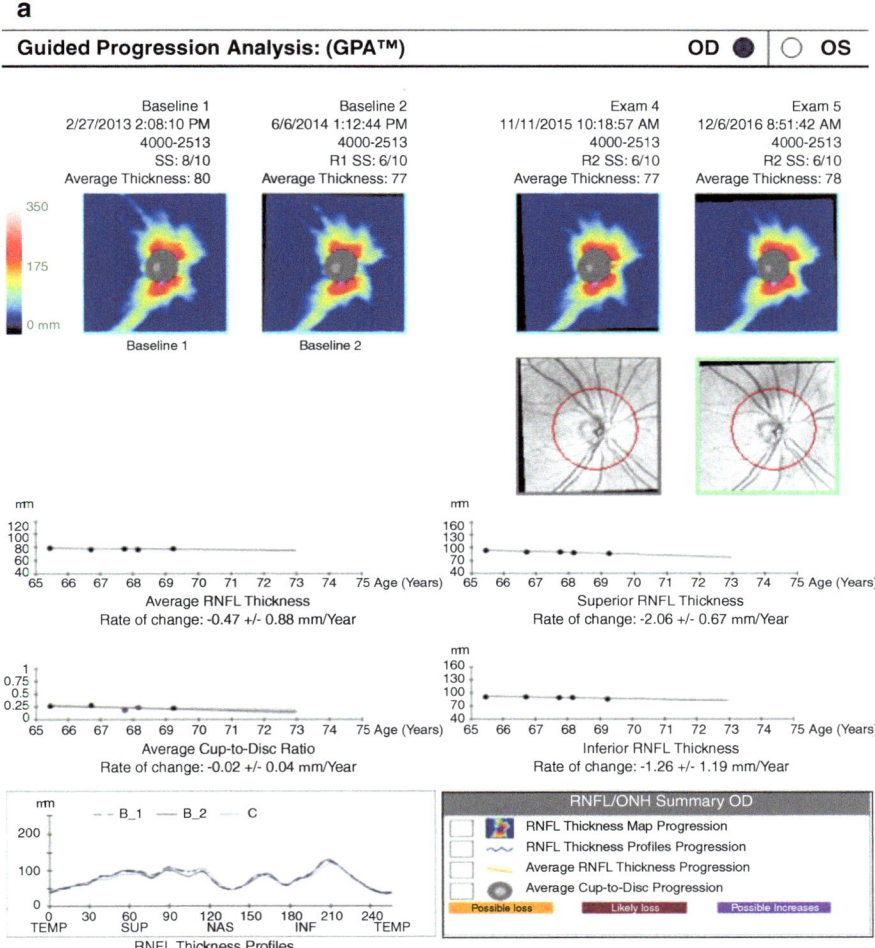

Fig. 15.11 Cirrus HD-OCT GPA, right eye (2013–2016). (**a, b**) In order to evaluate the progression after the trabeculectomy, we have to change the baseline to date of the trabeculectomy. With new baseline scans from 2013 and 2014, Cirrus HD-OCT's GPA shows stabilization of all parameters; no more progression is detected in any of the event and trend analyses and the average RNFL thickness is stable around 78 μm

b

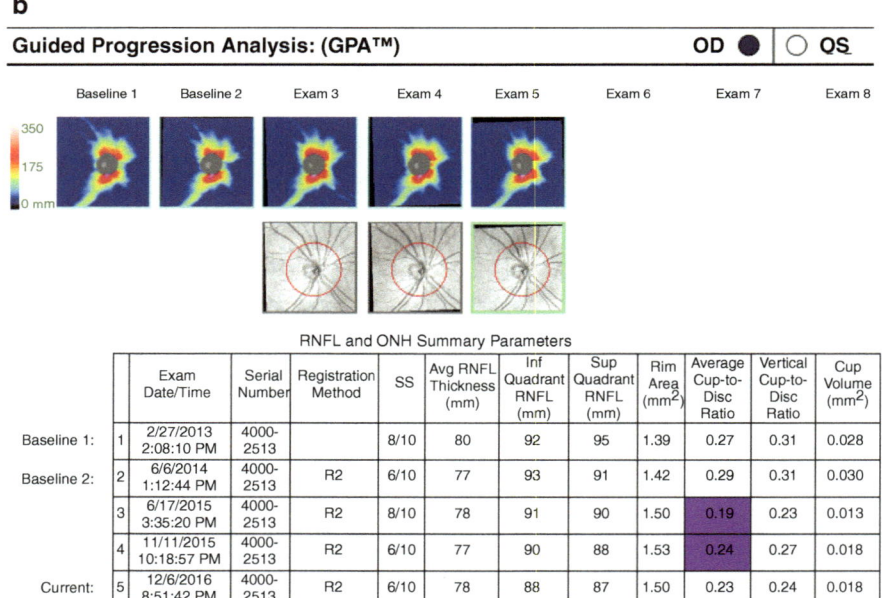

		Exam Date/Time	Serial Number	Registration Method	SS	Avg RNFL Thickness (mm)	Inf Quadrant RNFL (mm)	Sup Quadrant RNFL (mm)	Rim Area (mm²)	Average Cup-to-Disc Ratio	Vertical Cup-to-Disc Ratio	Cup Volume (mm²)
Baseline 1:	1	2/27/2013 2:08:10 PM	4000-2513		8/10	80	92	95	1.39	0.27	0.31	0.028
Baseline 2:	2	6/6/2014 1:12:44 PM	4000-2513	R2	6/10	77	93	91	1.42	0.29	0.31	0.030
	3	6/17/2015 3:35:20 PM	4000-2513	R2	8/10	78	91	90	1.50	0.19	0.23	0.013
	4	11/11/2015 10:18:57 PM	4000-2513	R2	6/10	77	90	88	1.53	0.24	0.27	0.018
Current:	5	12/6/2016 8:51:42 PM	4000-2513	R2	6/10	78	88	87	1.50	0.23	0.24	0.018

RNFL and ONH Summary Parameters

Fig. 15.11 (continued)

Conclusion: This case has two important features. First, Cirrus HD-OCT GPA can detect progression in early stages (progression in green), even before OCT results show out-of-range (red) values. In the OCT era, this possibility should be considered in order to detect early damage. Second, in order to detect progression after a therapeutic intervention like starting medications or surgery, baseline images must be set to the date of the specific event.

15.3 Case 3: Early Glaucoma OCT Progression

A 78-year old female patient was first seen in 2011. She had lost her left eye in a traffic accident and was wearing eye prosthesis on the left side. Her IOP in the right eye was 22 mmHg in 2011. She was diagnosed with ocular hypertension and advised to have regular exams every 6 months. After 3 years of follow-up with intervals of 6 months without any findings of OCT progression and IOP values ranging between 18 and 21 mmHg, the patient moved away and missed exams between years 2014 and 2016. She was seen again in 2016 with an IOP of 26 mmHg. A fixed combination of a prostaglandin analog with a beta blocker was prescribed, which lowered the IOP to 17 mmHg (Figs. 15.12, 15.13, 15.14, 15.15, and 15.16).

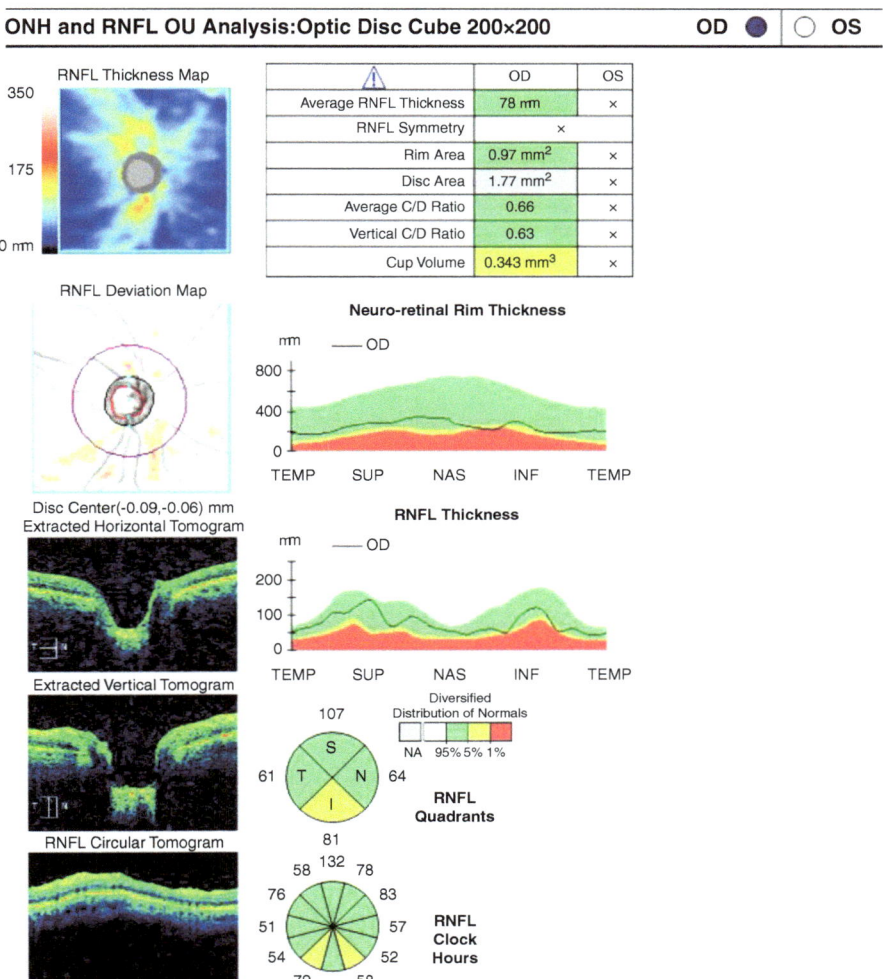

Fig. 15.12 Cirrus-HD OCT scan of patient's right eye in 2017. Average RNFL thickness is 78 μm, which is in the green normal range. RNFL deviation map shows few areas of RNFL thinning and the TSNIT plot shows an area of thinning in the inferior quadrant, clock hour pie graph shows borderline abnormal values for the 5 and 7 o'clock sectors. Overall, this OCT printout shows only very mild damage and average RNFL is still in the normal range

a

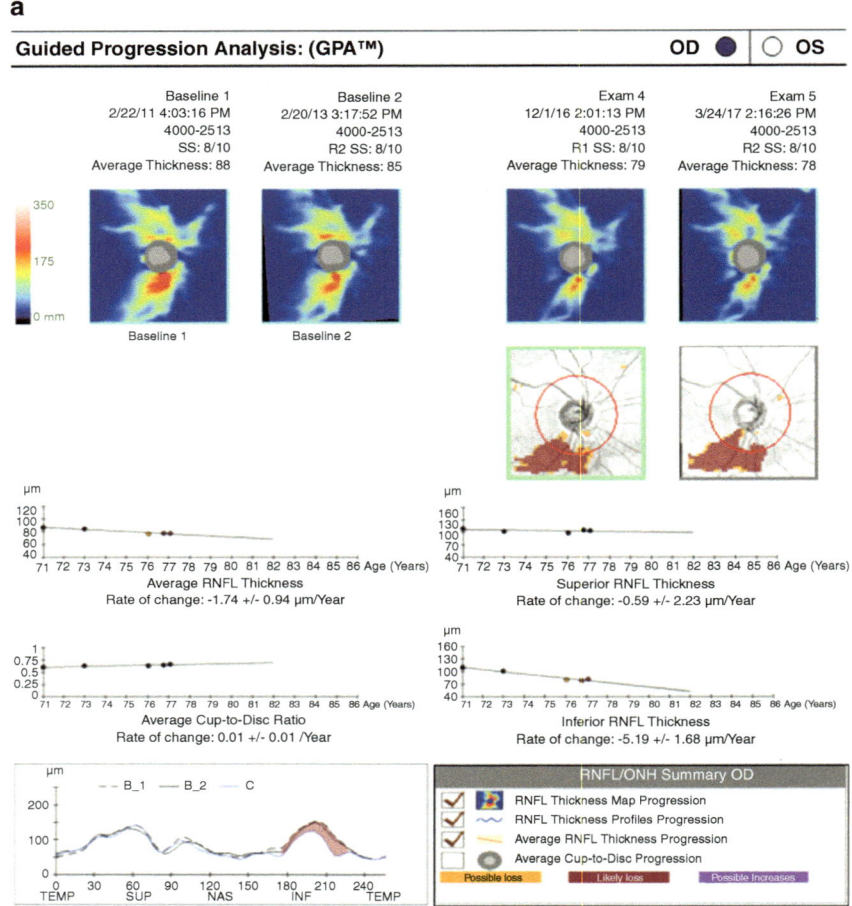

Fig. 15.13 Cirrus HD-OCT GPA, right eye (2011–2017). (**a**) *RNFL thickness map progression analysis* shows significant RNFL thinning in the inferior quadrant. As the thinning is present in consecutive scans, GPA marked these areas as "likely loss" and a red checkmark is present in the summary box. *RNFL thickness profile progression plot* also shows RNFL thinning in the inferior quadrant and areas with significant progression are displayed in red. The trend analysis based *RNFL thickness plots* detected statistically significant progression with estimation of linear regression slopes and yearly loss values. The rate of progression is fastest in the inferior quadrant (−5.19 ± 1.68 μm/year). *Average cup-to-disc ratio progression* is not statistically significant, so the average cup-to-disc progression check box is not checked. (**b**) *RNFL and ONH summary parameters* table on page two demonstrates worsening of the average and inferior RNFL thickness measurements. Reviewing this table is very important as we can see that the average and inferior RNFL thickness decreased between the baseline and 2016 measurements but the values stabilized after the start of the treatment in 2016. Like in the previous example, if we chose year 2016 as the baseline, GPA would not show any progression

b

	Exam Date/Time	Serial Number	Registration Method	SS	Avg RNFL Thickness (μm)	Inf Quadrant RNFL (μm)	Sup Quadrant RNFL (μm)	Rim Area (mm²)	Average Cup-to-Disc Ratio	Vertical Cup-to-Disc Ratio	Cup Volume (mm³)
Baseline 1:	2/22/11 4:03:06 PM	4000-2513		8/10	88	111	109	1.08	0.60	0.55	0.270
Baseline 2:	2/20/13 3:17:52 PM	4000-2513	R2	8/10	85	103	103	1.01	0.64	0.57	0.326
	3/1/16 2:51:08 PM	4000-2513	R2	6/10	77	82	100	0.93	0.64	0.61	0.314
	12/1/16 2:01:13 PM	4000-2513	R1	8/10	79	80	107	0.94	0.65	0.63	0.331
Current:	3/24/17 2:16:26 PM	4000-2513	R2	8/10	78	83	105	0.97	0.66	0.63	0.343

Fig. 15.13 (continued)

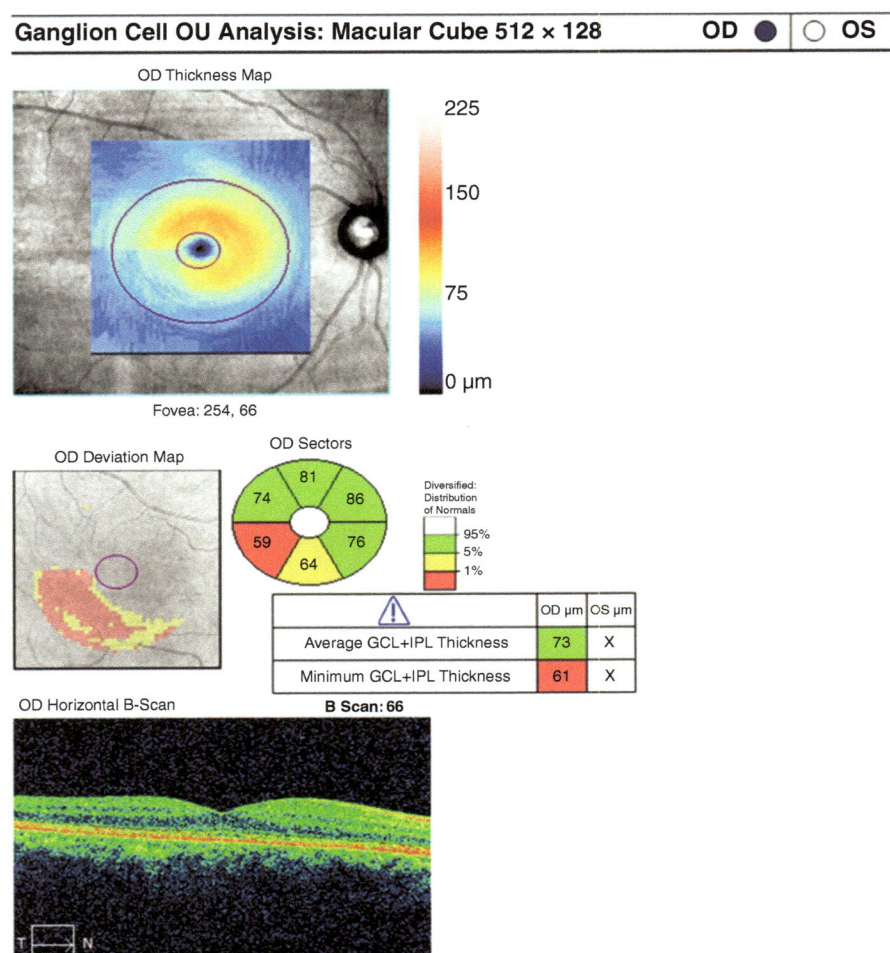

Fig. 15.14 Cirrus HD-OCT Macula GCL + IPL analysis in 2017 shows the thinned area in the infero-temporal and inferior sectors. Compare this figure to the RNFL findings in Fig. 15.12; unlike the macular OCT, the peripapillary OCT shows few clues about the ongoing RNFL loss in this eye

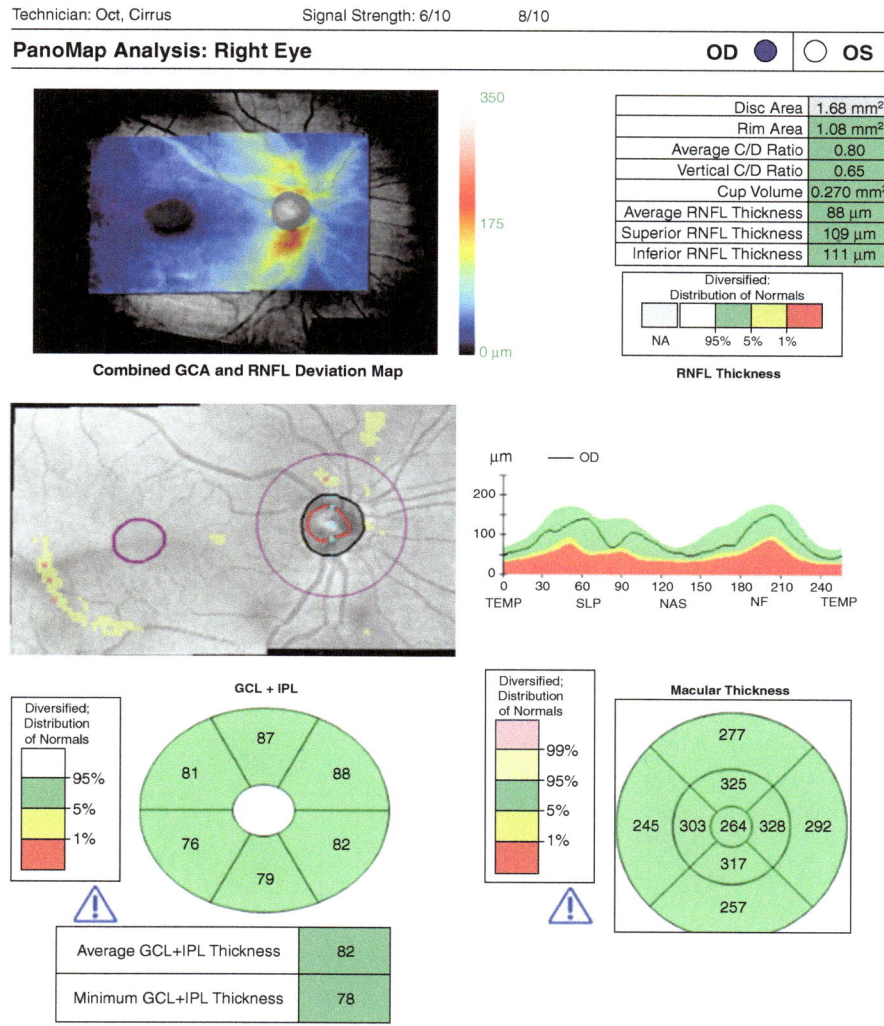

Fig. 15.15 The Cirrus HD-OCT Panomap analysis in 2011 is essentially within normal limits

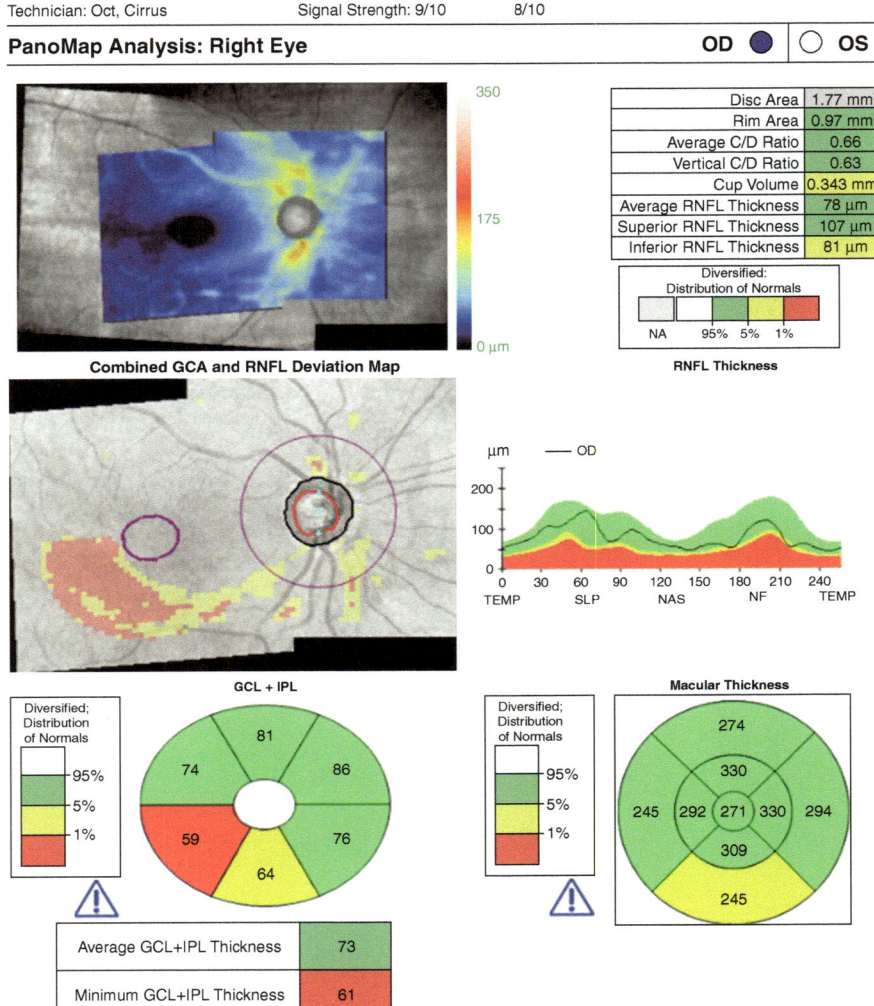

Fig. 15.16 Cirrus HD-OCT Panomap analysis in 2017 shows the extent of the RNFL and GCL + IPL damage. There was only one macular scan available from 2011 and without two baseline scans, macular GPA could not be performed

Conclusion: This case has similarities with the previous case. If one had seen this patient in 2017 and only checked the peripapillary OCT printout, he/she might have missed the extent of glaucomatous damage as none of the peripapillary OCT parameters were outside normal limits and the average RNFL was still in the green, normal range. On the contrary, peripapillary GPA shows that the patient's average RNFL thickness decreased from 88 to 77 μm between years 2011 and 2016; the reduction in the inferior quadrant is more dramatic, where RNFL thickness decreased from 111 to 82 μm. These data show that the peripapillary GPA can identify RNFL loss even in the average RNFL thickness while most of the peripapillary RNFL OCT is still within normal limits compared to the normative database.

In addition, the macular GCL + IPL analysis demonstrates another important point in this case. The macular OCT and Panomap analysis of the case show that significant damage is present at the GCL + IPL level in the macula although the peripapillary RNFL damage is minimal on the RNFL thickness maps. This case is a very good example of the importance of the macular analysis and the utility of progression analysis.

15.4 Case 4: Structural and Functional Progression in Advanced Glaucoma

A 60-year old female patient with primary open angle glaucoma was referred for trabeculectomy in 2006. Her IOP was 18 mmHg in the right eye and 26 mmHg in the left eye with the maximally tolerated medical treatment. Her vision was 20/20 in both eyes. She had early glaucoma in the right eye and advanced glaucomatous damage in the left eye. After an uneventful trabeculectomy, her IOP in the left eye decreased to 10 mmHg and has remained stable to date. Her right eye has been monitored on medical treatment. Her IOPs were between 20 and 23 mmHg between years 2006 and 2012. In 2012, possible progression was detected in the OCT reports and medical therapy was intensified, which resulted in IOP values between 16 and 20 mmHg. Cirrus HD-OCT became available in our clinic in 2010, so the OCT data of the patient begin from 2010 whereas VF data are available from 2006 (Figs. 15.17, 15.18, 15.19, 15.20, 15.21, and 15.22).

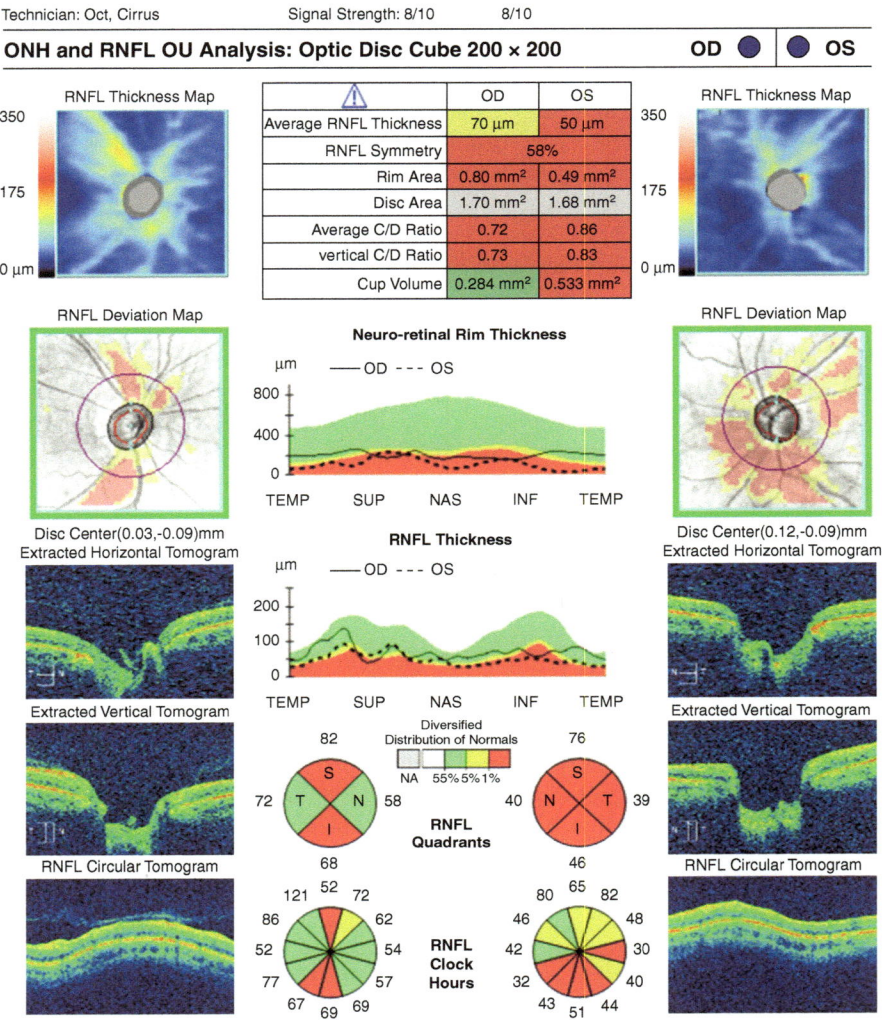

Fig. 15.17 Current Cirrus HD-OCT report of the patient shows moderate RNFL damage in the right eye and advanced RNFL damage in the left eye

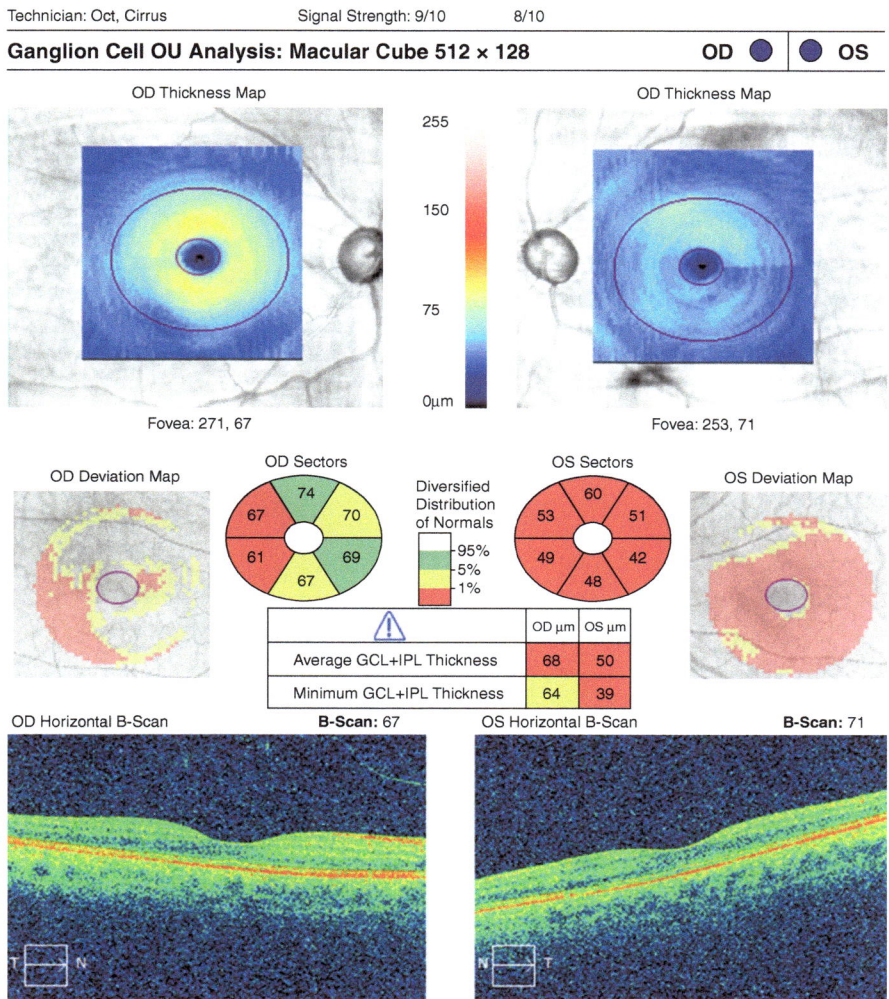

Fig. 15.18 Current macular GCL + IPL analysis also demonstrates moderate damage in the right eye and advanced damage in the left eye

a

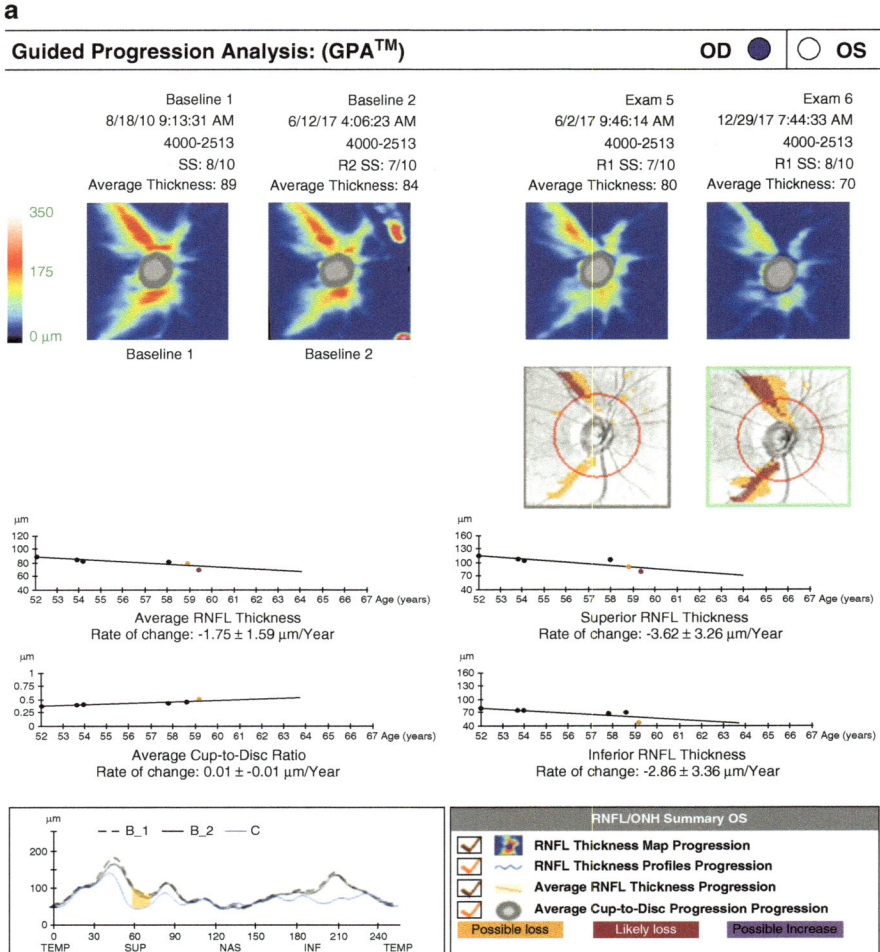

Fig. 15.19 Cirrus HD-OCT GPA, right eye (2010–2017). (**a**) The *RNFL/ONH Summary box* in the first page of the GPA report has red or orange check marks for all four progression analysis methods. *RNFL thickness map progression analysis* shows areas of "possible loss" in the fifth scan. RNFL thinning progressed to a wider area in the sixth scan leading to flagging of these superpixels in red denoting "likely loss". *RNFL thickness profile progression plot* shows that the current TSNIT graph is thinner in the superior and inferior quadrants. But only the superior RNFL thinning goes beyond the test retest variability so only this area is colored in orange. The *average, inferior and superior RNFL thickness plots* and the *ONH average cup-to-disc ratio plot* show progression and the circles for specific scans are displayed in orange and red color starting from the fifth scans. One can see the rate of progression under each plot and can use the estimated regression line for predicting future loss until the RNFL thickness reaches its measurement floor at about 40 µm. (**b**) In the second page, the *RNFL and ONH parameter summary* table shows all the measurements used in the GPA and values progressing more than test-retest variability are also flagged in orange and red in this table

b

Guided Progression Analysis: (GPA™)   OD ● ○ OS

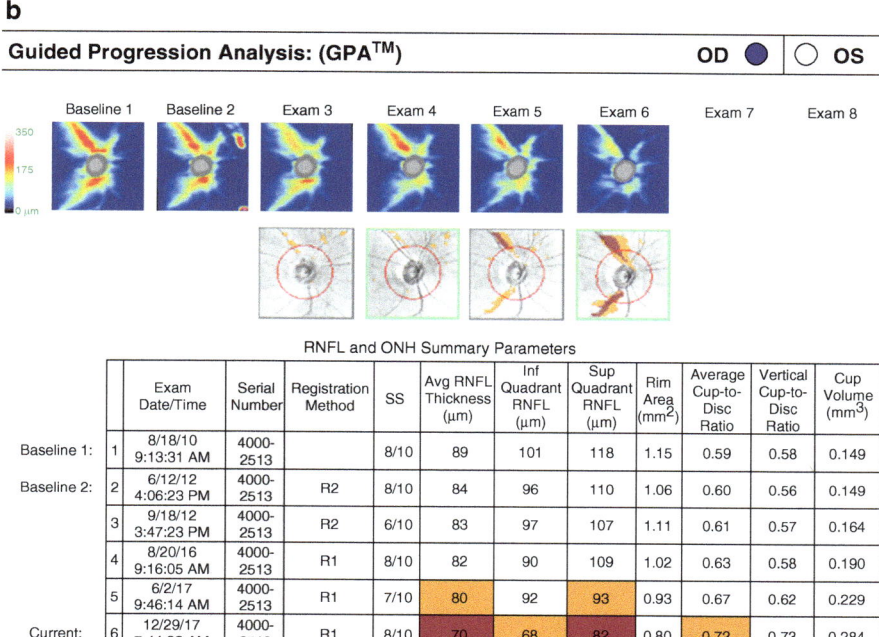

RNFL and ONH Summary Parameters

		Exam Date/Time	Serial Number	Registration Method	SS	Avg RNFL Thickness (μm)	Inf Quadrant RNFL (μm)	Sup Quadrant RNFL (μm)	Rim Area (mm²)	Average Cup-to-Disc Ratio	Vertical Cup-to-Disc Ratio	Cup Volume (mm³)
Baseline 1:	1	8/18/10 9:13:31 AM	4000-2513		8/10	89	101	118	1.15	0.59	0.58	0.149
Baseline 2:	2	6/12/12 4:06:23 PM	4000-2513	R2	8/10	84	96	110	1.06	0.60	0.56	0.149
	3	9/18/12 3:47:23 PM	4000-2513	R2	6/10	83	97	107	1.11	0.61	0.57	0.164
	4	8/20/16 9:16:05 AM	4000-2513	R1	8/10	82	90	109	1.02	0.63	0.58	0.190
	5	6/2/17 9:46:14 AM	4000-2513	R1	7/10	80	92	93	0.93	0.67	0.62	0.229
Current:	6	12/29/17 7:44:33 AM	4000-2513	R1	8/10	70	68	82	0.80	0.72	0.73	0.284

Fig. 15.19 (continued)

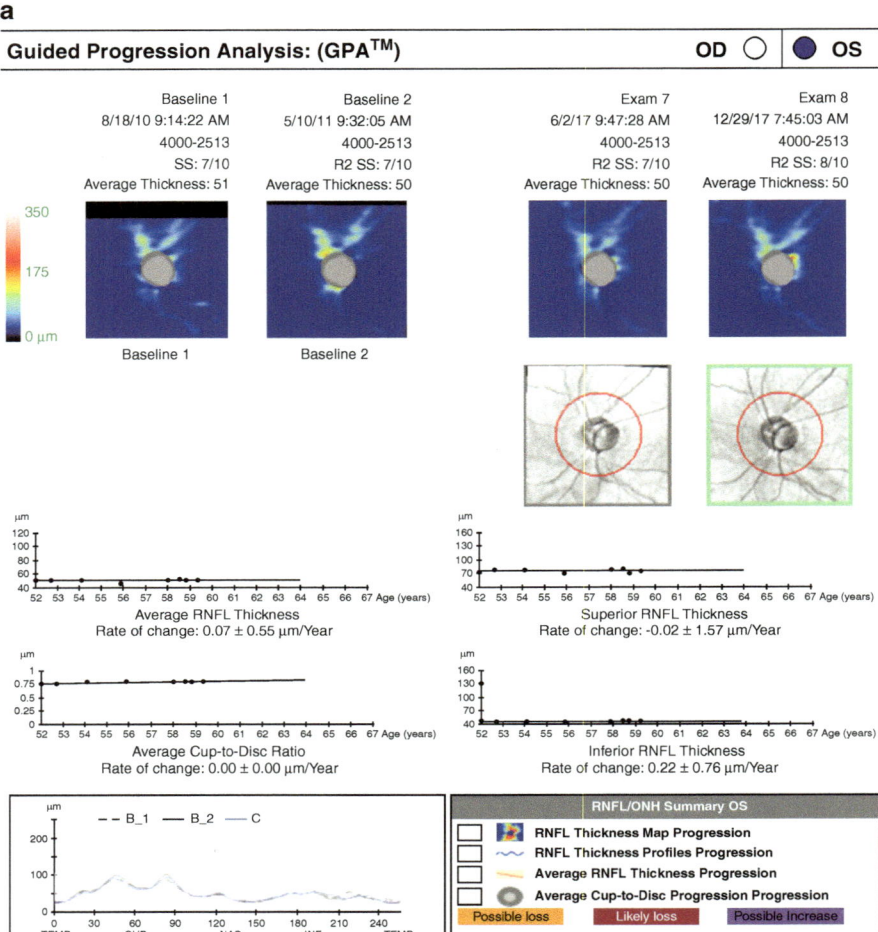

Fig. 15.20 Cirrus HD-OCT GPA, left eye (2010–2017). (**a, b**) *RNFL/ONH Summary box* on the first page of the GPA report is unchecked for all four progression analysis methods. There can be two reasons for not observing progression in this GPA report. Firstly, as the patient had trabeculectomy in 2006 and IOP is kept around 10 mmHg for the last eleven years. We do not expect progression in this patient and this GPA report can be reliable. Secondly, as the inferior RNFL and possibly the average RNFL thickness reached their measurement floor, detection of progression is not anymore possible. The left eye is a good example for advanced structural damage in RNFL and OCT progression analysis is not helpful for the inferior quadrant. VF progression analysis can be a good option in these advanced cases

b

Guided Progression Analysis: (GPA™)   OD ⃝ | ⬤ OS

RNFL and ONH Summary Parameters

		Exam Date/Time	Serial Number	Registration Method	SS	Avg RNFL Thickness (µm)	Inf Quadrant RNFL (µm)	Sup Quadrant RNFL (µm)	Rim Area (mm²)	Average Cup-to-Disc Ratio	Vertical Cup-to-Disc Ratio	Cup Volume (mm³)
Baseline 1:	1	8/18/10 9:14:22 AM	4000-2513		7/10	51	48	75	0.55	0.82	0.80	0.446
Baseline 2:	2	5/10/11 9:32:05 AM	4000-2513	R2	7/10	50	44	79	0.58	0.82	0.77	0.457
	3	9/18/12 3:48:55 PM	4000-2513	R2	7/10	50	45	78	0.50	0.85	0.83	0.541
	4	7/1/14 7:59:16 PM	4000-2513	R1	7/10	47	43	70	0.42	0.87	0.83	0.513
	5	8/20/16 9:16:57 AM	4000-2513	R1	7/10	50	44	79	0.50	0.85	0.82	0.505
	6	3/3/17 9:37:32 AM	4000-2513	R2	8/10	53	49	83	0.52	0.84	0.81	0.508
	7	6/2/17 9:47:28 AM	4000-2513	R2	7/10	50	49	71	0.51	0.84	0.86	0.524
Current:	8	12/29/17 7:45:03 AM	4000-2513	R2	8/10	50	46	75	0.49	0.86	0.83	0.533

Fig. 15.20 (continued)

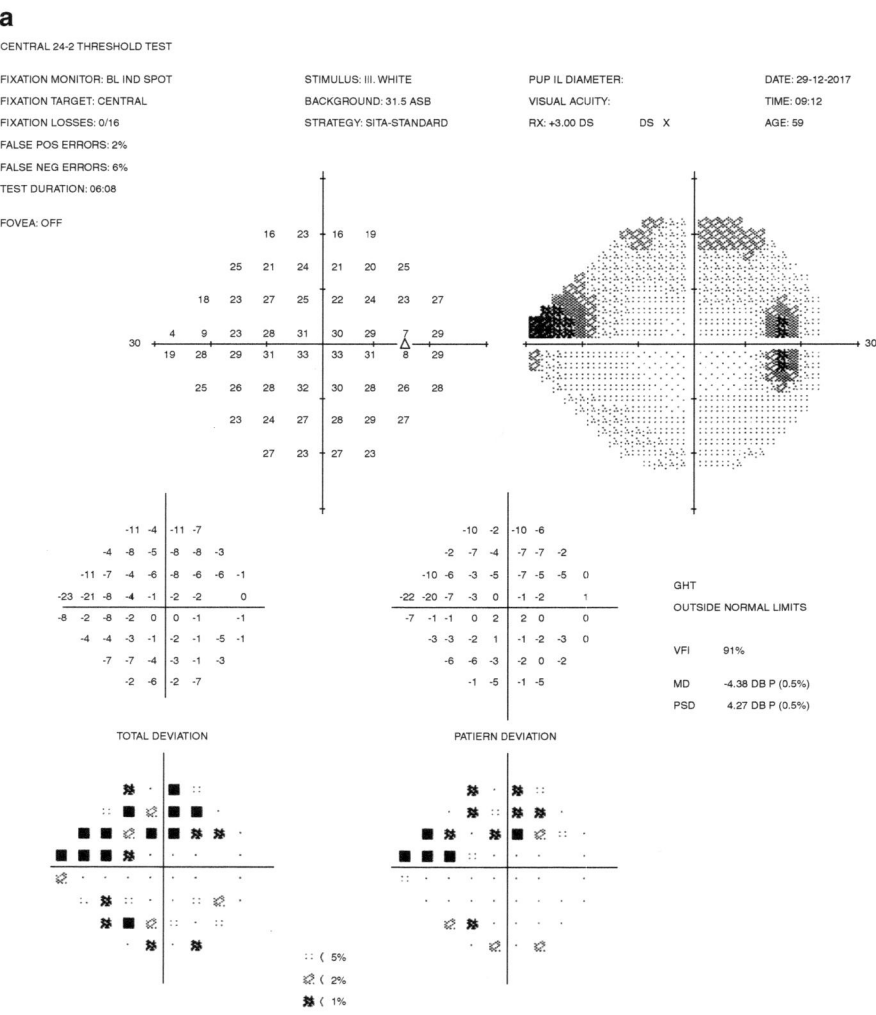

Fig. 15.21 (**a**) VF printouts show moderate damage in the right eye. (**b**) Humphrey Field Analyzer GPA report shows likely progression with worsening test locations in both hemifields although the deteriorating points are more numerous in the superior hemifield. VFI trend analysis shows that rate of progression started to increase in 2017, in agreement with the OCT GPA which demonstrates significant RNFL loss in last 6 months

b

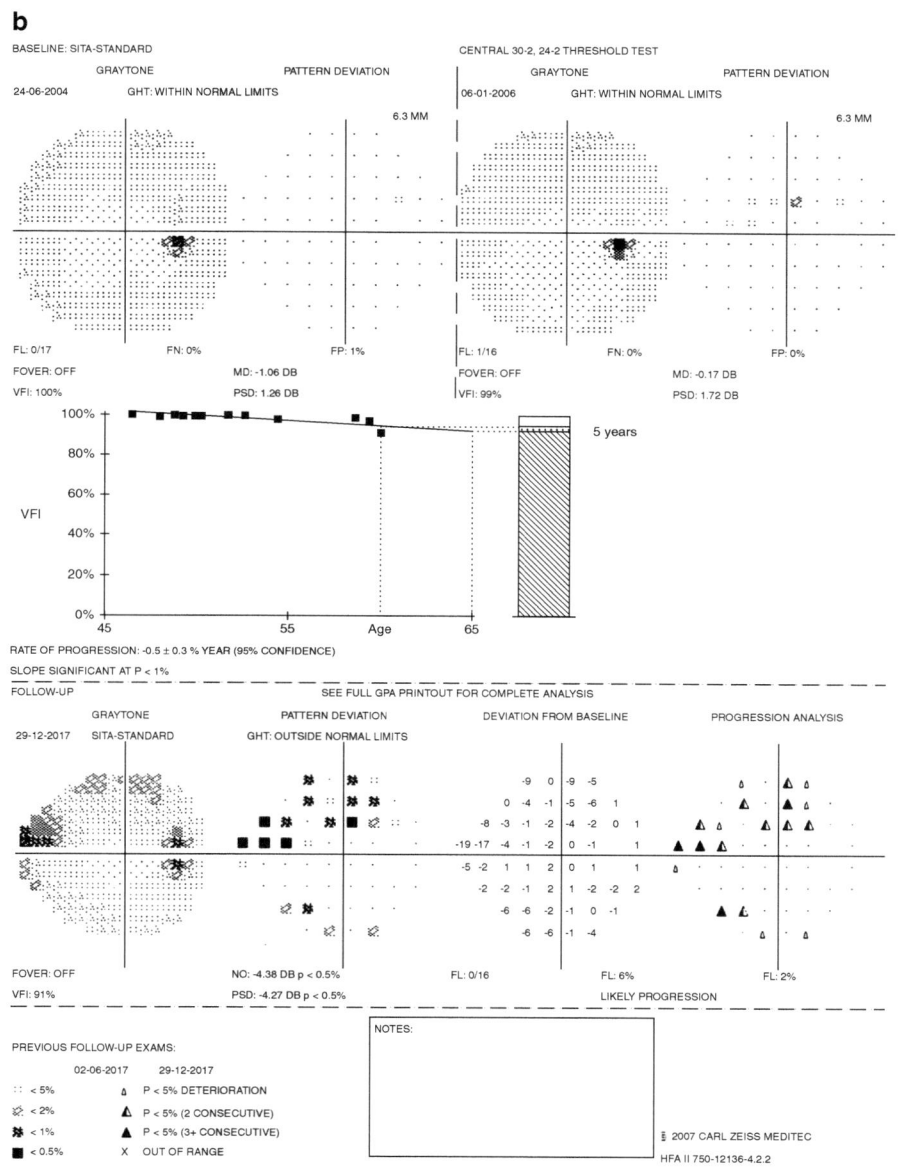

Fig. 15.21 (continued)

a

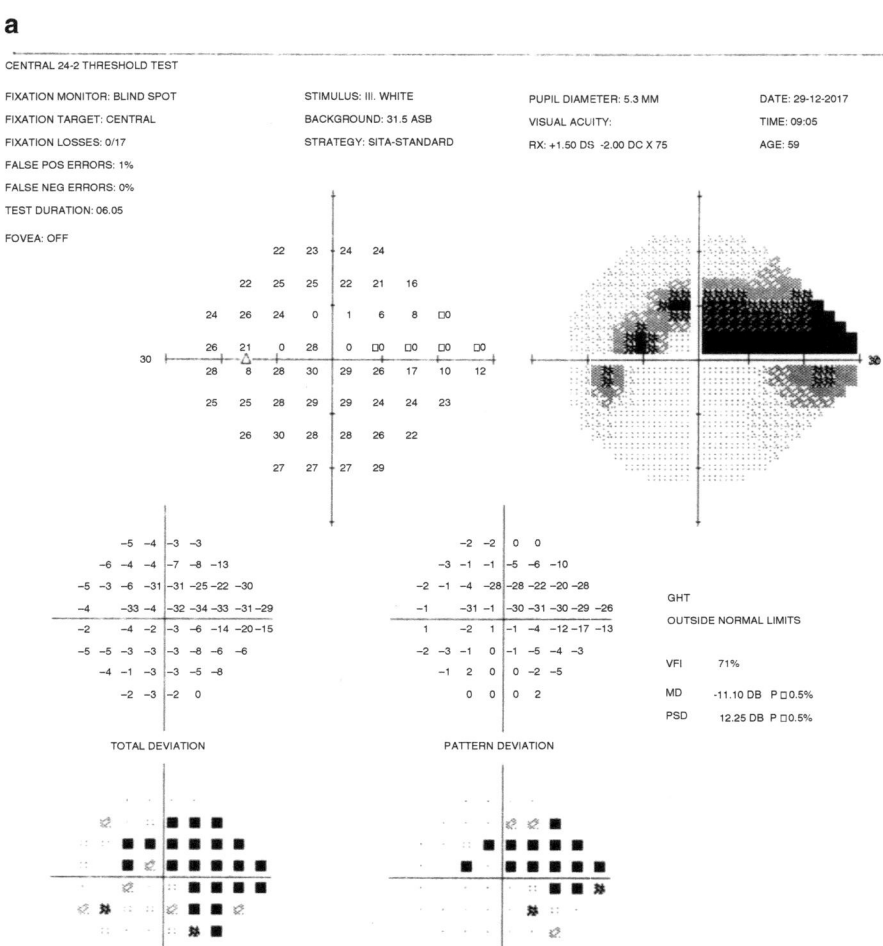

Fig. 15.22 (a) VF printout show advanced damage in the superior hemifield of the left eye, which is consistent with the RNFL damage in the inferior quadrant. (b) Humphrey field analyzer GPA detected no progression between years 2006 and 2017

b

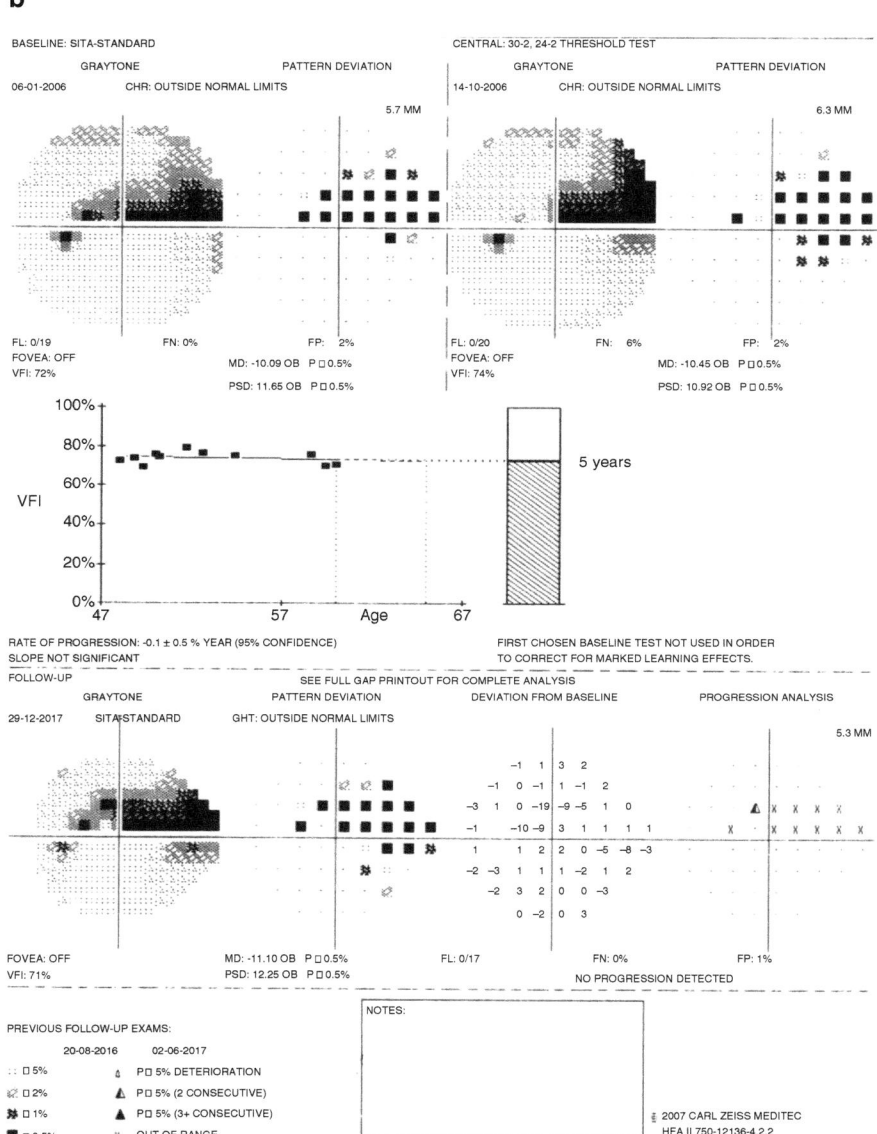

Fig. 15.22 (continued)

Conclusion: Both the structural and functional tests remained stable for many years with medical treatment in the right eye of this patient until very recently. As both functional and structural tests started to show progression on maximal medical treatment on last two visits, a trabeculectomy surgery was scheduled for IOP control.

The left eye of this patient is also a good example for issues with structural progression analysis in advanced glaucoma. As the RNFL thickness reaches the measurement floor (see Sect. 8.2.1), structural tests can no longer detect worsening damage, so functional progression analysis becomes more important. Due to the good IOP control resulting from successful trabeculectomy, Humphrey field analyzer GPA also does not show any progression in this case.

15.5   Case 5: Cirrus HD–OCT Guided Progression Analysis of a Fast Progressor

An 82-year old female patient with bilateral exfoliative glaucoma was monitored on medical treatment. Her BCVA was 20/80 in the right eye and counting fingers in the left eye. The anterior segment exam revealed pseudophakia and exfoliative material at the pupil margins bilaterally. Age-related macular degeneration was observed in both eyes on fundus exams. In 2015, her IOP was 18 mmHg in both eyes with maximum medical treatment. Her right eye had moderate damage and the left eye demonstrated advanced glaucomatous damage. The patient refused the proposed surgery for the right eye and preferred to remain on medical treatment. She was hospitalized for cardiac problems in early 2016 and missed her scheduled visits. The patient came back in October 2016 with IOPs of 28 mmHg on maximal medical treatment in both eyes (Figs. 15.23 and 15.24).

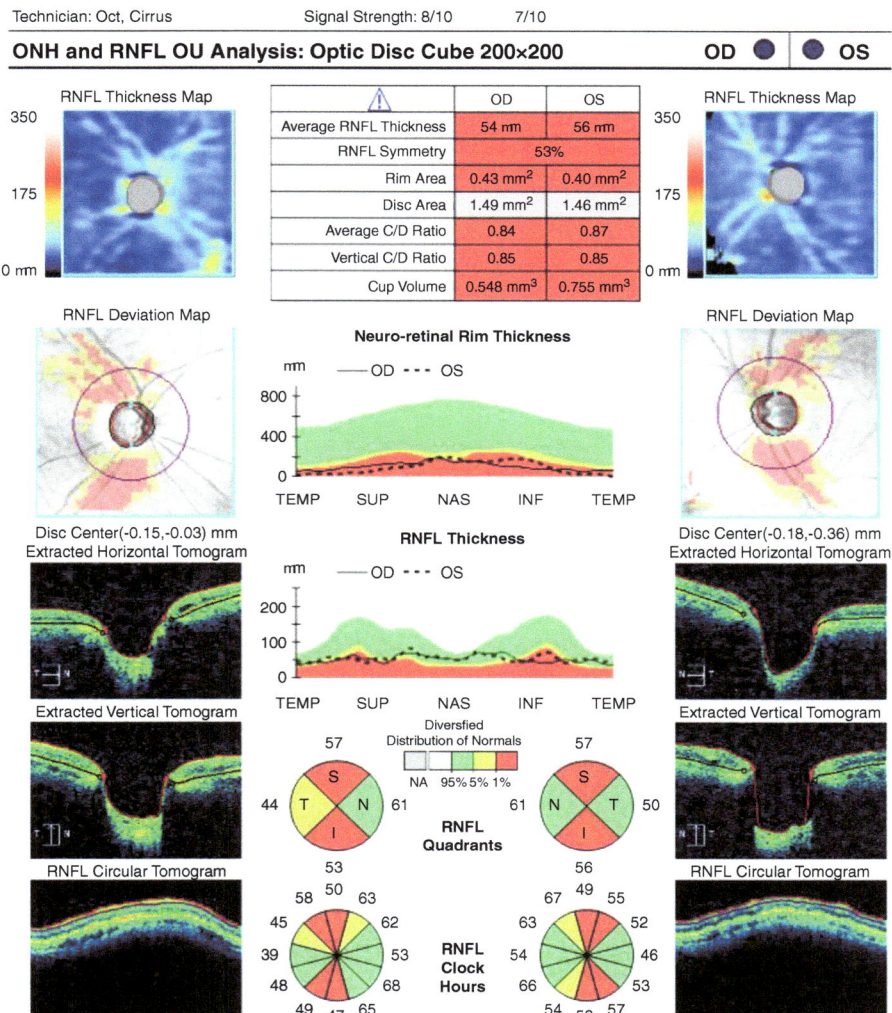

Fig. 15.23 The Cirrus HD-OCT scan shows advanced glaucomatous damage in both eyes. The left eye already had significant damage for the last few years. The right eye is the patient's only eye with useful vision

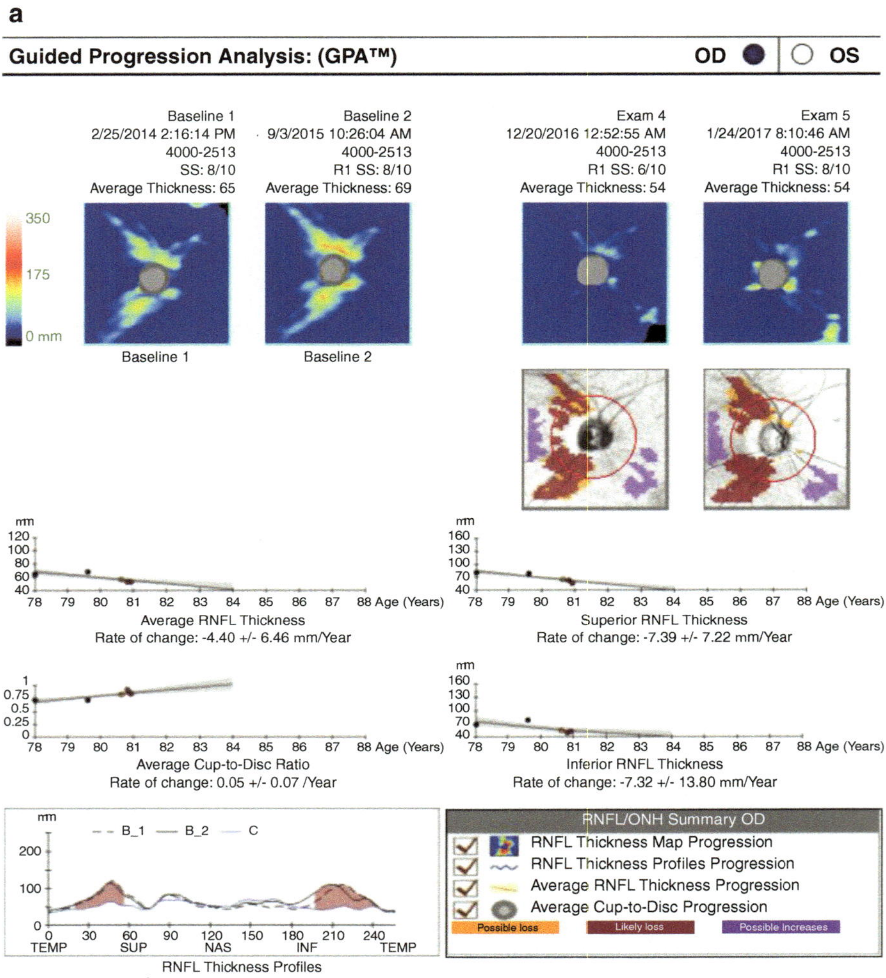

a

Fig. 15.24 Cirrus HD-OCT GPA right eye. (**a**) *RNFL/ONH Summary box* on the first page of the GPA report has red check marks for all four progression analysis methods. *RNFL thickness map progression analysis* shows likely loss in both the superior and inferior quadrants on the 200 × 200 cube. As progression is present in the same areas in the repeated scans, GPA marked these areas as "likely loss". *RNFL thickness profile progression plot* demonstrates that the current TSNIT graph is significantly thinner than the baseline scans and areas with statistically significant progression are displayed in red. Trend analysis based *average, inferior and superior RNFL thickness plots* detected statistically significant deterioration leading to estimation of yearly linear regression slopes. (**b**) The detailed analysis of RNFL measurements in these graphs is present in the second page. Changes in the average, superior, and inferior quadrant RNFL thickness measurements and the average cup-to-disc ratios can be seen with possible loss and likely loss flags in the table. The average cup-to-disc ratio progression is also statistically significant

b

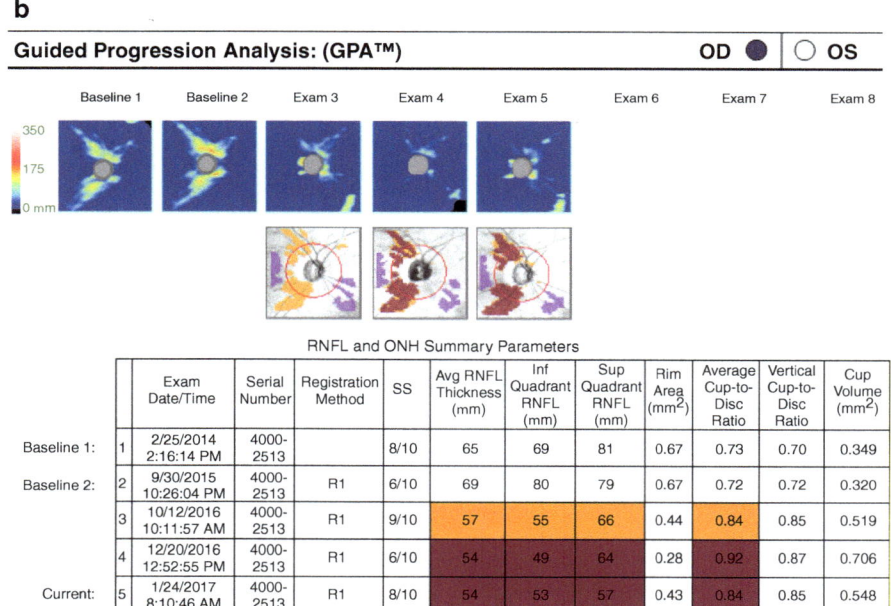

		Exam Date/Time	Serial Number	Registration Method	SS	Avg RNFL Thickness (mm)	Inf Quadrant RNFL (mm)	Sup Quadrant RNFL (mm)	Rim Area (mm²)	Average Cup-to-Disc Ratio	Vertical Cup-to-Disc Ratio	Cup Volume (mm²)
Baseline 1:	1	2/25/2014 2:16:14 PM	4000-2513		8/10	65	69	81	0.67	0.73	0.70	0.349
Baseline 2:	2	9/30/2015 10:26:04 PM	4000-2513	R1	6/10	69	80	79	0.67	0.72	0.72	0.320
	3	10/12/2016 10:11:57 AM	4000-2513	R1	9/10	57	55	66	0.44	0.84	0.85	0.519
	4	12/20/2016 12:52:55 PM	4000-2513	R1	6/10	54	49	64	0.28	0.92	0.87	0.706
Current:	5	1/24/2017 8:10:46 AM	4000-2513	R1	8/10	54	53	57	0.43	0.84	0.85	0.548

Fig. 15.24 (continued)

Conclusion: This is a very illustrative case demonstrating how rapid optic nerve damage can progress in exfoliative glaucoma. The patient had systemic health problems and missed the follow-up visits for more than a year. During this period, very fast deterioration occurred in her right eye. The patient was not able to perform VF tests because of neck problems and VF test results are not available during this period. Later, a Xen implant (Allergan, Dublin, Ireland) procedure was performed in the right eye. Although IOP decreased to 14 mmHg during the early postoperative period, the procedure later failed due to conjunctival fibrosis. Uneventful trabeculectomy procedure was performed in both eyes and now IOP is 8 mmHg in both eyes.

15.6 Case 6: OCT Progression in Pre-perimetric Glaucoma with Spectralis OCT Progression Analysis

This 69-year old female patient was diagnosed with ocular hypertension in 2009. She had exfoliation syndrome in the left eye and pre-treatment IOP values were 24 and 27 mmHg in the right and left eyes respectively. Medical treatment was started and her IOP was measured between 17 and 20 mmHg in both eyes during the follow-up. Her Humphrey field analyzer 24–2 VF test results are within normal limits OU. Following are the Spectralis OCT data of the left eye of the patient, between years 2012 and 2017 (Figs. 15.25, 15.26, 15.27, and 15.28).

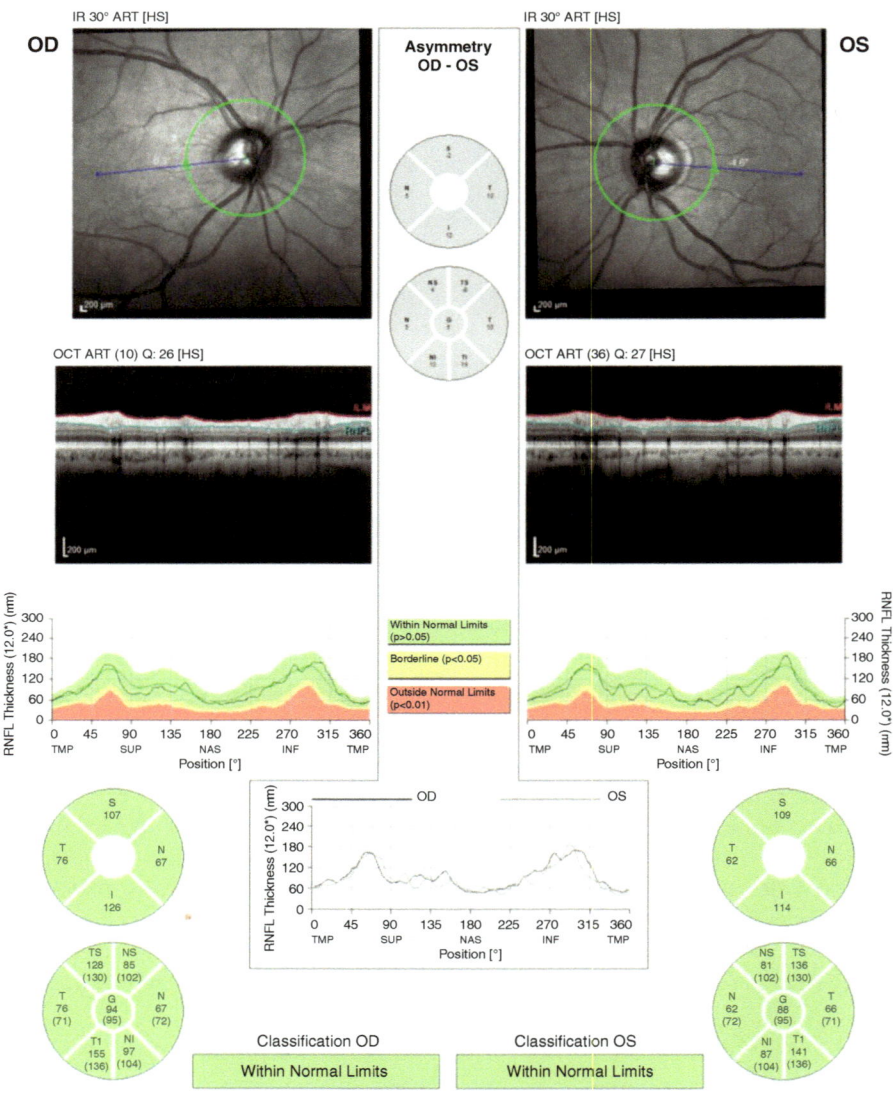

Fig. 15.25 Spectralis OCT RNFL report of the patient at the end of year 2017 is classified as "within normal limits" in both eyes although global average RNFL thickness value is lower in the left eye, compared to the right eye

Fig. 15.26 Spectralis OCT
RNFL Change Report of
the left eye from years
2012 to 2017 shows
depression of the TSNIT
plot in most sectors,
prominently in the nasal
superior sector in 2017
compared to 2012. Note
that all the sectors are
classified as "within
normal limits" during the
follow-up tests

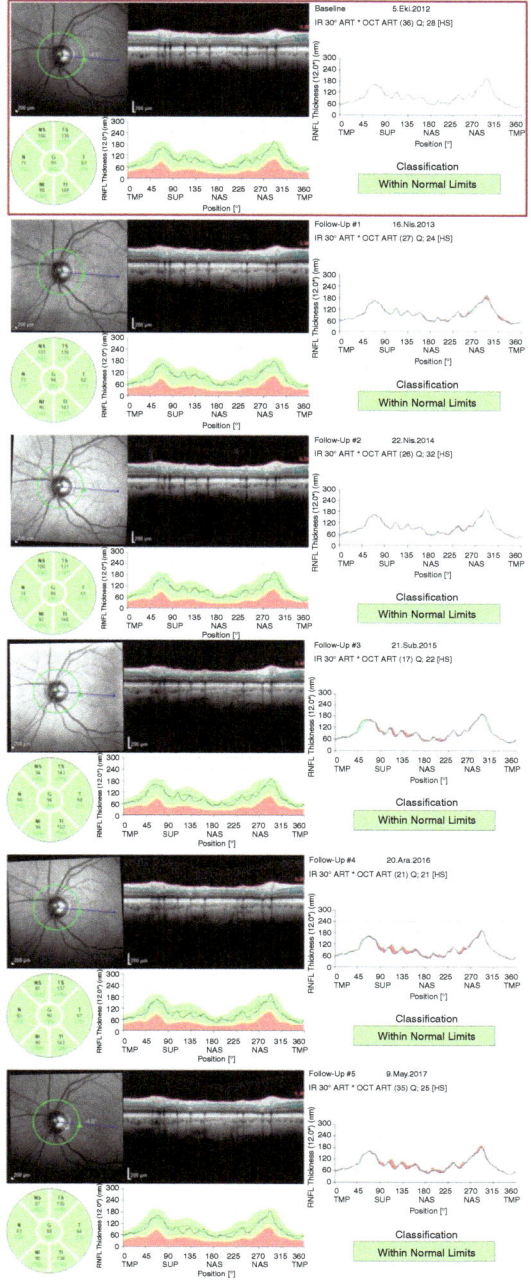

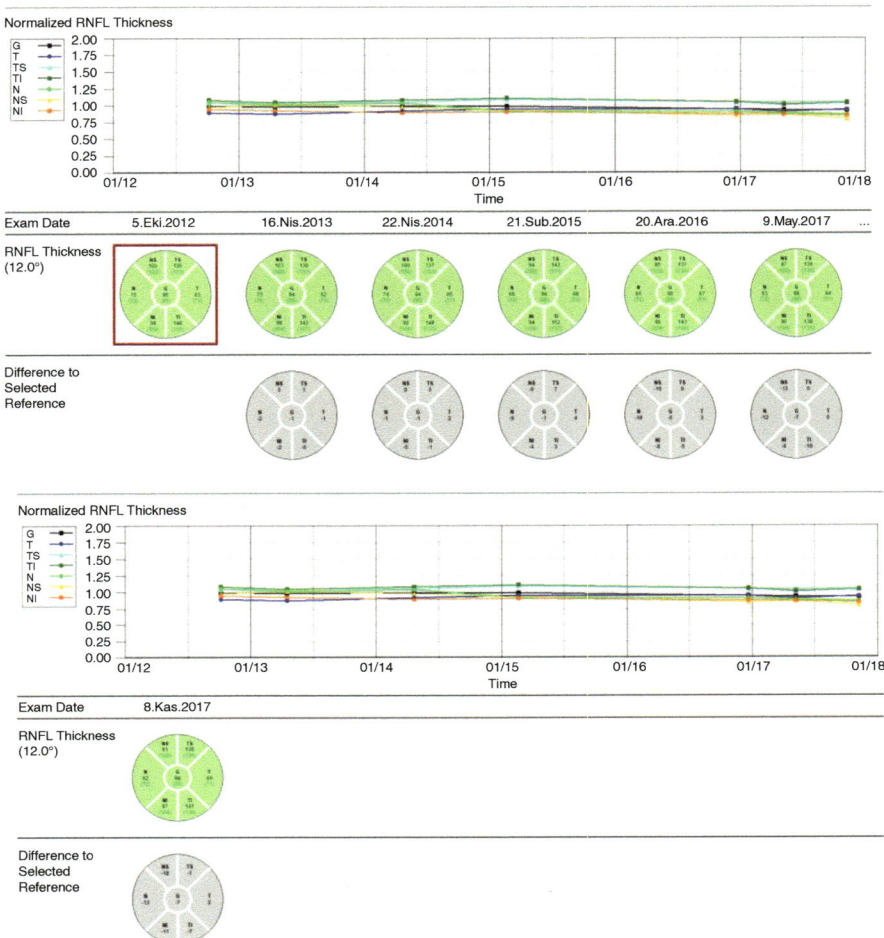

Fig. 15.27 Spectralis OCT RNFL Trend Report of the left eye from 2012 to 2017 shows 19 µm thinning of the nasal superior sector although still classified as "within normal limits"

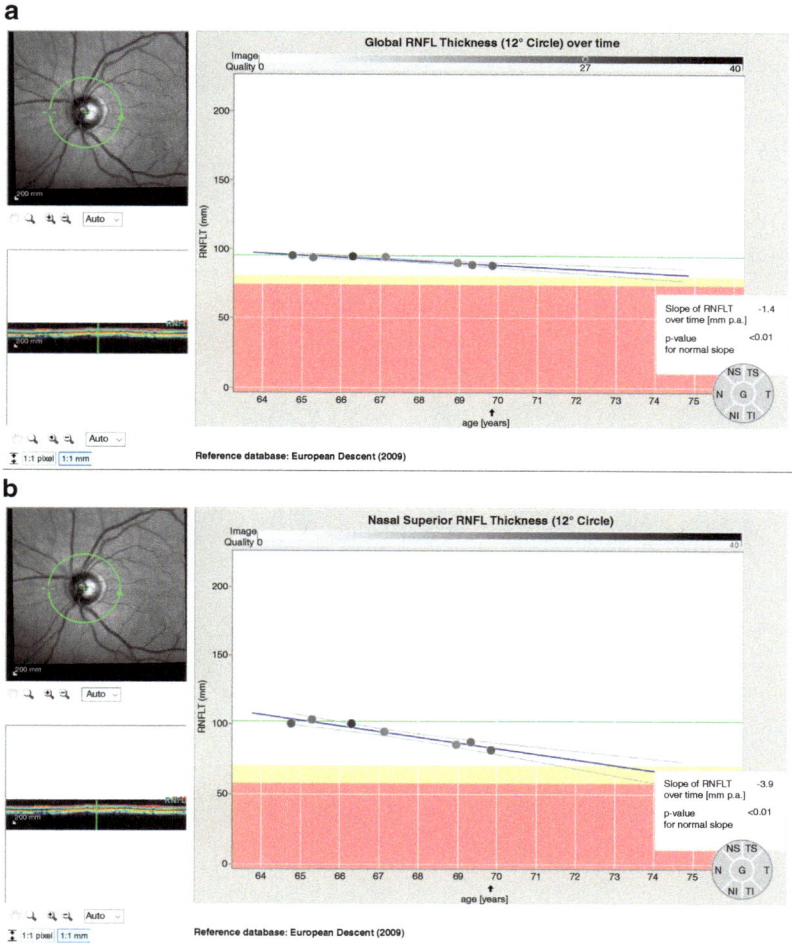

Fig. 15.28 (**a**) Spectralis OCT Global RNFL Thickness trend analysis of the left eye between years 2012 and 2017 shows that the slope of RNFL is −1.4 μm/year with a p-value of <0.01. (**b**) Nasal Superior RNFL Thickness trend analysis of the left eye during the same time interval shows that the slope of RNFL is −3.9 μm/year with a p-value of <0.01. Regression line for predicting future loss shows that this sector will probably be classified as "borderline" after couple years, if the treatment is not changed

Conclusion: This case is an example showing the importance of OCT progression analysis in detecting early glaucomatous progression, which is more evident in the sectorial analysis although present in the global progression analysis. OCT progression analysis in such a patient with exfoliation syndrome and ocular hypertension enables the clinician to identify eyes that are progressing structurally. Treatment modifications in these eyes can prevent further structural and functional damage. Note that nasal superior sector is not the frequent area for glaucomatous damage.

15.7 Case 7: Artifact in Guided Progression Analysis

A 77-year old female patient with ocular hypertension had been under supervision without medications. Her IOP was 22 mmHg in both eyes and OCT GPA showed possible progression (Fig. 15.29).

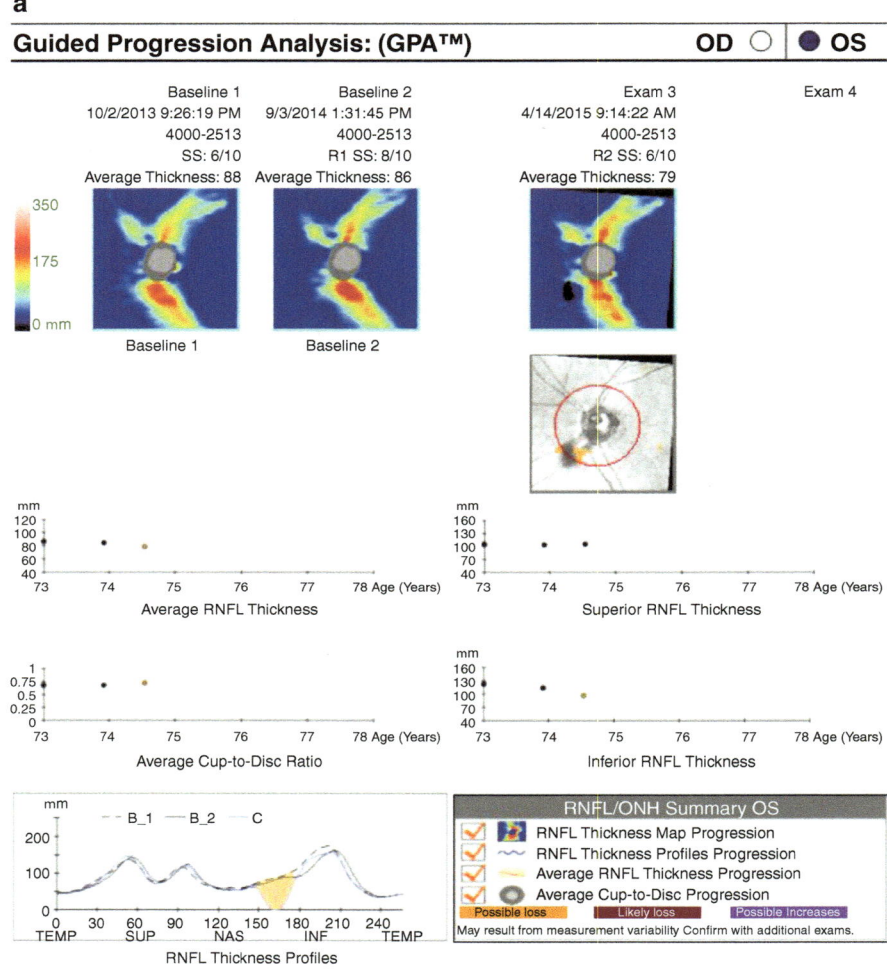

Fig. 15.29 Cirrus HD-OCT GPA, left eye. (**a, b**) OCT scanning artifacts, which were explained in Chap. 8 can cause errors in GPA. This case is an example of a vitreous opacity related scanning error in the last scan. Due to the Weiss ring coinciding with the calculation circle, it was not possible to obtain a high quality image for that quadrant during the last OCT scan. GPA flagged this area as having lost all RNFL with a zero RNFL thickness value in the *RNFL thickness profile plot*, which is clinically impossible due to the floor effect. All of the four criteria in the summary box show orange (possible loss) check marks. Careful inspection of the RNFL maps demonstrating an area of missing data and the impossibility of zero RNFL thickness in *RNFL thickness profile plot* are keys to understanding the artifact in this GPA output

b

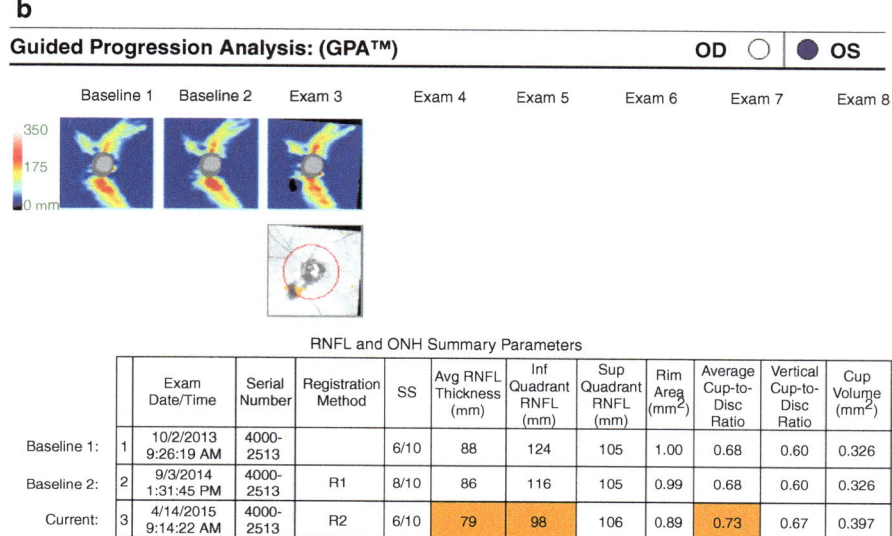

		Exam Date/Time	Serial Number	Registration Method	SS	Avg RNFL Thickness (mm)	Inf Quadrant RNFL (mm)	Sup Quadrant RNFL (mm)	Rim Area (mm²)	Average Cup-to-Disc Ratio	Vertical Cup-to-Disc Ratio	Cup Volume (mm²)
Baseline 1:	1	10/2/2013 9:26:19 AM	4000-2513		6/10	88	124	105	1.00	0.68	0.60	0.326
Baseline 2:	2	9/3/2014 1:31:45 PM	4000-2513	R1	8/10	86	116	105	0.99	0.68	0.60	0.326
Current:	3	4/14/2015 9:14:22 AM	4000-2513	R2	6/10	79	98	106	0.89	0.73	0.67	0.397

Fig. 15.29 (continued)

Conclusion: Many scanning artifacts can cause errors in the GPA report. Before reaching a conclusion, physician must carefully evaluate all parts of the report to identify artifacts that can influence GPA results.

15.8   Key Points

- Good quality images with signal strength of 6 or higher should be included in the Cirrus HD-OCT GPA.
- The RNFL maps, TSNIT graphs and other values must be checked for artifacts that can influence the results.
- The baseline images must be checked to see if they are relevant for the current exam, i.e., in case of a major change in treatment, the baseline must be updated accordingly to be able to observe the course of the disease after treatment.
- Cirrus HD-OCT GPA evaluates a maximum of two baseline and six follow-up reports of an individual patient. If more than eight scans are present, the sofware automotically selects the last six good quality scans.
- To see changes between the specific dates, manual selection of specific scans is possible.
- Cirrus HD-OCT Macular Ganglion Cell GPA must be evaluated in conjunction with the peripapillary RNFL GPA.

Part IV
Structure and Function

Chapter 16
Combining Structure and Function in Glaucoma

Atilla Bayer

16.1 Introduction

Glaucoma is a chronic ophthalmic disorder characterized by progressive neuroretinal rim thinning, excavation of the optic nerve head (ONH), and loss of the axons of the retinal ganglion cells. Accurate information about a patient's level of glaucoma damage and his/her risk of progression is of utmost importance for effective management of glaucoma. Structural changes observed in glaucoma are commonly accompanied by functional loss, which may ultimately result in a significant reduction in the patient's quality of life. The characteristic structural and functional changes seen are a direct result of axonal injury at the level of the lamina cribrosa and pathological loss of the retinal ganglion cells. Structural and functional measurements demonstrate varying degrees of noise or variability and such measurements have an imperfect relationship to one another. Currently, standard automatic perimetry (SAP) remains the established approach for monitoring functional changes in glaucoma patients. However, patients may present with structural alterations at the level of the ONH, retinal nerve fiber layer (RNFL), or macula before any changes are detected on visual field (VF) [1–5]. Some patients, on the other hand, can demonstrate evidence of functional damage or deterioration thereof without measurable changes on structural tests [2, 4]. This imperfect relationship between current structural and functional measurements is actually helpful clinically and seems to be a result of differences in measurement scale, magnitude of variability, measurement algorithms and most importantly stage of the disease.

Optical coherence tomography (OCT) devices have been evolving rapidly. There have been improvements in speed, resolution, and segmentation algorithms that

A. Bayer
Department of Glaucoma, Dünyagöz Eye Hospital, Ankara, Turkey

© Springer International Publishing AG, part of Springer Nature 2018   329
A. Akman et al. (eds.), *Optical Coherence Tomography in Glaucoma*,
https://doi.org/10.1007/978-3-319-94905-5_16

delineate various layers of the retina. It is now possible to obtain reliable measurements of RNFL thickness, valid topographic information with regard to the ONH structures and to detect evidence of macular damage in glaucoma eyes. However, it is not frequently clear to clinicians how to incorporate the information provided by OCT into their clinical practice. This is partly because combining structural and functional data can be challenging. To address this issue, recent platforms of some OCT devices provide clinicians with information on both structure and function. It seems logical that further evolution of OCT devices will eventually allow clinicians to routinely use combined structural and functional information at the level of individual patients.

16.2 How Much Damage Needs to Happen Before Detection Is Clinically Possible?

As mentioned above, the performance of OCT structural measures and functional tests in an individual patient depends on the stage of glaucomatous damage. Although there are some exceptions, VF tests frequently miss early retinal ganglion cell (RGC) loss in glaucoma. Quigley et al. reported that recognition of RGC loss based on disc or RNFL exam could be possible with loss of about 5% of RGC, but normally would require 15–40% RGC loss. Evidence of VF loss manifests with variable amounts of RGC loss, depending on the method and retinal eccentricity, with greater RGC loss required centrally. VF loss at 5% probability at a test location on the Humphrey Field Analyzer's (Carl Zeiss Meditec, Dublin, CA) 24-2 test usually occurs at about 25–35% RGC loss in a local area [6]. It is generally accepted that VF loss on SAP equates to moderate disease. By the time VF loss is detected by SAP, substantial structural damage frequently exists although there are some selective functional tests (e.g., frequency doubling technology perimetry or short-wave automated perimetry) that specifically were developed for earlier detection of the disease [7, 8].

Structural and functional tests should be considered complementary to each other (Fig. 16.1); in many respects, each compensates for the shortcomings of the other approach. SAP tends to underestimate the magnitude of neural damage in the early stages of glaucoma; as a result, it also underestimates the rate of progression in the earlier stages of glaucoma. On the other hand, early structural damage can be assessed with OCT. Therefore, rates of change can be more accurately estimated with OCT in such eyes, alerting the clinician to progression at a time when VFs demonstrate little or no evidence of damage. As expected, as the disease becomes more advanced, OCT becomes less useful due to a floor effect. Beyond its measurement floor, OCT can no longer detect evidence of further progression (Fig. 16.2) [9].

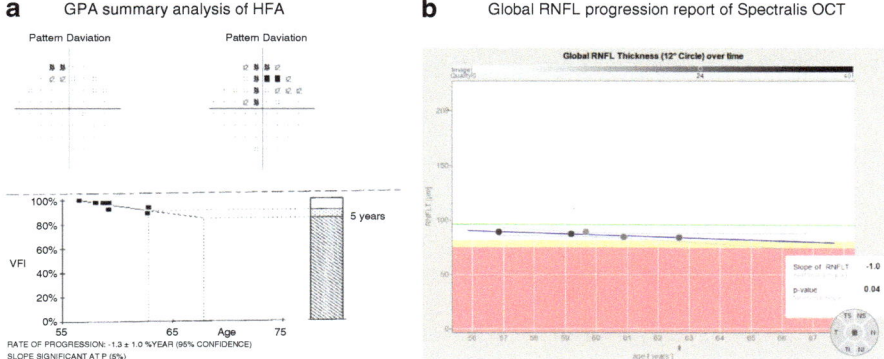

Fig. 16.1 A case of moderately severe glaucoma with structural and functional loss in the right eye. (**a**) The pattern deviation map and trend analysis of Visual Field Index of Humphrey Field Analyzer demonstrate significant deterioration. (**b**) Spectralis OCT's global RNFL progression report also displays a significant downward slope over time

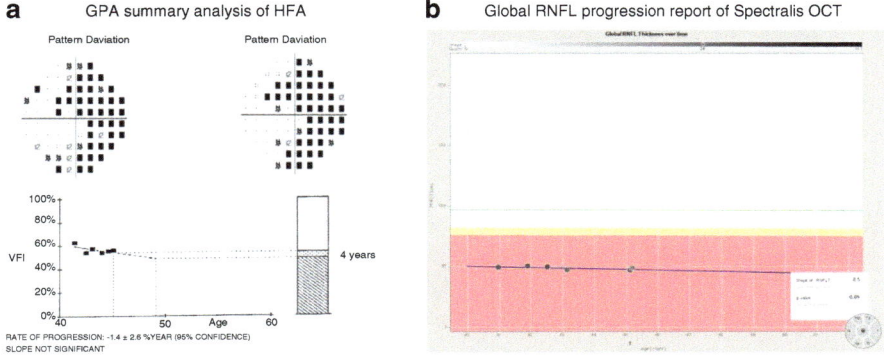

Fig. 16.2 (**a**) A case of advanced glaucoma with evidence of severe structural and functional loss in the left eye; VF testing with Humphrey Field Analyzer can still detect progression in this setting. (**b**) Spectralis OCT's global RNFL progression report shows advanced damage at baseline (floor effect) and therefore, it is much less likely to demonstrate progression

16.3   Detection of Glaucoma Deterioration with Structural vs. Functional Outcomes

Nouri-Mahdavi et al. have addressed issues related to measurement of rates with structural vs. functional outcomes [10]. These issues are the subjective vs. objective nature of the tests, sources of noise, measurement scale, and magnitude of variability. Since structural tests are objective, they are less dependent on patient's performance. Sources of noise in structural tests are mostly technical and these exams are in general less time consuming, whereas sources of noise in functional tests are mostly subjective, they take more time to carry out and fatigue makes repetition of the test onerous. Structural tests are ordinarily measured in linear scale; on the other hand, functional tests (specifically perimetric measurements) are expressed in logarithmic scale (dB). Variability of functional tests is higher, and increases with worse baseline damage as compared to the structural tests [10].

16.4   Which Test, When, Why to Combine?

A combination of structural measurements and functional testing may provide more definitive evidence of glaucoma, so both are needed for detection and confirmation of the early stages of the disease or for detection of progression [11]. There is an inverse relationship between the utility of structure and function in detecting progression as a function of disease severity. As mentioned above, structural and functional tests provide more useful information at different stages of the disease and can actually be complementary; in many respects each compensates for the weaknesses of the other technology. However, it is difficult to estimate the exact point at which one test might perform better than the other for monitoring an individual patient. Hence combining these two approaches is advisable so that one can evaluate progression and measure rates of change throughout all the stages of the disease. If the clinician relies on the information provided by either VF or OCT alone, he/she may not be able to detect progression in a timely fashion in every patient. Practically, this means changing emphasis on the two modalities depending on the stage of the disease in individual patients [12]. In early disease, clinicians should rely more on structural tools such as OCT, which is able to evaluate the RNFL thickness [7, 8, 12], Bruch's Membrane-based minimal rim width [13] or macular thickness parameters [14]. Structural scans need be acquired repeatedly over time and the rates of change estimated. If the rates of structural change are fast, the patient may be at high risk of future visual loss. It has been shown that the rates of glaucomatous change, measured with OCT, are predictive of future VF loss [15–17]. It has also been demonstrated that structural measurements are predictive of functional impairment such as patient-reported disability and difficulty with everyday tasks [18]. Harwerth et al. reported that estimates of RGC loss obtained from VF exam agreed closely with estimates of RGC loss from RNFL assessment with OCT [19]. Medeiros et al. developed a new index to estimate glaucoma severity based on a combination of functional measurements (SAP) and structural assessment with spectral domain OCT [17]. The weighted RGC estimate was used to develop a combined structure-function index (CSFI) [12, 20]. The CSFI is an estimate of the percentage of RGC loss compared with the age-adjusted RGC count in normal individuals. Therefore, an eye with a CSFI of 10%

has an estimated RGC count equal to 90% of that expected for patient's age, whereas an eye with a CSFI of 50% has an estimated RGC count half of that expected for age.

16.5   Structure and Function Correlation

The anatomical relationship between VF regions and corresponding sectors of the ONH and retina need be established as accurately as possible. However, there is significant variability in the correspondence of ONH or RNFL sectors to VF sectors. Garway-Heath et al. superimposed the 24-2 VF test pattern on RNFL photographs from NTG patients and created a map that related VF clusters to regions of the ONH neuroretinal rim [21]. The relationship between a test point and the ONH was determined by identifying points adjacent to the edge of an RNFL defect and tracing the defect, or missing bundle, back to the ONH.

The VF sector size should represent a compromise between a minimum practical sector size and the number of VF test points for each sector. A clinically useful map, relating VF regions to ONH and corresponding peripapillary RNFL sectors (Garway-Heath Sectors), has been frequently used for correlating structure and function [21]. Some device manufacturers provide an output that juxtaposes the VF sectoral results with the corresponding Garway-Heath RNFL sectors (Fig. 16.3).

Clinicians should keep in mind that structural and functional tests may not seem to be correlated in every case. There are instances where the two may disagree; however this should not be construed to suggest that one of them might be incorrect. As mentioned above, there are many sources of variability for the two types of measurements, which can lead to apparent lack of agreement.

16.6   Available OCT Systems for Structure and Function Evaluation

The FORUM Glaucoma Workplace (Carl Zeiss Meditec Inc., Dublin, CA) can automatically combine relevant information from Humphrey Field Analyzer (HFA), the Cirrus HD-OCT, and fundus images. The HFA and Cirrus HD-OCT Combined Report of FORUM summarizes patient structure and function analyses on a single printout. This combined report provides patient information, VF test type and data, Cirrus HD-OCT results, HFA and Cirrus HD-OCT combined structure and function output, an optional fundus photograph, and the RNFL and ganglion cell/inner plexiform layer (GCL + IPL) thickness deviation maps. The Cirrus HD-OCT ONH/RNFL data summary table is also provided (Figs. 16.4, 16.5, and 16.6).

The Heidelberg Structure-Function map provides a combined report of data from Spectralis OCT and Heidelberg Edge Perimeter (HEP) devices (Fig. 16.7). The HEP

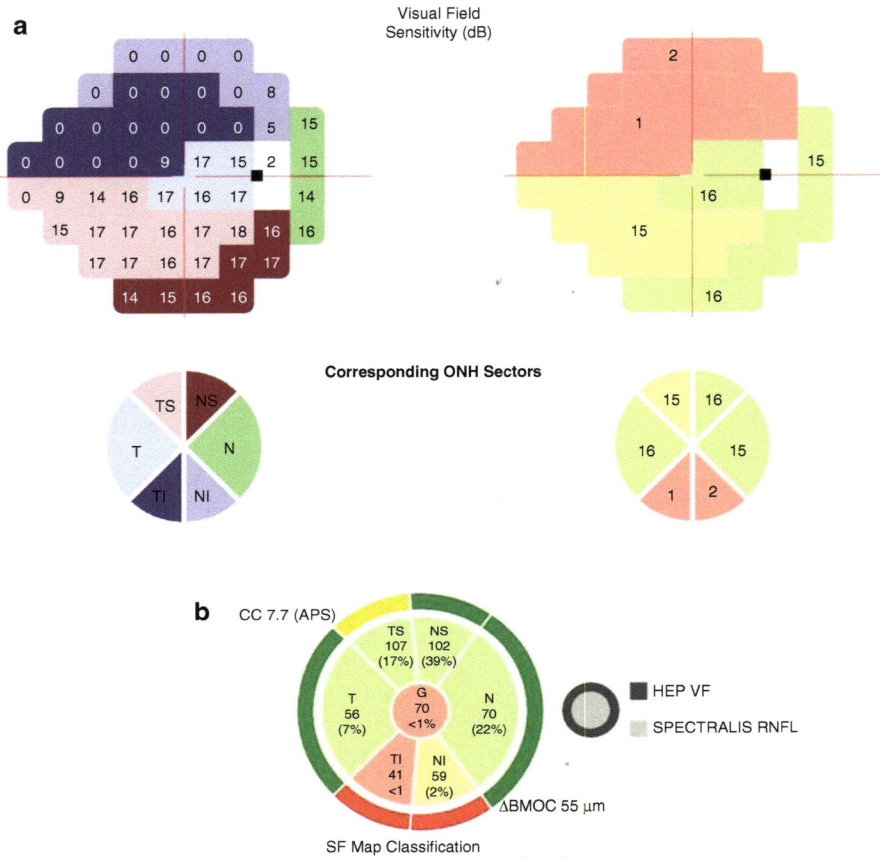

Fig. 16.3 (**a**) Heidelberg Edge Perimeter sector map report provides the opportunity to correlate VF sensitivities within predefined sectors with the corresponding RNFL sectors from Spectralis OCT as defined by Garway-Heath et al. [21]. (**b**) The RNFL and VF structure-function map report of the same patient are also displayed

performs VF testing using either white-on-white (SAP) or Flicker-Defined-Form (FDF) perimetry algorithms. The device provides various ways to observe the combined structure-function results. The Glaucoma Module Premium Edition (GMPE) software can combine the structure-function data for 3.5, 4.1, and 4.7 mm circle scans and the minimum rim width (Figs. 16.8 and 16.9). On the structure-function output, in addition to patient data, conventional Spectralis OCT test results such as the infrared image and the RNFL thickness profile are shown on the left side. The VF part of the report includes the grayscale, total and pattern deviation maps, global indices, the Glaucoma Hemifield Test result and patient performance indices. The OCT and HEP results are conjointly displayed on the structure-function classification map. Global and sectorial RNFL values are presented in the center and the

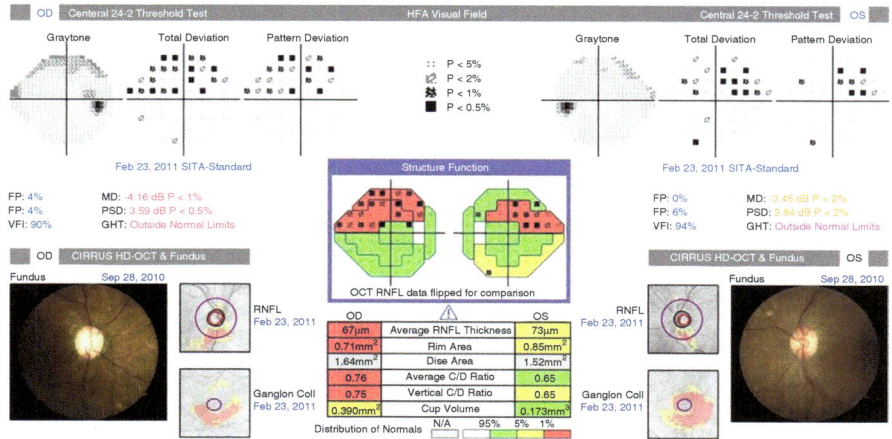

Fig. 16.4 The Humphrey Visual Field Analyzer and Cirrus HD-OCT RNFL combined report of the FORUM platform in a patient with moderate glaucomatous damage in both eyes. Superior VF defects can be observed in both eyes on the central 24-2 test. RNFL and GCA results show loss of RNFL and GCL + IPL inferiorly in both eyes. The Structure-Function report in the central part of the output provides combined information about RNFL and VF data both graphically and numerically (with permission from Carl Zeiss Meditec)

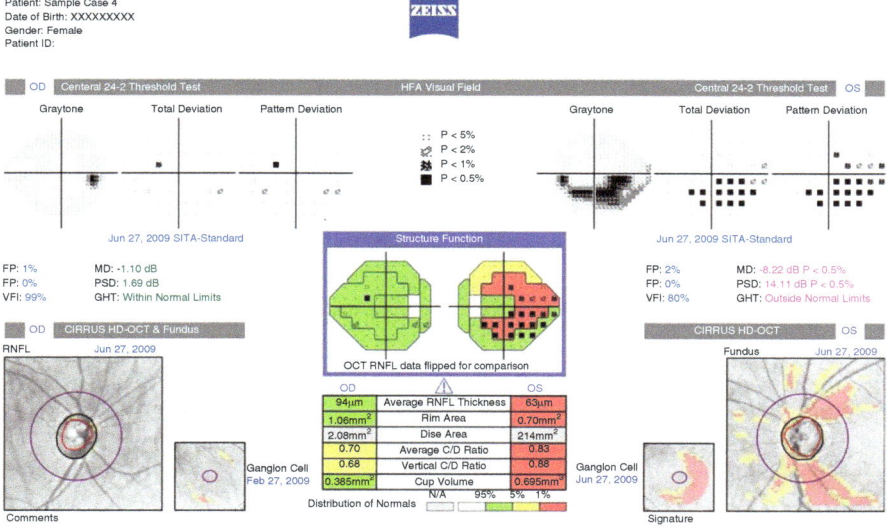

Fig. 16.5 Humphrey Visual Field Analyzer 24-2 and Cirrus HD-OCT RNFL combined report of FORUM. In this example, while the right eye's VF and RNFL measurements seem healthy, there are definitive signs of RNFL damage and VF loss in the patient's left eye, which correspond especially in the areas where the RNFL has been severely damaged and in the regions with dense VF loss (with permission from Carl Zeiss Meditec)

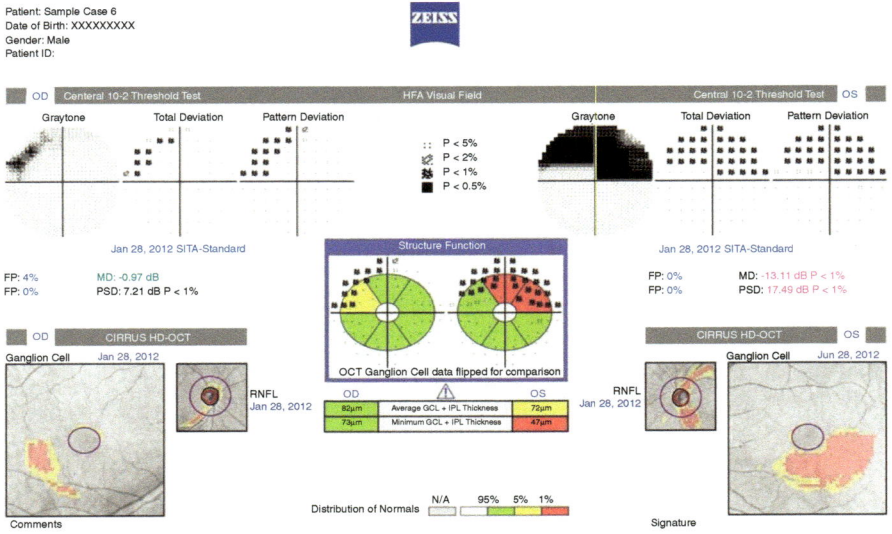

Fig. 16.6 Humphrey Visual Field Analyzer (HFA) 10-2 and Cirrus HD-OCT GCL + IPL combined report of FORUM. In this example, the left eye's GCL + IPL thickness is flagged as Outside Normal Limits. The Structure Function box indicates that two GCL + IPL sectors are abnormal at 1% significance level (red). As in the RNFL output, the GCL + IPL data are flipped for comparison to functional data in the Structure Function box. The pattern deviation probability plot from the HFA shows much of the superior VF flagged at the p < 1% significance level. The right eye demonstrates GCL + IPL thinning in one sector, which is significant at the p < 5% level. This sector corresponds to the abnormal area on the HFA's pattern deviation plot flagged at mostly p < 1% level (with permission from Carl Zeiss Meditec)

outer ring provides the HEP results. Both the OCT and HEP results are color-coded. A green color represents "within normal limits"; a yellow color represents "borderline" significance (i.e. p <5% but > 1% compared to the normative database); and a red color represents results that are "outside normal limits" (i.e., p < 1%). HEP's color-coded upper graph displays the eye's threshold sensitivity values in decibel scale. The lower graph can be chosen to show either the grayscale, or the probability maps of the total or pattern deviation.

The 3D Wide Glaucoma Report with VF test points (Hood report) of Topcon (Topcon medical Systems, Oakland, NJ) provides a one-page commercial report based upon a single wide-field (9X12mm) swept-source OCT cube scan. VF view with the 24-2 and 10-2 test locations are superimposed onto the RNFL and GCL + IPL maps also called the RGC+ map (Figs. 16.10 and 16.11).

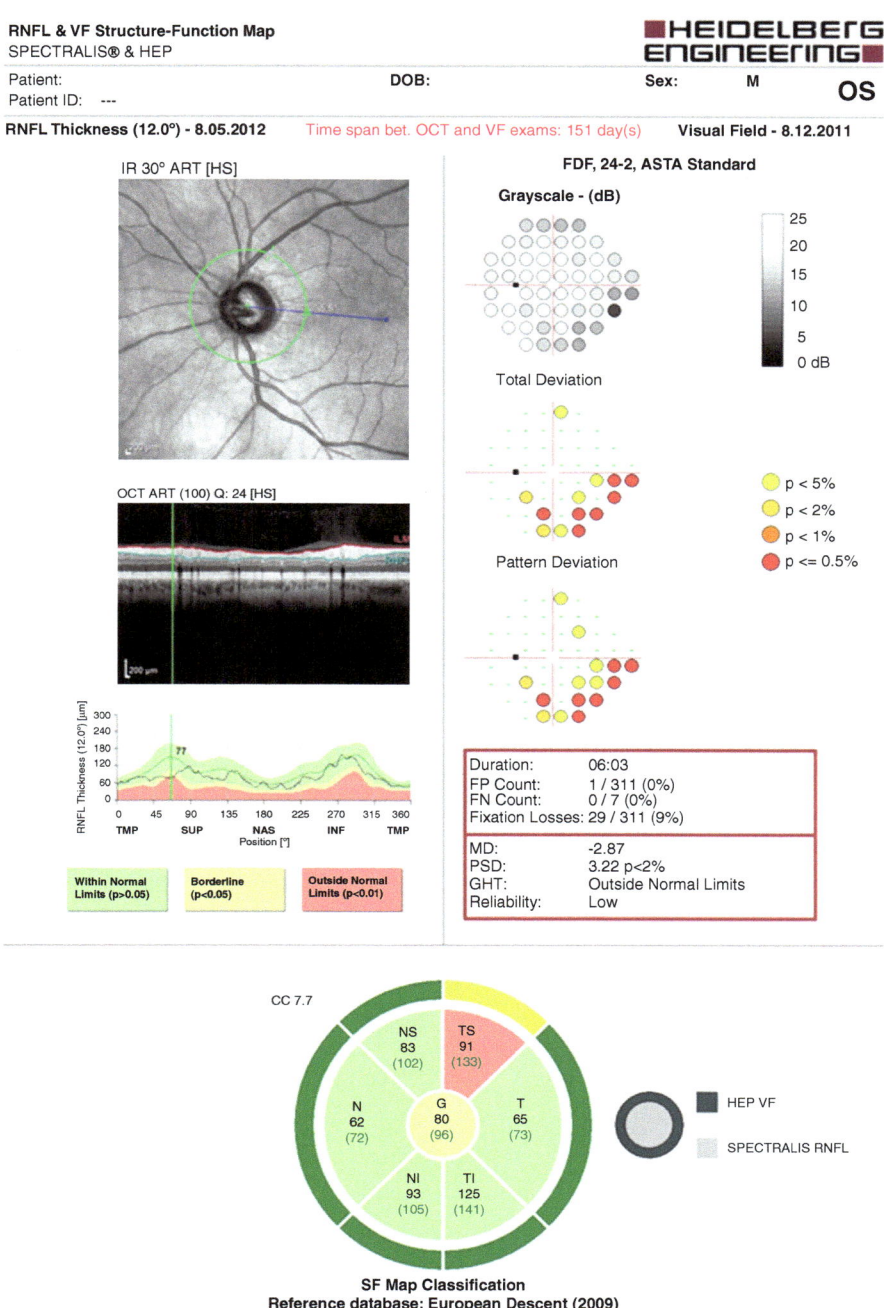

Fig. 16.7 The RNFL and VF structure-function map provided by Spectralis OCT and Heidelberg Edge Perimeter. The patient has inferior nasal field loss in the left eye as seen on the total and pattern deviation maps. The RNFL thickness profile demonstrates thinning in the temporal superior area, which is also flagged as red in the temporal superior sector of the structure-function map classification. The location and extent of VF loss is consistent with the RNFL loss and is flagged as yellow in the outer ring

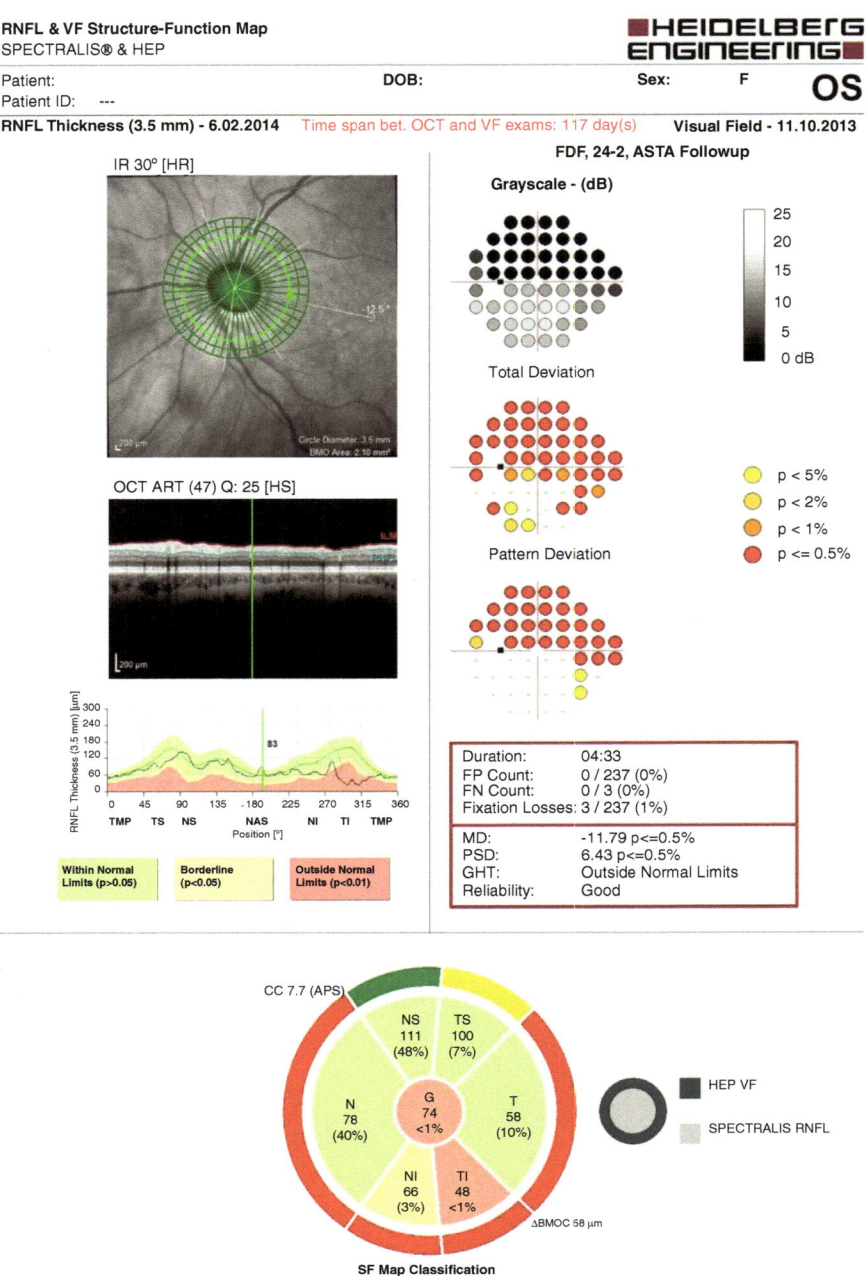

Fig. 16.8 The RNFL and VF structure-function map provided by the Glaucoma Module Premium Edition (GMPE) module of Spectralis OCT and Heidelberg Edge Perimeter. This eye demonstrates superior hemifield and inferior nasal VF loss in the left eye as observed on the total and pattern deviation maps. The RNFL thickness on the 3.5 mm circle scan profile shows thinning in the temporal inferior and nasal inferior sectors, which are flagged as red and yellow in the structure-function map classification. The outer ring, displaying VF data, is outside normal limits in all except superior temporal and superior nasal sectors

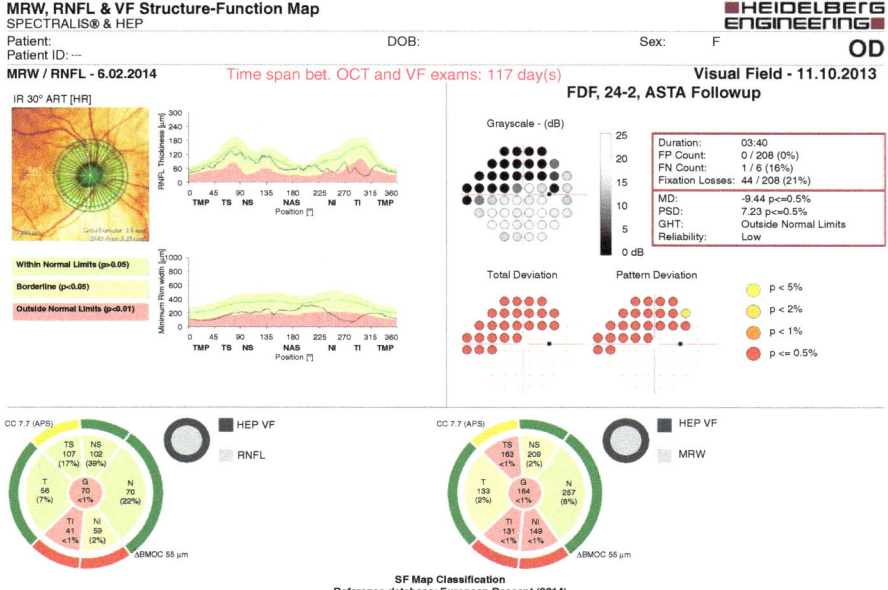

Fig. 16.9 The Bruch's membrane opening minimum rim width (BMO-MRW), RNFL and VF structure-function maps as provided by the GMPE software of Spectralis OCT and Heidelberg Edge Perimeter. Superior hemifield and inferior nasal VF defects can be observed in the right eye on the total and pattern deviation maps. The 3.5 mm RNFL thickness profile shows thinning in the temporal and nasal inferior sectors, which are flagged as red and yellow sectors in the temporal inferior and nasal inferior sectors on the structure-function map classification. The global average RNFL thickness is also outside normal limits. The BMO-MRW sector classification shows more advanced damage compared to the RNFL. The outer ring representing the VF sectors is outside normal limits in the inferior sectors and is classified as borderline abnormal in the temporal superior sector. The VF is in partial agreement with the RNFL loss but seems more consistent with the BMO-MRW findings

16.7   Key Points

- Combining structural and functional information is not always straightforward clinically. It can be challenging for clinicians to correlate the information from VF and OCT tests as these two tests may disagree on presence, location, and magnitude of damage. Varying degrees of disagreement are not infrequent.
- In an eye without established VF loss, clinicians should rely more heavily on structural information such as that provided by OCT imaging for diagnosis or detection of disease progression. In eyes with early to moderate VF loss, both structural and functional information can be used to monitor the disease course. As the disease progresses and becomes more advanced, structural measurements may reach their floor and therefore, OCT imaging will not be able to measure any further change, at which point, VF testing becomes the only modality for detection of disease progression.
- Additional risk factors for presence or progression of glaucoma must be taken into consideration as this changes the pre-test probability of presence of glaucoma or its progression. If the patient has high IOPs or if VF progression is suspected,

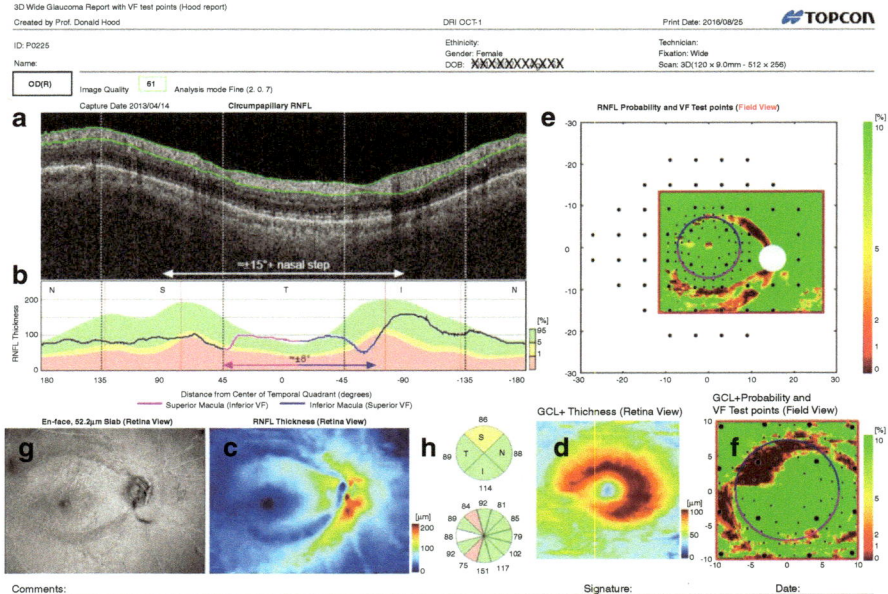

Fig. 16.10 An example of the one-page commercial (Hood) report based upon a single wide-field (9 × 12mm) swept-source OCT cube scan [v1.16beta (IMAGEnet6), Topcon Inc., Tokyo, Japan]. (**a**) A circumpapillary image derived from the wide-field cube scan. (**b**) The circumpapillary retinal nerve fiber layer (RNFL) thickness plot (black) obtained from (**a**) and shown in NSTIN (nasal-superior-temporal-inferior-nasal) orientation [22]. (**c**) The RNFL thickness map. (**d**) The retinal ganglion cell plus inner plexiform layer (called RGC+) thickness map from the central (6 × 6mm) portion of the wide-field cube scan centered on the fovea. (**e**) The RNFL probability maps based upon the thickness map in panel (**c**) shown in VF view with the 24-2 (large black filled circles) and 10-2 (small black circles) VF locations superimposed. (**f**) The RGC+ probability map based upon the thickness maps in panel (**d**) with the 10-2 and central 24-2 VF test locations superimposed. The circles in panels (**e**) and (**f**) show the borders (±8°) of the macula and, the scale to the right indicates the probability range for OCT thickness measurements. (**g**) An en-face slab image as described in Hood et al. [23]. (**h**) Pie charts showing the thickness values and probabilities for quadrants (top) and clock hour sectors (bottom). Green, yellow and red colors indicate within normal limits, $0.01 \leq p \leq 0.05$ and $p \leq 0.01$. See Hood et al. [24] and Hood [25] for details (This figure and caption is provided by Donald C. Hood, PhD)

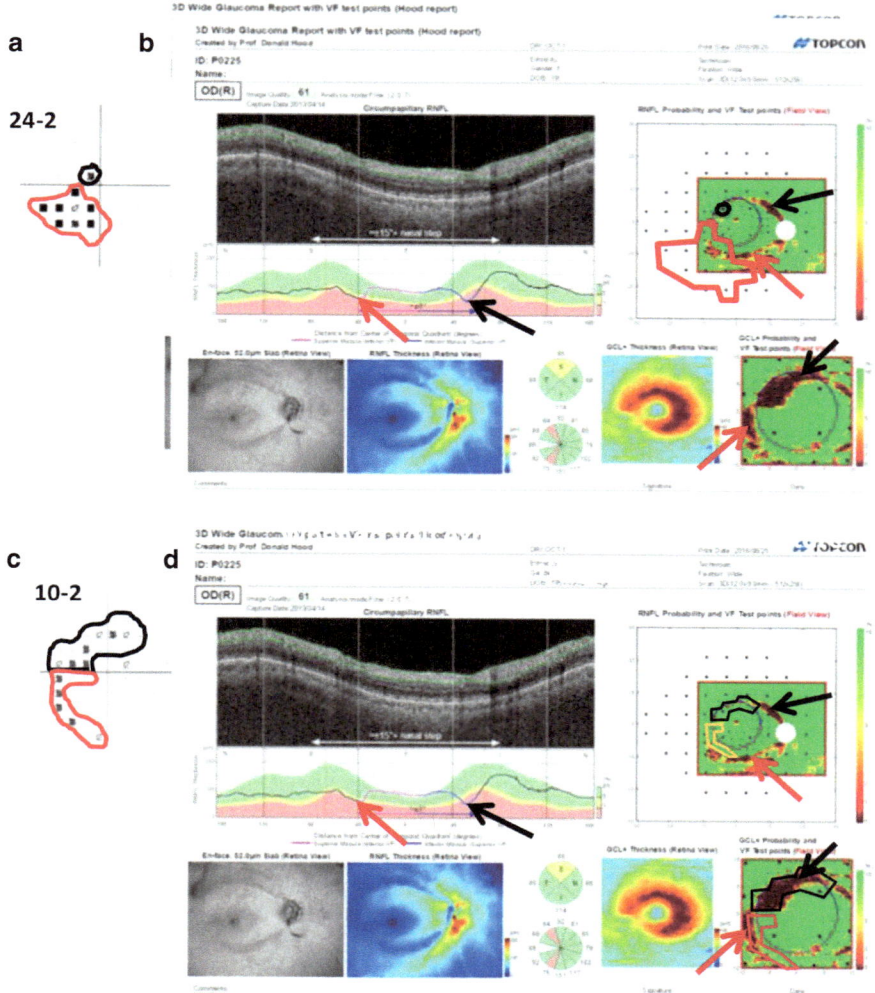

Fig. 16.11 (**a**) The 24-2 Total Deviation plot for the same eye as in Fig. 16.10 with the abnormal field points marked in black (superior VF) and red (inferior VF). (**b**) The same Hood report as in Fig. 16.10, but with abnormal points on 24-2 in panel (**a**) flagged in red and black. (**c**) 10-2 Total Deviation plot for the same eye with the abnormal VF points encircled in black (superior VF) and red (inferior VF). (**d**) Same as in Fig. 16.10, but with abnormal points on 10-2 in panel (**c**) enclosed within the red and black borders. The arrows in panels (**b**) and (**d**) indicate corresponding defects in the upper VF/inferior retina/disc (black) and in the lower VF/superior retina/disc (red). See Hood [25] for details (This figure and caption is provided by Donald C. Hood, PhD)

a structural change is more likely to be real. On the other hand, in an eye with well-controlled glaucoma, a suspicious change in OCT results is less likely to represent true progression. In general, the more tests are available, the higher the power for detection of disease progression as the estimates of rates of change will be less noisy. Under ideal settings, with very frequent structural and functional testing (i.e., every 3–4 months), it may be possible to measure a treatment effect on rates of change within a period of 2–3 years [10].

• Clinicians need to be aware of false positive results. OCT provides a huge amount of information that needs to be processed by the machine or human observers. The multiplicity of data and numerous comparisons to the normative database increase the chances of false positive results and drawing wrong conclusions from the data. Given the numerous analyses, one or more of OCT or VF parameters would be expected to be abnormal or show a progression by chance. This is called "the red disease," where OCT printouts demonstrate abnormalities in a healthy eye. A combined index of structural and functional damage could decrease the likelihood of false positive results.

References

1. Strouthidis NG, Scott A, Peter NM, Garway-Heath DF. Optic disc and visual field progression in ocular hypertensive subjects: detection rates, specificity, and agreement. Invest Ophthalmol Vis Sci. 2006;47:2904–10.
2. Miglior S, Zeyen T, Pfeiffer N, Cunha-Vaz J, Torri V, Adamsons I. Results of the European Glaucoma Prevention Study. Ophthalmology. 2005;112:366–75.
3. Medeiros FA, Alencar LM, Zangwill LM, Bowd C, Sample PA, Weinreb RN. Prediction of functional loss in glaucoma from progressive optic disc damage. Arch Ophthalmol. 2009;127:1250–6.
4. Kass MA, Heuer DK, Higginbotham EJ, Johnson CA, Keltner JL, Miller JP, et al. The Ocular Hypertension Treatment Study: a randomized trial determines that topical ocular hypotensive medication delays or prevents the onset of primary open-angle glaucoma. Arch Ophthalmol. 2002;120:701–13. discussion 729–730
5. Hood DC, Kardon RH. A framework for comparing structural and functional measures of glaucomatous damage. Prog Retin Eye Res. 2007;26:688–710.
6. Quigley HA, Addicks EM, Green WR. Optic nerve damage in human glaucoma. III. Quantitative correlation of nerve fiber loss and visual field defect in glaucoma, ischemic neuropathy, papilledema, and toxic neuropathy. Arch Ophthalmol. 1982;100:135–46.
7. Sommer A, Katz J, Quigley HA, Miller NR, Robin AL, Richter RC, Witt KA. Clinically detectable nerve fiber atrophy precedes the onset of glaucomatous field loss. Arch Ophthalmol. 1991;109:77–83.
8. Bowd C, Zangwill LM, Berry CC, Blumenthal EZ, Vasile C, Sanchez-Galeana C, Bosworth CF, Sample PA, Weinreb RN. Detecting early glaucoma by assessment of retinal nerve fiber layer thickness and visual function. Invest Ophthalmol Vis Sci. 2001;42:1993–2003.
9. Medeiros FA, Zangwill LM, Bowd C, Mansouri K, Weinreb RN. The structure and function relationship in glaucoma: implications for detection of progression and measurement of rates of change. Invest Ophthalmol Vis Sci. 2012;53(11):6939–46.
10. Nouri-Mahdavi K, Caprioli J. Measuring rates of structural and functional change in glaucoma. Br J Ophthalmol. 2015;99:893–8.

11. Weinreb RN, Greve EL, editors. Glaucoma diagnosis: structure and function. San Diego, CA., November 13-14: Kugler Publications; 2003.
12. Medeiros FA, Zangwill LM, Anderson DR, et al. Estimating the rate of retinal ganglion cell loss in glaucoma. Am J Ophthalmol. 2012;154(5):814–24.
13. Danthurebandara VM, Sharpe GP, Hutchison DM, Denniss J, Nicolela MT, McKendrick AM, Turpin A, Chauhan BC. Enhanced structure-function relationship in glaucoma with an anatomically and geometrically accurate neuroretinal rim measurement. Invest Ophthalmol Vis Sci. 2014;56:98–105.
14. Raza AS, Cho J, de Moraes CG. Retinal ganglion cell layer thickness and local visual field sensitivity in glaucoma. Arch Ophthalmol. 2011;129:1529–36.
15. Meira-Freitas D, Lisboa R, Tatham A, Zangwill LM, Weinreb RN, Girkin CA, Liebmann JM, Medeiros FA. Predicting progression in glaucoma suspects with longitudinal estimates of retinal ganglion cell counts. Invest Ophthalmol Vis Sci. 2013;54(6):4174–83.
16. Miki A, Medeiros FA, Weinreb RN, Jain S, He F, Sharpsten L, Khachatryan N, Hammel N, Liebmann JM, Girkin CA, Sample PA, Zangwill LM. Rates of retinal nerve fiber layer thinning in glaucoma suspect eyes. Ophthalmology. 2014;121(7):1350–8.
17. Medeiros FA, Lisboa R, Weinreb RN, Girkin CA, Liebmann JM, Zangwill LM. A combined index of structure and function for staging glaucomatous damage. Arch Ophthalmol. 2012;130:107–16.
18. Gracitelli CP, Abe RY, Tatham AJ, Rosen PN, Zangwill LM, Boer ER, Weinreb RN, Medeiros FA. Association between progressive retinal nerve fiber layer loss and longitudinal change in quality of life in glaucoma. JAMA Ophthalmol. 2015;133(4):384–90.
19. Harwerth RS, Wheat JL, Fredette MJ, Anderson DR. Linking structure and function in glaucoma. Prog Retin Eye Res. 2010;29:249–71.
20. Medeiros FA, Lisboa R, Zangwill LM, Liebmann JM, Girkin CA, Bowd C, Weinreb RN. Evaluation of progressive neuroretinal rim loss as a surrogate end point for development of visual field loss in glaucoma. Ophthalmology. 2014;121(1):100–9.
21. Garway-Heath DF, Poinoosawmy D, Fitzke FW, Hitchings RA. Mapping the visual field to the optic disc in normal tension glaucoma eyes. Ophthalmology. 2000;107:1809–15.
22. Hood DC, Raza AS. On improving the use of OCT imaging for detecting glaucomatous damage. Br J Ophthalmol. 2014;98(Suppl 2):ii1–9.
23. Hood DC, Fortune B, Mavrommatis MA, Reynaud J, Ramachandran R, Ritch R, Rosen RB, Muhammad H, Dubra A, Chui TY. Details of glaucomatous damage are better seen on OCT en face images than on OCT retinal nerve fiber layer thickness maps. Investig Ophthalmol Vis Sci. 2015;56:6208–16.
24. Hood DC, De Cuir N, Blumberg DM, Liebmann J, Jarukasetphon R, Ritch R, De Moraes CG. A single wide-field OCT protocol can provide compelling information for the diagnosis of early glaucoma. Transl Vis Sci Technol. 2016;5:4.
25. Hood DC. Improving our understanding, and detection, of glaucomatous damage: An approach based upon optical coherence tomography (OCT). Prog Retin Eye Res. 2017;57:46–75.

Part V
Optical Coherence Tomography
Angiography in Glaucoma

Chapter 17
Optical Coherence Tomography Angiography (OCTA)

Ramin Daneshvar and Kouros Nouri-Mahdavi

17.1 Introduction

Glaucoma is a multifactorial disease and many risk factors contribute to its pathophysiology. Despite the long debate on mechanical and ischemic mechanisms as explanations for development of the disease, it is likely that both mechanisms are at work to varying degrees in different patients. There are several pieces of evidence that point to a vascular mechanism for the disease. Clinical findings such as disc hemorrhage and peripapillary atrophy in glaucomatous eyes and comorbidities such as migraine, Raynaud's syndrome and nocturnal hypotension have been interpreted as evidence of the role of disturbed blood supply in the development or progression of glaucoma [1–4]. However, direct study of vascular changes in glaucoma patients was technically impractical until recently. Various technologies have been used to explore retinal and optic nerve circulatory changes in glaucoma. These include retinal fluorescein and indocyanine green angiography [5, 6], Heidelberg retinal flowmeter [7–9], laser Doppler flowmetry [10], laser speckle flowgraphy [11], and ultrasonic Doppler imaging of retrobulbar blood flow [12]. However, drawbacks like necessity of intravenous dye injection and possible allergic and anaphylactic reactions, inability to differentiate different vascular layers, limited ability to detect small vessels and capillaries, and low repeatability and reproducibility limited the usefulness of the above diagnostic tests in clinical practice and glaucoma research. Recently, optical coherence tomography angiography (OCTA) has been introduced as a promising technology for imaging vascular networks and discriminating various vascular layers in the retina and optic

R. Daneshvar
Mashad University of Medical Sciences, Mashad, Iran

K. Nouri-Mahdavi (⊠)
Stein Eye Institute, University of California Los Angeles, Los Angeles, CA, USA
e-mail: nouri-mahdavi@jsei.ucla.edu

© Springer International Publishing AG, part of Springer Nature 2018   347
A. Akman et al. (eds.), *Optical Coherence Tomography in Glaucoma*,
https://doi.org/10.1007/978-3-319-94905-5_17

nerve head (ONH). Moreover, this technology is fast and noninvasive and could be potentially incorporated into daily clinical practice. There is growing evidence regarding altered circulation of the optic nerve, peripapillary retina and macula in glaucoma patients and an association between the magnitude of hemodynamic disturbance and severity of glaucomatous damage has been demonstrated [13–19].

17.2 Principles

Optical coherence tomography angiography is still in evolution and the technology and its implementation in optical coherence tomography (OCT) devices is changing rapidly; the basic principles though remain the same. OCT uses a highly coherent laser source to measure the delay in the returning light reaching the sensor and to calculate the distance the light traveled. A topographic map is generated based on multiple A-scans carried out during the imaging session. To produce high quality images, each point is measured several times (between 10 and 100 times, based on the device) and an averaged value is used to produce a high-quality image. OCTA not only measures the distance to a point of interest, but also measures the variation of the amplitude and other characteristics of the returning signal over time. The device takes advantage of its ultrahigh scanning speed to scan any single point multiple times in a very short period of time and compares the timing and intensity of the returning signals. For static tissues such as various retinal layers and neural elements in the optic nerve, the amplitude of the returning signal has little variability and is constant. In contrast, moving elements like blood cells in the vascular network cause variations in the amplitude of the returning signals. Statistically, the correlation between successive measurements of static tissue is high whereas it is low for dynamic, moving tissue. Decorrelation is defined as 1—correlation and therefore, it has a higher value in dynamic tissues [20]. To increase the quality of image and vessel detection, averaging of several measurements at any given point is necessary; this mandates a very high scanning speed or some alternative algorithms. There are non-commercial OCT prototypes with ultrahigh scanning speeds in the range of 400–1000 KHz, which are capable of capturing high quality angiographic images in a very short time with minimal artifacts [13, 21]. To compensate for the lower scanning speed (70–150 KHz) of commercially available OCT devices, some alternative algorithms are available. One of the first and most popular algorithms is the Split-Spectrum Amplitude Decorrelation Angiography (SSADA) [20]. In this approach, each full width spectrum wavelength is divided into multiple (between 4 and 12) smaller bandwidths, which multiplies the number of possible comparisons and improves image quality [20, 22]. As a result of 'splitting the spectrum' to narrower bands, the axial resolution of the scan diminishes. However, the transverse resolution is almost unaffected; this is a desired side-effect which can reduce the motion artifact of axial eye movement secondary to pulsation of large retrobulbar blood vessels. Additionally, most devices use multiple scanning in orthogonal, mostly horizontal and vertical directions, and average the data to enhance the quality of image.

Other, less popular algorithms such as phase variance, speckle variance and optical microangiography (OMAG) approaches have been used in some commercially available devices. The phase variance analyzes phase variations of the OCT laser beam and sometimes uses dual beam-scanning OCT. The speckle variance, uses alterations in signal amplitude like SSADA and OMAG analyzes changes in complex signals by taking into account both intensity and phase changes [23–25].

Currently available technologies capture high quality angiograms in less than 3 seconds. The technique does not require any contrast media and has very good repeatability and reproducibility [13, 26–28]. Moreover, OCTA can segment the vasculature into slabs with different thickness and provide depth information [13]. Because of these advantages, OCTA is being used in many research and clinical settings and can be easily fit into everyday clinical practice.

17.3   OCTA in Glaucoma Diagnosis and Management

There has been a surge of published articles on the role of OCTA in the field of ophthalmology and specifically glaucoma. The technology has been used to better understand the disease pathophysiology and also as a potential diagnostic tool. Many researchers have investigated alterations in blood circulation in the ONH, peripapillary retina and macula and applied various segmentation algorithms to further explore differential hemodynamic changes at various levels in the ONH and retina. Generally, all published studies demonstrated some degree of reduced circulation or vascular drop-out in glaucoma patients and several studies confirmed vascular-structural and vascular-functional correlations.

One of the first reports on the application of OCTA in glaucoma patients was a short case series published in 2012 by Jia and colleagues [20]. The authors reported significantly lower ONH perfusion in three preperimetric glaucomatous eyes compared to three normal eyes. Later studies confirmed the findings and also demonstrated correlations between vascular attenuation and drop-off and visual field (VF) pattern standard deviation [13, 27, 29] or mean deviation [14, 16, 29, 30] or corresponding VF loss and mean sensitivity [15, 18]. Moreover, vascular changes coincide with various structural changes in the ONH, peripapillary retina and macula [14, 16, 17, 26, 31–40] Several studies demonstrated spatial and temporal correspondence between decreased vascular density and perfusion and VF defects and retinal nerve fiber layer loss [16, 18, 32, 34]. Two studies found vascular alterations on OCTA to have stronger correlations with VF measures compared to structural parameters [13, 17]. Macular foveal avascular zone (FAZ) circularity and size were recently reported to correlate with the presence and severity of central VF loss [26].

Although some studies suggested a higher diagnostic accuracy for OCTA for detection of glaucoma [15–17, 19], other studies have failed to confirm these results and reported a better diagnostic performance for structural OCT parameters [44, 45]. Shin and colleagues investigated regional vascular changes in glaucoma and normal eyes [19]. Superficial peripapillary vasculature (i.e. radial peripapillary capillaries; RPC) in the temporal-inferior region (7 o'clock in right eye) had the highest diagnostic performance. Notably, the zone immediately adjacent to the disc border had a lower area under receiver operating curve (AUC) and the zone with the most discriminating vascular alterations was located between 2.7 and 5.5 mm diameter circles around the ONH. Rao and colleagues similarly found the highest vascular-structural and vascular-functional correlations were in the inferotemporal region [41]. The current OCTA technology allows differentiation of capillaries and medium-to-large vessels and also provides a global vascular density index. However, Zeboulon and colleagues suggested a preferential loss of capillaries compared to larger vessels by observing density color maps [42]. Some investigators studied the effect of intraocular pressure changes on peripapillary and macular vasculature as detected by OCTA [42, 43]; however, the results have not been consistent so far. Although some studies suggested that vascular changes may precede structural changes in glaucoma [15, 30], others have found the opposite [18] and this question remains to be addressed. As a diagnostic tool, reproducibility and repeatability of the results are of outmost importance and these indices are highly promising for OCTA in glaucoma patients [28].

17.4 OCTA Limitations and Future Horizons

Currently, OCTA uses motion-detection as the cornerstone of all algorithms to detect vascular structures. Because of this, the images are highly vulnerable to motion artifacts. Various movements, including saccadic eye movement, ocular pulsations, patient's tremor and lid twitching or blinking can deteriorate the image quality, even when the signal strength is high. To reduce motion artifact, different approaches have been implemented in the OCTA devices, including increasing scanning speed, decreasing imaging area and using image registration. With available scanning speeds, the best image resolution of most OCTA devices is for a 3 × 3 mm area. With enlarging measurement area, the noise usually increases leading to worse image quality; however, with post-processing of smaller imaging areas, montage wide-field images can be created [22]. There are also some other sources of artifact, which can reduce image quality; these include shadow artifacts from any kind of media opacity like posterior vitreous detachment, shadowing of more superficial vessels, blinking artifact, and artifact caused by moving pigment epithelial detachments. When there is a suspicion of vascular leakage, one has to rely on alternative angiographic approaches as OCTA cannot detect leaks.

Despite these limitations, with ongoing technological improvements, it is antici-pated that future OCTA devices will have ultra-high scanning speeds in the MHz range resulting in enhanced image quality and less artifacts. Having more than one laser source in a single device, such as in swept-source laser, and using adaptive optics are also promising approaches. In addition, ongoing research aims to incor-porate some no injection, 'inducible' contrast enhancement for OCTA. An example of an inducible contrast is acoustic shock waves [46]. With the current pace of inno-vation in OCTA technology, one can predict that, in near future, it could become a fundamental part of ophthalmological evaluation in many patients.

17.5   Sample OCTA Reports

17.5.1   OCTA—Normal Eye

See Fig. 17.1.

17.5.1.1   OCTA—Glaucomatous Eyes

See Fig. 17.2.

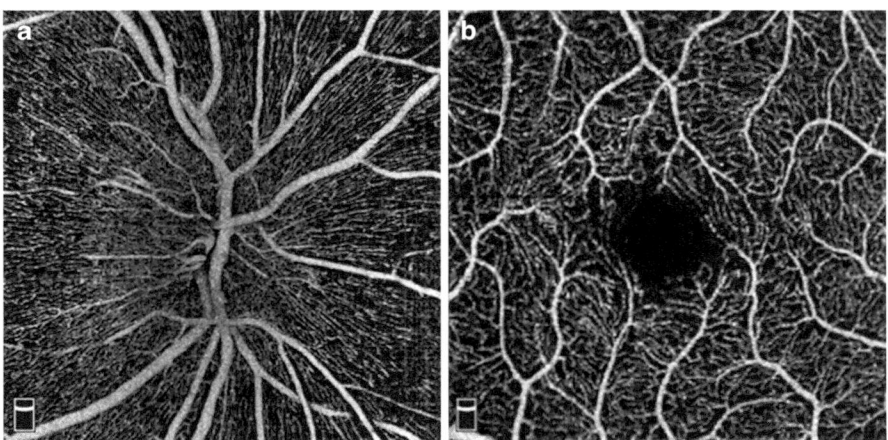

Fig. 17.1 Examples of optical coherence tomography angiography (OCTA) images. (**a**) Radial peripapillary capillary (RPC) network. (**b**) Superficial retinal vascular network in the macular region. (Images obtained with OCT RT XR Avanti with the AngioVue software, OptoVue Inc. Fremont, CA, USA.)

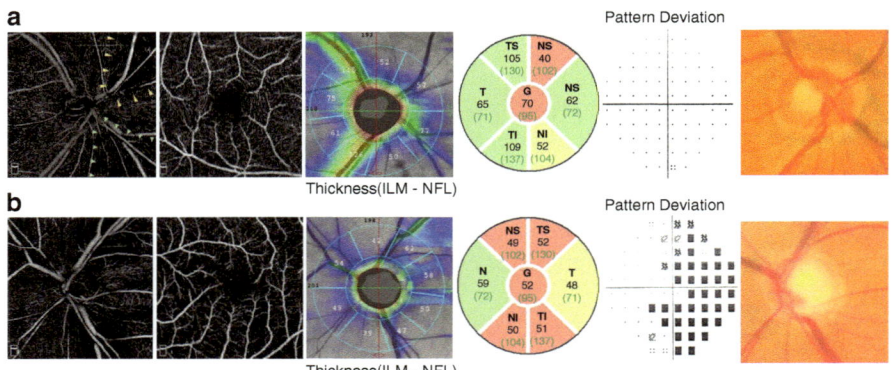

Thickness(ILM - NFL)

Fig. 17.2 Representative vascular, structural, and functional images in two eyes with mild-to-moderate and severe glaucomatous damage. (**a**) Glaucomatous eye (right eye) with mild neuroretinal rim loss, normal VF, and obvious, localized vascular drop-off of the radial peripapillary capillaries (RPCs) (yellow and green arrowheads), enlargement of foveal avascular zone (FAZ) and peripapillary retinal nerve fiber layer (pRNFL) thinning. (**b**) Glaucomatous eye (left eye) with advanced cupping, severe VF loss and wide-spread vascular drop-off of the RPC and macular region, irregular, enlarged FAZ and diffuse pRNFL loss

References

1. Yanagi M, Kawasaki R, Wang JJ, Wong TY, Crowston J, Kiuchi Y. Vascular risk factors in glaucoma: a review. Clin Exp Ophthalmol. 2011;39:252–8.
2. Nicolela MT. Clinical clues of vascular dysregulation and its association with glaucoma. Can J Ophthalmol. 2008;43:337–41.
3. Ster AM, Popp RA, Petrisor FM, Stan C, Pop VI. The role of oxidative stress and vascular insufficiency in primary open angle glaucoma. Clujul Med. 2014;87:143–6.
4. Pasquale LR. Vascular and autonomic dysregulation in primary open-angle glaucoma. Curr Opin Ophthalmol. 2016;27:94–101.
5. Schwartz B, Rieser JC, Fishbein SL. Fluorescein angiographic defects of the optic disc in glaucoma. Arch Ophthalmol. 1977;95:1961–74.
6. Plange N, Kaup M, Weber A, Remky A, Arend O. Fluorescein filling defects and quantitative morphologic analysis of the optic nerve head in glaucoma. Arch Ophthalmol. 2004;122:195–201.
7. Michelson G, Groh MJ, Langhans M. Perfusion of the juxtapapillary retina and optic nerve head in acute ocular hypertension. Ger J Ophthalmol. 1996;5:315–21.
8. Michelson G, Langhans MJ, Groh MJ. Perfusion of the juxtapapillary retina and the neuroretinal rim area in primary open angle glaucoma. J Glaucoma. 1996;5:91–8.
9. Michelson G, Schmauss B, Langhans MJ, Harazny J, Groh MJ. Principle, validity, and reliability of scanning laser Doppler flowmetry. J Glaucoma. 1996;5:99–105.
10. Yoshida A, Feke GT, Mori F, Nagaoka T, Fujio N, Ogasawara H, Konno S, Mcmeel JW. Reproducibility and clinical application of a newly developed stabilized retinal laser Doppler instrument. Am J Ophthalmol. 2003;135:356–61.
11. Sugiyama T, Araie M, Riva CE, Schmetterer L, Orgul S. Use of laser speckle flowgraphy in ocular blood flow research. Acta Ophthalmol. 2010;88:723–9.
12. Siesky B, Harris A, Carr J, Verticchio Vercellin A, Hussain RM, Parekh Hembree P, Wentz S, Isaacs M, Eckert G, Moore NA. Reductions in retrobulbar and retinal capillary blood flow

strongly correlate with changes in optic nerve head and retinal morphology over 4 years in open-angle glaucoma patients of african descent compared with patients of european descent. J Glaucoma. 2016;25:750–7.

13. Jia Y, Wei E, Wang X, Morrison JC, Parikh M, Lombardi LH, Gattey DM, Armour RL, Edmunds B, Kraus MF, Fujimoto JG, Huang D. Optical coherence tomography angiography of optic disc perfusion in glaucoma. Ophthalmology. 2014;121:1322–32.

14. Wang X, Jiang C, Ko T, Kong X, Yu X, Min W, Shi G, Sun X. Correlation between optic disc perfusion and glaucomatous severity in patients with open-angle glaucoma: an optical coherence tomography angiography study. Graefes Arch Clin Exp Ophthalmol. 2015;253: 1557–64.

15. Yarmohammadi A, Zangwill LM, Diniz-Filho A, Saunders LJ, Suh MH, Wu Z, Manalastas PIC, Akagi T, Medeiros FA, Peripapillary WRN. Macular vessel density in patients with glaucoma and single-hemifield visual field defect. Ophthalmology. 2017;124:709–19.

16. Yarmohammadi A, Zangwill LM, Diniz-Filho A, Saunders LJ, Suh MH, Wu Z, Manalastas PIC, Akagi T, Medeiros FA, Weinreb RN. Optical coherence tomography angiography vessel density in healthy, glaucoma suspect, and glaucoma eyes. Invest Ophthalmol Vis Sci. 2016;57:OCT451–9.

17. Yarmohammadi A, Zangwill LM, Diniz-Filho A, Suh MH, Yousefi S, Saunders LJ, Belghith A, Manalastas PI, Medeiros FA, Weinreb RN. Relationship between optical coherence tomography angiography vessel density and severity of visual field loss in glaucoma. Ophthalmology. 2016;123:2498–508.

18. Akagi T, Iida Y, Nakanishi H, Terada N, Morooka S, Yamada H, Hasegawa T, Yokota S, Yoshikawa M, Yoshimura N. Microvascular density in glaucomatous eyes with hemifield visual field defects: an optical coherence tomography angiography study. Am J Ophthalmol. 2016;168:237–49.

19. Shin JW, Lee J, Kwon J, Choi J, Kook MS. Regional vascular density-visual field sensitivity relationship in glaucoma according to disease severity. Br J Ophthalmol. 2017;101: 1666–72.

20. Jia Y, Tan O, Tokayer J, Potsaid B, Wang Y, Liu JJ, Kraus MF, Subhash H, Fujimoto JG, Hornegger J, Huang D. Split-spectrum amplitude-decorrelation angiography with optical coherence tomography. Opt Express. 2012;20:4710–25.

21. Choi W, Waheed NK, Moult EM, Adhi M, Lee B, De Carlo T, Jayaraman V, Baumal CR, Duker JS, Fujimoto JG. Ultrahigh speed swept source optical coherence tomography angiography of retinal and choriocapillaris alterations in diabetic patients with and without retinopathy. Retina. 2017;37:11–21.

22. de Carlo TE, Romano A, Waheed NK, Duker JS. A review of optical coherence tomography angiography (OCTA). Int J Retina Vitreous. 2015;1:5.

23. Shin JW, Sung KR, Lee JY, Kwon J, Seong M. Optical coherence tomography angiography vessel density mapping at various retinal layers in healthy and normal tension glaucoma eyes. Graefes Arch Clin Exp Ophthalmol. 2017;255:1193–202.

24. Wylegala A, Teper S, Dobrowolski D, Wylegala E. Optical coherence angiography: a review. Medicine (Baltimore). 2016;95:e4907.

25. Zhang A, Zhang Q, Chen CL, Wang RK. Methods and algorithms for optical coherence tomography-based angiography: a review and comparison. J Biomed Opt. 2015;20:100901.

26. Kwon J, Choi J, Shin JW, Lee J, Kook MS. Alterations of the foveal avascular zone measured by optical coherence tomography angiography in glaucoma patients with central visual field defects. Invest Ophthalmol Vis Sci. 2017;58:1637–45.

27. Liu L, Jia Y, Takusagawa HL, Pechauer AD, Edmunds B, Lombardi L, Davis E, Morrison JC, Huang D. Optical coherence tomography angiography of the peripapillary retina in glaucoma. JAMA Ophthalmol. 2015;133:1045–52.

28. Venugopal JP, Rao HL, Weinreb RN, Pradhan ZS, Dasari S, Riyazuddin M, Puttiah NK, DAS R, Devi S, Mansouri K, Webers CA. Repeatability of vessel density measurements of optical coherence tomography angiography in normal and glaucoma eyes. Br J Ophthalmol. 2018;102:325–57.

29. Bojikian KD, Chen CL, Wen JC, Zhang Q, Xin C, Gupta D, Mudumbai RC, Johnstone MA, Wang RK, Chen PP. Optic disc perfusion in primary open angle and normal tension glaucoma eyes using optical coherence tomography-based microangiography. PLoS One. 2016;11:e0154691.
30. Leveque PM, Zeboulon P, Brasnu E, Baudouin C, Labbe A. Optic disc vascularization in glaucoma: value of spectral-domain optical coherence tomography angiography. J Ophthalmol. 2016;2016:6956717.
31. Chen CL, Bojikian KD, Gupta D, Wen JC, Zhang Q, Xin C, Kono R, Mudumbai RC, Johnstone MA, Chen PP, Wang RK. Optic nerve head perfusion in normal eyes and eyes with glaucoma using optical coherence tomography-based microangiography. Quant Imaging Med Surg. 2016;6:125–33.
32. Ichiyama Y, Minamikawa T, Niwa Y, Ohji M. Capillary dropout at the retinal nerve fiber layer defect in glaucoma: an optical coherence tomography angiography study. J Glaucoma. 2017;26:e142–5.
33. Lee EJ, Choi YJ, Kim TW, Hwang JM. Comparison of the deep optic nerve head structure between normal-tension glaucoma and nonarteritic anterior ischemic optic neuropathy. PLoS One. 2016;11:e0150242.
34. Rao HL, Pradhan ZS, Weinreb RN, Reddy HB, Riyazuddin M, Dasari S, Palakurthy M, Puttaiah NK, Rao DA, Webers CA. Regional comparisons of optical coherence tomography angiography vessel density in primary open-angle glaucoma. Am J Ophthalmol. 2016;171:75–83.
35. Scripsema NK, Garcia PM, Bavier RD, Chui TY, Krawitz BD, Mo S, Agemy SA, Xu L, Lin YB, Panarelli JF, Sidoti PA, Tsai JC, Rosen RB. Optical coherence tomography angiography analysis of perfused peripapillary capillaries in primary open-angle glaucoma and normal-tension glaucoma. Invest Ophthalmol Vis Sci. 2016;57:OCT611–20.
36. Suh MH, Zangwill LM, Manalastas PI, Belghith A, Yarmohammadi A, Medeiros FA, Diniz-Filho A, Saunders LJ, Weinreb RN. Deep retinal layer microvasculature dropout detected by the optical coherence tomography angiography in glaucoma. Ophthalmology. 2016;123:2509–18.
37. Suh MH, Zangwill LM, Manalastas PI, Belghith A, Yarmohammadi A, Medeiros FA, Diniz-Filho A, Saunders LJ, Yousefi S, Weinreb RN. Optical coherence tomography angiography vessel density in glaucomatous eyes with focal lamina cribrosa defects. Ophthalmology. 2016;123:2309–17.
38. Chihara E. Myopic cleavage of retinal nerve fiber layer assessed by split-spectrum amplitude-decorrelation angiography optical coherence tomography. JAMA Ophthalmol. 2015;133:e152143.
39. Lee EJ, Kim S, Hwang S, Han JC, Kee C. Microvascular compromise develops following nerve fiber layer damage in normal-tension glaucoma without choroidal vasculature involvement. J Glaucoma. 2017;26:216–22.
40. Lee EJ, Lee KM, Lee SH, Kim TW. OCT angiography of the peripapillary retina in primary open-angle glaucoma. Invest Ophthalmol Vis Sci. 2016;57:6265–70.
41. Rao HL, Pradhan ZS, Weinreb RN, Dasari S, Riyazuddin M, Raveendran S, Puttaiah NK, Venugopal JP, Rao DAS, Devi S, Mansouri K, Webers CAB. Relationship of optic nerve structure and function to peripapillary vessel density measurements of optical coherence tomography angiography in glaucoma. J Glaucoma. 2017;26:548–54.
42. Zeboulon P, Leveque PM, Brasnu E, Aragno V, Hamard P, Baudouin C, Labbé A. Effect of surgical intraocular pressure lowering on peripapillary and macular vessel density in glaucoma patients: an optical coherence tomography angiography study. J Glaucoma. 2017;26:466–72.
43. Hollo G. Influence of large intraocular pressure reduction on peripapillary OCT vessel density in ocular hypertensive and glaucoma eyes. J Glaucoma. 2017;26:e7–e10.

44. Rao HL, Pradhan ZS, Weinreb RN, Riyazuddin M, Dasari S, Venugopal JP, Puttaiah NK, Rao DA, Devi S, Mansouri K, Webers CA. A comparison of the diagnostic ability of vessel density and structural measurements of optical coherence tomography in primary open angle glaucoma. PLoS One. 2017;12:e0173930.
45. Rao HL, Pradhan ZS, Weinreb RN, Riyazuddin M, Dasari S, Venugopal JP, Puttaiah NK, Rao DAS, Devi S, Mansouri K, CAB W. Vessel density and structural measurements of optical coherence tomography in primary angle closure and primary angle closure glaucoma. Am J Ophthalmol. 2017;177:106–15.
46. Tsai MT, Zhang JW, Liu YH, Yeh CK, Wei KC, Liu HL. Acoustic-actuated optical coherence angiography. Opt Lett. 2016;41:5813–6.

Index

© Springer International Publishing AG, part of Springer Nature 2018   357
A. Akman et al. (eds.), *Optical Coherence Tomography in Glaucoma*,
https://doi.org/10.1007/978-3-319-94905-5

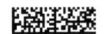